Editors

ASIF M. ILYAS
SHITAL N. PARIKH
SAQIB REHMAN
GILES R. SCUDERI
FELASFA WODAJO

ORTHOPEDIC CLINICS OF NORTH AMERICA

www.orthopedic.theclinics.com

July 2013 • Volume 44 • Number 3

ELSEVIER

1600 John F. Kennedy Boulevard • Suite 1800 • Philadelphia, Pennsylvania, 19103-2899.

http://www.orthopedic.theclinics.com

ORTHOPEDIC CLINICS OF NORTH AMERICA Volume 44, Number 3
July 2013 ISSN 0030-5898, ISBN-13: 978-1-4557-7602-3

Editor: Jennifer Flynn-Briggs

Orthopedic Clinics of North America (ISSN 0030-5898) is published quarterly by Elsevier Inc., 360 Park Avenue South, New York, NY 10010-1710. Months of issue are January, April, July, and October. Business and Editorial Offices: 1600 John F. Kennedy Blvd., Suite 1800, Philadelphia, PA 19103-2899. Customer Service Office: 3251 Riverport Lane, Maryland Heights, MO 63043. Periodicals postage paid at New York, NY and additional mailing offices. Subscription prices are $293.00 per year for (US individuals), $554.00 per year for (US institutions), $347.00 per year (Canadian individuals), $664.00 per year (Canadian institutions), $427.00 per year (international individuals), $689.00 per year (international institutions), $144.00 per year (US students), $208.00 per year (Canadian and international students). Foreign air speed delivery is included in all *Clinics* subscription prices. All prices are subject to change without notice. **POSTMASTER:** Send change of address to *Orthopedic Clinics of North America,* **Elsevier Health Sciences Division, Subscription Customer Service, 3251 Riverport Lane, Maryland Heights, MO 63043. Customer Service (orders, claims, online, change of address): Elsevier Health Sciences Division, Subscription Customer Service, 3251 Riverport Lane, Maryland Heights, MO 63043. Tel: 1-800-654-2452 (U.S. and Canada); 314-447-8871 (outside U.S. and Canada). Fax: 314-447-8029. E-mail: journalscustomerservice-usa@elsevier. com (for print support); journalsonlinesupport-usa@elsevier.com (for online support).**

Reprints. For copies of 100 or more, of articles in this publication, please contact the Commercial Reprints Department, Elsevier Inc., 360 Park Avenue South, New York, NY 10010-1710. Tel.: 212-633-3812; Fax: 212-462-1935; E-mail: reprints@elsevier. com.

Orthopedic Clinics of North America is covered in *MEDLINE/PubMed (Index Medicus), Cinahl, Excerpta Medica,* and *Cumulative Index to Nursing and Allied Health Literature.*

Printed and bound by CPI Group (UK) Ltd, Croydon, CR0 4YY

Transferred to digital print 2013

Contributors

EDITORS

ASIF M. ILYAS, MD - *Upper Extremity*
Program Director, Hand and Upper Extremity
Surgery, Rothman Institute, Associate
Professor of Orthopaedic Surgery, Thomas
Jefferson University, Philadelphia,
Pennsylvania

SHITAL N. PARIKH, MD, FACS - *Pediatrics*
Associate Professor of Orthopaedic Surgery,
Cincinnati Children's Hospital Medical Center,
University of Cincinnati School of Medicine,
Cincinnati, Ohio

SAQIB REHMAN, MD - *Trauma*
Associate Professor, Department of
Orthopaedic Surgery, Director of Orthopaedic

Trauma, Temple University Hospital,
Philadelphia, Pennsylvania

**GILES R. SCUDERI, MD - *Adult
Reconstruction***
Vice President, Orthopedic Service Line,
Northshore LIJ Health System; Director, ISK
Institute, New York, New York

**FELASFA WODAJO, MD - *Musculoskeletal
Oncology***
Musculoskeletal Tumor Surgery, Virginia
Hospital Center, Assistant Professor,
Orthopedic Surgery, Georgetown University
Hospital; Assistant Professor, VCU School of
Medicine, Inova Campus, Virginia

AUTHORS

IRFAN AHMED, MD
Assistant Professor, Department of
Orthopaedics, UMDNJ-New Jersey Medical
School, New Jersey Orthopaedic Institute,
Newark, New Jersey

LOUIS F. AMOROSA, MD
Orthopaedic Surgeon, Westchester Medical
Center, New York Medical College, Valhalla,
New York

JENNIFER HARMS AMOROSA, MD, MAT
Resident, Department of Obstetrics and
Gynecology, Columbia University Medical
Center, New York, New York

JEAN-NOËL ARGENSON, MD, PhD
Institute for Locomotion, Center for Arthritis
Surgery, Sainte-Marguerite Hospital,
Aix-Marseille University, Marseille, France

MICHAEL R. BLOOMFIELD, MD
Adult Reconstruction Fellow, Rothman
Institute, Thomas Jefferson University
Hospital, Philadelphia, Pennsylvania

BRANDON T. BROWN, BS
Swanson School of Mechanical Engineering
and Material Science, University of Pittsburgh,
Pittsburgh, Pennsylvania

PETER A. COLE, MD
Department Chief, Department of Orthopaedic
Surgery, Regions Hospital, St Paul; Professor,
Department of Orthopaedic Surgery, University
of Minnesota, Minneapolis, Minnesota

ALVIN H. CRAWFORD, MD, FACS
Professor Emeritus, Division of Orthopaedic
Surgery, Cincinnati Children's Hospital Medical
Center, Cincinnati, Ohio

LORI J. DESIMONE, PA-C
Physician Assistant, Department of Orthopedic
Surgery, Mayo Clinic, Rochester, Minnesota

CHRISTOPHER A.F. DODD, FRCS
Consultant Orthopaedic Surgeon, Nuffield
Department of Orthopaedic Surgery, Nuffield
Orthopaedic Centre, Oxford, United Kingdom

JONATHAN R. DUBIN, MD
Trauma Fellow, Department of Orthopaedic
Surgery, Regions Hospital, St Paul, Minnesota

JOHN R. FOWLER, MD
Division of Hand, Upper Extremity, and
Microvascular Surgery, Department of
Orthopaedic Surgery, University of Pittsburgh,
Pittsburgh, Pennsylvania

GIL FREEMAN, MD
Trauma Fellow, Department of Orthopaedic
Surgery, Regions Hospital, St Paul, Minnesota

ROBERT J. GOITZ, MD
Chief, Division of Hand, Upper Extremity, and
Microvascular Surgery, Professor Department
of Orthopaedic Surgery, University of
Pittsburgh, Pittsburgh, Pennsylvania

DAVID L. HELFET, MD
Attending Orthopaedic Surgeon, Chief of
Combined Orthopaedic Trauma, Hospital for
Special Surgery, Professor of Surgery
(Orthopaedics), Weill Cornell Medical College,
New York, New York

JAMES P. HIGGINS, MD
Chief, Curtis National Hand Center, MedStar
Union Memorial Hospital, Baltimore, Maryland

ASIF M. ILYAS, MD
Program Director, Hand and Upper Extremity
Surgery, Rothman Institute, Associate
Professor of Orthopaedic Surgery, Thomas
Jefferson University, Philadelphia,
Pennsylvania

VIRAL V. JAIN, MD
Division of Orthopaedic Surgery, Cincinnati
Children's Hospital Medical Center, Cincinnati,
Ohio

CLAUDIUS D. JARRETT, MD
Upper Extremity Reconstructive Surgery;
Department of Orthopaedic Surgery, The
Emory Orthopaedic Center, Emory University
School of Medicine, Atlanta, Georgia

ALEXANDER D. LIDDLE, BSc, MRCS
Clinical Research Fellow, Nuffield Department
of Orthopaedics, Rheumatology and
Musculoskeletal Sciences, Botnar Research
Centre, Oxford, United Kingdom

JESS H. LONNER, MD
Attending Orthopaedic Surgeon, Rothman
Institute, Associate Professor, Thomas
Jefferson University, Philadelphia,
Pennsylvania

DEAN G. LORICH, MD
Associate Director of Orthopaedic Trauma
Service, Hospital for Special Surgery,
Associate Professor of Orthopaedic Surgery,
Weill Cornell Medical College, New York,
New York

MARIOS G. LYKISSAS, MD, PhD
Spine and Scoliosis Service, Hospital for
Special Surgery, Weill Cornell Medical College,
New York, New York

DAVID W. MURRAY, MD, FRCS(Orth)
Professor of Orthopaedic Surgery, Nuffield
Department of Orthopaedics, Rheumatology
and Musculoskeletal Sciences, Botnar
Research Centre, Oxford, United Kingdom

SAMEER NAGDA, MD
Clinical Assistant Professor of Orthopaedic
Surgery, Georgetown University School of
Medicine and Surgeon, Anderson Orthopaedic
Clinic, Inova Mount Vernon Hospital,
Alexandria, Virginia

GENGHIS E. NIVER, MD
Fellow, Hand and Upper Extremity Surgery,
Rothman Institute, Thomas Jefferson
University, Philadelphia, Pennsylvania

SHADE OGUNRO, MD
Fellow in Hand, Upper Extremity and
Microvascular Surgery, Department of
Orthopaedics, UMDNJ-New Jersey Medical
School, Newark, New Jersey

MATTHIEU OLLIVIER, MD
Institute for Locomotion, Center for Arthritis
Surgery, Sainte-Marguerite Hospital,
Aix-Marseille University, Marseille, France

LAURA LYNN ONDERKO, BS
Department of Orthopaedic Surgery, Temple
University, Philadelphia, Pennsylvania

HEMANT PANDIT, DPhil, FRCS(Orth)
Orthopaedic Surgeon and Honorary Senior
Lecturer, Nuffield Department of Orthopaedics,
Rheumatology and Musculoskeletal Sciences,
Botnar Research Centre, Oxford,
United Kingdom

SEBASTIEN PARRATTE, MD, PhD
Institute for Locomotion, Center for Arthritis
Surgery, Sainte-Marguerite Hospital,
Aix-Marseille University, Marseille, France

KETAN M. PATEL, MD
Curtis National Hand Center, MedStar Union
Memorial Hospital, Baltimore, Maryland

SAQIB REHMAN, MD
Associate Professor, Department of
Orthopaedic Surgery, Director of Orthopaedic
Trauma, Temple University, Philadelphia,
Pennsylvania

JOAQUIN SANCHEZ-SOTELO, MD, PhD
Consultant and Professor, Director, Shoulder
and Elbow Fellowship Program, Department of
Orthopedic Surgery, Mayo Clinic, Rochester,
Minnesota

CHRISTOPHER C. SCHMIDT, MD
Director of Shoulder Surgery, Orthopedic
Specialist, UPMC, Pittsburgh, Pennsylvania

VIRAK TAN, MD
Professor, Department of Orthopaedics,
UMDNJ-New Jersey Medical School,
New Jersey Orthopaedic Institute, Newark,
New Jersey

MIHIR M. THACKER, MD
Department of Orthopedic Surgery, Nemours -
Alfred I duPont Hospital for Children,
Wilmington, Delaware

ALFRED J. TRIA Jr, MD
Clinical Professor of Orthopaedic Surgery,
Robert Wood Johnson Medical School,
New Brunswick, New Jersey

DAVID S. WELLMAN, MD
Assistant Attending Orthopaedic Surgeon,
Hospital for Special Surgery, Instructor of
Orthopaedic Surgery, Weill Cornell Medical
College, New York, New York

BRENT B. WIESEL, MD
Assistant Professor of Orthopaedic Surgery,
Georgetown University School of Medicine
and Chief Shoulder Service, Department of
Orthopaedic Surgery, Medstar Georgetown
University Hospital, Washington, DC

GERALD R. WILLIAMS, MD
Professor of Orthopaedic Surgery, Chief
Shoulder and Elbow Surgery, Rothman
Institute, Thomas Jefferson University,
Philadelphia, Pennsylvania

Contents

Adult Reconstruction

Cementless fixation is an increasingly popular option in unicondylar knee arthroplasty (UKA). Early cementless UKAs suffered from unreliable fixation and uptake of cementless UKA was limited. However, modern designs of cementless UKA have demonstrated excellent results with improved radiographic appearances when compared with cemented implants. This is supported by early joint registry data, which demonstrate a survival advantage with cementless fixation in one design of UKA. This review explains the rationale for cementless UKA, summarizes the results from published trials, and highlights technical aspects points to be aware of when implanting cementless UKA.

Patellofemoral arthroplasty has a long record of use in the treatment of isolated patellofemoral arthritis, with outcomes influenced by patient selection, surgical technique, and trochlear implant design. The trochlear components have evolved from inlay-style to onlay-style designs, which have reduced the incidence of patellar instability. Minimizing the risk of patellar instability with onlay-design patellofemoral arthroplasties has enhanced mid-term and long-term results and leaves progressive tibiofemoral arthritis as the primary failure mechanism beyond 10 to 15 years.

Replacement of the patellofemoral and medial tibiofemoral joints has been performed since the 1980s. Bicompartmental replacement was modified. Two different designs were developed: one custom implant and one with multiple predetermined sizes. The surgical technique and instruments are unique and training is helpful. There are no clinical reports for the custom design as of yet. The standard implant has several reports in the literature with only fair to good results and has subsequently been withdrawn from the market. Bicompartmental arthroplasty remains a questionable area of knee surgery. At present, the two separate implant technique is the best choice.

Precise outcome evaluation is mandatory to improve analysis of the results of knee replacement procedures. Patients' expectations toward surgery and activity levels have increased with changes in patient populations and improvement of surgical results. It is difficult, however, to accurately assess outcomes because objective evaluation of patient function performed only by a surgeon remains highly inaccurate. New methods of objective evaluation after unicompartmental knee arthroplasty have been developed. These devices provide information about range of motion and patient function during daily activities. This article provides up-to-date information concerning the different tools of function evaluation after unicompartmental knee arthroplasty.

Trauma

Management of Pelvic Injuries in Pregnancy

Louis F. Amorosa, Jennifer Harms Amorosa, David S. Wellman, Dean G. Lorich, and David L. Helfet

Pelvic fractures in pregnant women are usually high-energy injuries associated with risk of mortality to both mother and fetus. The mother's life always takes priority in the acute setting as it offers the best chance of survival to both the mother and the fetus. Indications for operative intervention of acute pubic symphysis rupture depend on presence of an open disruption, amount of displacement, and degree of disability. Chronic symphyseal instability related to pregnancy is a challenging problem and the first line of treatment is nonoperative care. A previous pelvic fracture is not a contraindication by itself to vaginal delivery.

Technical Pitfalls of Shoulder Hemiarthroplasty for Fracture Management

Brent B. Wiesel, Sameer Nagda, and Gerald R. Williams

Although most proximal humerus fractures can be treated nonoperatively, 4-part fractures and 3-part fractures/dislocations in elderly patients often require management with prosthetic arthroplasty. Reverse arthroplasty is gaining in popularity, but hemiarthroplasty still has a role in the management of 4-part and some 3-part fractures and dislocations. The 2 most important technical factors influencing functional outcome in hemiarthroplasty patients are the restoration of the patient's correct humeral head height and version, and healing of the greater and lesser tuberosities in an anatomic position. Hemiarthroplasty for proximal humerus fracture provides predictable pain relief, but functional recovery is much less predictable.

Operative Techniques in the Management of Scapular Fractures

Peter A. Cole, Jonathan R. Dubin, and Gil Freeman

Operative fixation of the scapula is associated with good outcomes. Techniques have been developed to facilitate surgical exposure of the osseous anatomy so that stability can be achieved. Although the familiar deltopectoral approach can be used for anterior glenoid fractures, the more common exposure is a posterior approach for fractures involving the neck and body of the scapula. The posterior approach has been nuanced to match needs related to fracture pattern and timing of surgery. Reducing the fragments and stabilizing them can be challenging but, a satisfactory reduction and stable fixation can be achieved, which allows immediate motion and rehabilitation.

This article presents a review of the basic science and current research on the use of continuous passive motion therapy after surgery for an intra-articular fracture. This information is useful for surgeons in the postoperative management of intra-articular fractures in determining the best course of treatment to reduce complications and facilitate quicker recovery.

Pediatrics

Surgery in a child with spinal deformity is challenging. Although current orthopedic practice ensures good long-term surgical results, complications occur. Idiopathic scoliosis represents the most extensively investigated deformity of the pediatric spine. Nonidiopathic deformities of the spine are at higher risk for perioperative and long-term complications, mainly because of underlying comorbidities. A multidisciplinary treatment strategy is helpful to assure optimization of medical conditions before surgery. Awareness of complications that occur during or after spine surgery is essential to avoid a poor outcome and for future surgical decision making. This article summarizes the complications of surgical treatment of the growing spine.

Upper Extremity

This article reviews the current indications and clinical outcomes of total wrist arthroplasty. The section on indications reviews both rheumatoid and nonrheumatoid arthritic conditions. The section on clinical outcomes examines the data regarding the 3 current total wrist implants approved by the Food and Drug Administration.

Total elbow arthroplasty has become increasingly popular for the treatment of distal humerus fractures in elderly patients with poor bone quality, comminution, and/or pre-existent elbow abnormalities. The procedure is performed without violating the extensor mechanism; the fractured fragments are exposed and resected on both sides of the triceps, and the components can be implanted through the same exposure. Early outcomes are satisfactory in most elbows and compare favorably with internal fixation in this same group of elderly patients. Advances in elbow arthroplasty for fractures will likely combine refinement of the indications and development of implants with lower rates of failure.

The reverse shoulder arthroplasty is considered to be one of the most significant technological advancements in shoulder reconstructive surgery over the past 30 years. It is able to successfully decrease pain and improve function for patients with rotator cuff–deficient shoulders. The glenoid is transformed into a sphere that articulates with a humeral socket. The current reverse prosthesis shifts the center of rotation more medial and distal, improving the deltoid's mechanical advantage. This design has resulted in successful improvement in both active shoulder elevation and in quality of life.

Many options exist for reconstruction of the posterior elbow/olecranon area following wound formation. Careful early wound management is crucial to ensure successful outcomes following reconstruction. Local and regional options are preferred methods for soft tissue coverage in this region. Common flap options include the reversed lateral arm flap, the radial forearm flap, posterior interosseous artery flap, brachioradialis muscle flap, flexor carpi ulnaris flap, and the latissimus flap. The advantages and disadvantages of these flap options are discussed in this review.

Radial nerve palsy is the most common peripheral nerve injury following a humerus fracture, occurring in 2% to 17% of cases. Radial nerve palsies associated with closed humerus fractures have traditionally been treated with observation, with late exploration restricted to cases without spontaneous nerve recovery at 3 to 6 months. Advocates for early exploration believe that late exploration can result in increased muscular atrophy, motor endplate loss, compromised nerve recovery upon delayed repair, and significant interval loss of patient function and livelihood. In contrast, early exploration can hasten nerve injury characterization and repair, and facilitate early fracture stabilization and rehabilitation.

Radial head fractures without associated bony or ligamentous injury can be safely treated with internal fixation, if possible, or arthroplasty if nonreconstructable. However, nonreconstructable radial head fractures in association with elbow dislocation and/or ligamentous injury in the elbow or forearm represent a specific subset of injuries that requires restoration of the radiocapitellar articulation for optimal function. The purpose of this article was to summarize the indications for radial head arthroplasty and discuss the reported outcomes.

Musculoskeletal Oncology

ORTHOPEDIC CLINICS OF NORTH AMERICA

FORTHCOMING ISSUES

Beginning with this issue, *Orthopedic Clinics of North America* appear in this new format. Rather than focusing on a single topic, each issue will contain articles on key areas in orthopedics—adult reconstruction, upper extremity, trauma, pediatrics and oncology. Articles on sports medicine and foot and ankle will also be included on a regular basis. As the practice of orthopedics has become more specialized, the format of one topic per issue is no longer fulfilling our readers' needs. The new format is intended to address these changing needs.

Orthopedic Clinics of North America will continue to publish a print issue four times a year, in January, April, July, and October. However, it will also include online-only articles that will be published on a rolling basis (not in accordance with our quarterly publication dates). These articles, along with articles from our print issues, will be available on http://www.orthopedic.theclinics.com/.

RECENT ISSUES

April 2013
Osteoporosis and Fragility Fractures
Jason A. Lowe and Gary E. Friedlaender, *Editors*

January 2013
Emerging Concepts in Upper Extremity Trauma
Michael P. Leslie, DO and Seth D. Dodds, MD, *Editors*

October 2012
Management of Compressive Neuropathies of the Upper Extremity
Asif M. Ilyas, MD, *Editor*

DOWNLOAD
Free App!

Review Articles
THE CLINICS

YOUR iPhone and iPad

ADULT RECONSTRUCTION

Preface
Adult Reconstruction

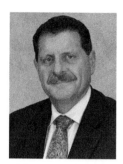

Giles R. Scuderi, MD
Editor

After years of publication, *Orthopedic Clinics of North America* has a new format with the inclusion of multiple contemporary topics in each issue. As the Section Editor for Adult Reconstruction, it is my plan, along with the other members of the editorial board, to keep each issue current with topics that are relevant to the orthopedic community.

One current challenge is the rising number of baby boomers who present with a painful knee. The prevalence of knee osteoarthritis has been increasing, placing a challenge on the orthopedic community on how to manage these patients. While total knee arthroplasty remains the primary surgical treatment for those patients who fail nonoperative modalities, partial knee arthroplasty provides an option for those patients who have limited arthritic changes. The attraction of unicompartmental knee arthroplasty and patellofemoral arthroplasty is that these are joint-preserving procedures, which have been shown to provide a viable functional outcome in a well-selected group of patients. The following articles on unicompartmental, bicompartmental, and patellofemoral arthroplasty report on the current outcomes with these implants. While there have been improvements in surgical technique and implant design, it is evident that these procedures, such as tissue-sparing surgery, still require careful placement of the components to maintain the function and durability of the knee.

Giles R. Scuderi, MD
Vice President
Orthopedic Service Line
Northshore LIJ Health System
New York, USA

Director
ISK Institute
New York, USA

E-mail address:
grscuderi@aol.com

http://dx.doi.org/10.1016/j.ocl.2013.05.002
0030-5898/13/$ – see front matter © 2013 Published by Elsevier Inc.

orthopedic.theclinics.com

Cementless Unicondylar Knee Arthroplasty

Alexander D. Liddle, BSc, MRCS[a],
Hemant Pandit, DPhil, FRCS(Orth)[a],
David W. Murray, MD, FRCS(Orth)[a],
Christopher A.F. Dodd, FRCS[b],*

KEYWORDS

- Cementless • Unicondylar knee arthroplasty • Revision rate

KEY POINTS

- Modern designs of cementless unicondylar knee arthroplasty (UKA) have demonstrated encouraging early results in follow-up studies.
- Cementless fixation provides radiologically superior fixation with fewer radiolucencies compared with cemented UKA.
- Avoidance of implantation errors and adequate clearing of peg and keel slots are important to ensure adequate early fixation and prevent periprosthetic fracture.
- Indications for cementless UKA seem to be similar to those for cemented prostheses.

INTRODUCTION

Unicondylar knee arthroplasty (UKA) is now an established treatment for end-stage osteoarthritis of the knee and accounts for around 10% of all primary knee replacements.[1] Very high early failure rates, largely caused by wear of polyethylene components, have been addressed by the use of improved polyethylene and developments in design, particularly the introduction of mobile bearings.[2–4] UKA has advantages over total knee arthroplasty (TKA), including faster recovery times,[5] reduced perioperative morbidity and mortality,[1,6] and improved returns to work and sport,[7] and there is now a significant body of literature supporting the use of UKA. Excellent outcomes (in terms of both implant survival and functional outcome) have been reported up to 20 years after implantation.[8–13]

However, the revision rate of UKA remains a concern. National Joint Registries (NJR) report around a threefold increase in crude cumulative revision rate at 8 to 10 years for UKA compared with TKA,[1,14,15] and this is supported by other observational studies that demonstrate significantly poorer survivorship for UKA.[16,17]

The difference in revision rate between UKA and TKA is likely to be multifactorial. The ease of revision of UKA lowers the threshold for revision when compared with TKA[18]; patients for UKA are likely to be younger with higher demands,[1] and UKA seems to be more sensitive to surgical inexperience.[19,20] Alongside a greater understanding of these factors, modifications to implant design, particularly in terms of the bone-implant interface, have the potential to improve the reproducibility of UKA and, in turn, to improve the survivorship.

RATIONALE FOR CEMENTLESS UKA

The commonest reason given for revision of UKA in NJR is aseptic loosening, accounting for up to

One or more of the authors has received personal/institutional support from Biomet.
[a] Nuffield Department of Orthopaedics, Rheumatology and Musculoskeletal Sciences, Botnar Research Centre, Windmill Road, Oxford OX3 7LD, UK; [b] Nuffield Department of Orthopaedic Surgery, Nuffield Orthopaedic Centre, Windmill Road, Oxford OX3 7HE, UK
* Corresponding author.
E-mail address: cafdodd@aol.com

Orthop Clin N Am 44 (2013) 261–269
http://dx.doi.org/10.1016/j.ocl.2013.03.001
0030-5898/13/$ – see front matter © 2013 Published by Elsevier Inc

48% of all UKA revisions.[1,14] This mechanism is significantly rarer in published series, and it seems to account for a significant proportion of the difference in UKA survival between these series and NJR data.

The higher rate of aseptic loosening in NJRs is replicated in series from lower volume centers and those at the beginning of their learning curve,[21–23] but not in high-volume centers with experienced surgeons.[9,10,12,13,24,25] Two main theories for this discrepancy have been suggested: errors in cementation technique and misdiagnosis of loosening.

Cementation is technically demanding, particularly in conjunction with the minimally invasive surgical (MIS) technique, which is now used commonly for UKA.[26] Analysis of failures from units new to MIS UKA demonstrates that a high proportion of failures are due to the inability to achieve an adequate cement mantle.[22,27] Cadaveric studies have demonstrated very poor cement penetration in UKAs implanted with inadequately prepared surfaces.[28,29] Removal of loose fragments of cement is particularly difficult with the MIS technique, and such fragments seem to cause intra-articular impingement, leading to excessive wear and subsequent implant loosening, which is apparent in specimens retrieved from revised UKAs.[30]

Misinterpretation of postoperative radiographs is a common problem. Radiolucent lines are a common finding adjacent to cemented UKAs.[31,32] These "physiologic" radiolucencies are narrow and nonprogressive and represent an incomplete layer of fibrocartilage at the cement-bone interface (Fig. 1).[33] Although they may indicate suboptimal fixation, they are not associated with symptoms, have a poor specificity and sensitivity for loosening, and do not affect survival.[34,35] Anteromedial tibial pain is an occasional finding following UKA (probably as a result of increased proximal tibial stress) and usually resolves within the first year with conservative treatment.[36] It has been hypothesized that the combination of radiolucent lines and anteromedial tibial pain may be misinterpreted as indicating loosening and precipitate unnecessary revision.[37] A reduction in the incidence of radiolucent lines in cementless UKA may be a mechanism of improving the revision rate.

Theoretically, UKA should be more suitable for cementless fixation than TKA. UKA aims to restore normal ligament tension with minimal implant constraint (to restore the normal ligament-driven kinematics of the native knee). This normal ligament tension is achieved by using either a congruent, unconstrained mobile bearing or a flat, nonconforming fixed-bearing tibial component.[4,38] The lack of tibiofemoral constraint ensures that

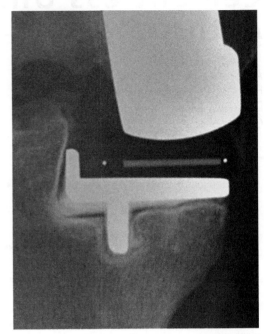

Fig. 1. Radiolucent line adjacent to a cemented UKA.

(aside from the effects of friction) all the force transfer through the components is compressive, with minimal shear forces.[37] In contrast, with TKA there is excision or release of the cruciate and collateral ligaments, thus requiring a degree of tibiofemoral joint constraint, either by dishing of the tibial plateaux or by the use of a cam-post mechanism. The use of a constrained tibiofemoral articulation leads to the generation of shear forces at the bone-implant interface. If there is eccentric loading in TKA, the tibial component may rock and cause tension and failure at the interface; this contrasts with the situation in UKA, where the forces remain compressive.

DEVELOPMENT OF CEMENTLESS UKA

Although UKA was developed in the mid-1970s, there are very few reports of the use of cementless fixation in the first 30 years of its use.[39] Swank and colleagues[40] reported a small series containing both cemented and cementless prostheses in 1993. The cementless prostheses were Fibremesh (Zimmer, Warsaw, IN, USA) and Microloc (Johnson and Johnson, Braintree, MA, USA). The cementless prostheses seemed to perform slightly better than their cemented comparators, although the overall results were poor with a 12% failure rate at 4 years (with a high rate of polyethylene wear).

Although studies of the cementless PCA arthroplasty in the mid-1990s were initially promising,[41] joint registry data demonstrated a very high failure rate, which was attributed to the high degree of tibiofemoral constraint in this design.[42] Similar problems led to the withdrawal of the cementless LCS/Preservation knee (de Puy Johnson and Johnson, Leeds, UK),[43,44] which had a mobile bearing running in a highly constrained track on the tibial component. Forsythe and colleagues reported encouraging survivorship of 98.2% using the Whiteside Ortholoc II cementless prosthesis (Wright Medical, Arlington, TN, USA). However, these results were presented with very short follow-up (mean follow-up of 40 [12–96] months). Until recent years, the vast majority of UKAs continued to use cemented fixation.

CLINICAL RESULTS OF MODERN CEMENTLESS UKA

Cementless UKA has become increasingly popular in recent years as more modern implants have been introduced (**Fig. 2**). Longer term results have been published for 4 cementless UKAs, which are currently in use (**Table 1**). These cementless UKAs are the Unix (Stryker, Marwah, NJ, USA), the AMC/Uniglide (Corin, Cirencester, UK), the Alpina, and the Oxford (both Biomet, Bridgend, UK).

The Unix is a modular cementless UKA with a fixed tibial bearing and a polyradial femoral component. Both components are fully hydroxyapatite

(HA)-coated. The tibial component has no keels or pegs, but there is a horizontal fin at the lateral corner of the tibial tray, and fixation can be augmented with screws. Hall and colleagues[45] report a series of 85 Unix UKAs, demonstrating 76% survivorship at 12 years (number at risk 11, 95% CI 60%–97%), which contrasts with a designer series demonstrating 98.4% survivorship at 5 years.[46]

The Alpina UKA is only on the market in France. It is a fixed-bearing implant with an HA-coated polyradial femoral component and a flat tibial component. The HA-coated tibial component has a keel below its lateral wall and a screw placed centrally. The single published series of 100 patients (90 medial, 10 lateral) demonstrates a 5-year survival of 95.7%.[47]

The AMC/Uniglide UKA is available in both cemented and cementless versions, with either a fixed or a mobile bearing. All versions have a polyradial femoral component, which articulates with either a flat, monoblock polyethylene tibial component (only available for cemented implantation) or a partially conforming mobile tibial bearing, which itself sits on a tibial baseplate that can be either cemented or cementless. Although the implant has been used for over 20 years, there is only one published series.[10] This series was a mixed series of medial and lateral UKA, with 260 cemented, 89 cementless, and 12 hybrid implants

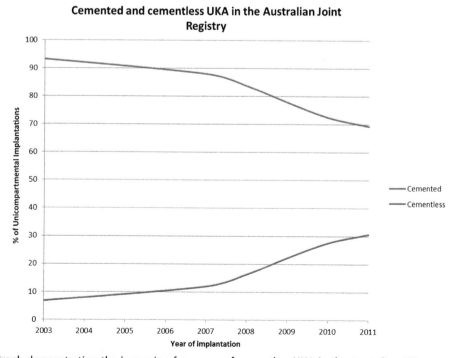

Fig. 2. Graph demonstrating the increasing frequency of cementless UKA in the Australian NJR.

Table 1
Series of cementless UKA

First Author, y	Implant	No.	Mean (and minimum) Follow-up (y)	Survivorship (%)	Functional Outcome	Radiological Outcome
Liddle,[37] 2013	Oxford	1000	3.2 (1)	97.2	1 y OKS 40.2	No loosening. Partial radiolucency in 8.9%
Pandit,[50] 2013	Oxford	30	5 (5)	100	5 y OKS 39.4, KSS(Fcn) 92	No loosening. Partial radiolucency in 7.4%
Hooper,[53] 2012	Oxford	321	2 (2)	99.6	2 y OKS 42.2, HAAS 10.4	1 incompletely seated and loose. Partial radiolucency in 1.5%
Bontemps,[48] 2012	AMC/Uniglide	79	Min 10	97.5	—	—
Saxler,[10] 2004	AMC/Uniglide	89	5.5 (2.3–12.5)	—	KSS(Obj) 93, KSS(Fcn) 89	Radiolucencies in 21.6% (includes cemented knees)
Lecuire,[47] 2008	Alpina	120	6.5	95.7	Combined KSS(O&F) 168.2	Radiolucencies in 4 (1 femoral, 3 tibial; 3.3%)
Hall,[45] 2013	UNIX	85	10 (8–13)	76	—	Tibial lysis in 5%–7%.
Epinette,[46] 2008	UNIX	125	5–13	98.4	KSS(Obj) 97.9, KSS(Fcn) 93.1	Partial tibial radiolucency in 2.3%

Abbreviations: HAAS, High Activity Arthroplasty Score; KSS(Fcn), Knee Society Score (functional component); KSS(Obj), Knee Society Score (objective component).

used; no results are given for the cementless subset. However, a recent conference presentation of 10-year results of 79 cementless knees from the same cohort reports 97.5% survival at 10 years, compared with 95.4% for the cemented version.[48]

The cementless Oxford UKA has generated much interest in recent years. It is the most frequently implanted UKA in New Zealand (accounting for 43.5% of all UKAs implanted) and accounts for 13.5% of all UKAs implanted in Australia (making it the third most commonly used device).[14,49] Like the cemented Oxford, the implant consists of a spherical femoral component that articulates with an unconstrained, fully congruent mobile bearing. The flat underside of the bearing articulates with a flat tibial component. The femoral and tibial components are covered with porous titanium with HA coating; the femoral component has 2 pegs and the tibial component has a keel (**Fig. 3**).

A randomized controlled trial of 62 knees comparing cemented and cementless Oxford UKA has demonstrated a greatly reduced incidence of tibial radiolucencies with similar functional outcomes at 1 year. Physiologic radiolucencies were seen in 75% (24/32) of the cemented cohort and only 7% (2/28) of the cementless cohort.[50] Of the patients in the cemented arm, 24% (11/32) had a radiolucency extending over the entire bone-implant interface on the anteroposterior radiograph (complete radiolucencies), whereas both of the radiolucencies in the cementless arm were partial. The difference in frequency of radiolucencies is preserved to 5 years, and a proportion of early radiolucencies seen around cementless implants initially were observed to "fill in" over the first year (**Fig. 4**). At 5 years, the cementless device demonstrates a significantly improved knee society functional score (92.0 vs 78.8, $P = .003$), whereas Oxford Knee Score (OKS) and knee society objective score remain similar.[51]

Two longitudinal series exist for the cementless Oxford UKA. The first, an independent series of 231 knees at a minimum of 2 years demonstrated excellent radiological evidence of fixation (with partial tibial radiolucencies in <2% of cases, no complete or femoral radiolucencies), and excellent functional scores (OKS 42.2 [score ranges from 0 to 48], high-activity arthroplasty score [HAAS] 10.4 [score ranges 0–18] at 2 years). The second study, a multicenter study of 1000 knees (including some of the 231 reported in the first study), was reported at a mean follow-up of 38.2 months (19–88), demonstrating 97.2% survival at 5 years.[37] Again there were no femoral radiolucencies; there were partial tibial radiolucencies in 8.9%, with no complete tibial radiolucencies. A comparison was made with a previous, single-center series of cemented Oxford UKA,[13] and similar functional results, survivorship, and complication rates were demonstrated, with superior radiological results. The authors suggest that the implantation in osteoporotic patients is not contraindicated, and that the indications for cementless UKA are no different from the indications for cemented UKA.

Given the recent introduction of the cementless Oxford, most NJRs have no separate survival figures for this device. However, the New Zealand Joint Registry suggests that the cementless Oxford may provide a survival advantage over the cemented prosthesis. The registry gives a revision rate (expressed as revisions per 100 implant-years) of 0.6 (95% CI 0.3–1.0) for the cementless Oxford, compared with 1.4 (95% CI 1.3–1.6) for the cemented Oxford,[49] which contrasts with the situation in TKA, where all joint registries demonstrate a poorer survival for cementless implants.[1,15,49,52]

SPECIAL CONSIDERATIONS IN CEMENTLESS UKA

Surgical technique for cementless implantation is very similar to that used for cemented UKA, but there are some important differences that need to be borne in mind when implanting cementless UKA. The quality of fixation depends on adequate seating of the implants. Although the HA-coated cementless implants seem to be relatively forgiving of incomplete seating, there is a threshold at which fixation will fail (**Fig. 5**).[37,53] Care should be taken to adequately clear keels and peg-holes before impaction, and the implant should be

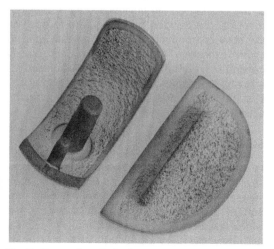

Fig. 3. Cementless Oxford UKA.

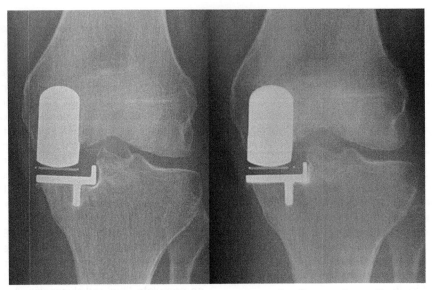

Fig. 4. Cementless Oxford UKA: Lateral tibial radiolucency at 6 months, disappearing at 5 years.

observed to be completely seated before the position is accepted.

Cementless implants and instrumentation are designed to fit more tightly than cemented designs, to achieve an adequate initial press-fit. As a result of this, cadaveric studies have demonstrated cementless implants to be more susceptible to peri-prosthetic tibial plateau fracture (PTPF), when implanted with errors known to predispose to PTPF.[54] Fracture is a rare complication and has been demonstrated in both cemented and cementless UKA.[55–57] Risk factors include making a deep posterior cortical cut in the tibia, as well as perforating the posterior cortex during keel preparation.[58,59] The risk of PTPF can be minimized by avoiding these known errors of implantation, by using a "keel cut" saw blade designed to avoid excessively deep keel preparation, by adequately

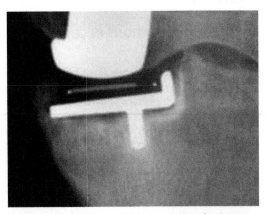

Fig. 5. Incompletely seated cemented Oxford UKA.

clearing peg and keel slots, and by careful impaction.

The final consideration concerns the interpretation of postoperative radiographs. Although radiolucent lines are uncommon in cementless UKA, they have different appearances to those in cemented UKA. They usually occur far medially or far laterally and are often present earlier than those seen in cemented UKA. In the case of the Oxford UKA, the vertical tibial wall is not coated with porous titanium, and lucency is often present adjacent to the wall: this may safely be ignored.[37,53] More concerning are reports of a few cases of early tibial subsidence into valgus. In the multicenter study of the cementless Oxford, 3 cases were identified where the tibial implant subsided into valgus, possibly as a result of impingement of the bearing on the tibial wall.[37] Wall impingement can be avoided by taking care to position the tibial component adequately laterally, and to avoid excessive femoral rotation. The cases described in the series became well-fixed secondarily and a period of watchful waiting is suggested in such cases, rather than early revision surgery, which is probably unnecessary.

SUMMARY

Modern designs of cementless UKA have demonstrated encouraging early results and have several potential advantages over cemented fixation. In countries where cementless devices are widely available, they have become very popular and may overtake cemented UKA in coming years. Although the available clinical studies are promising, they are generally short term and often have low numbers of patients. To determine whether cementless UKA fulfills its early promise, further studies with longer follow-up are necessary. In the interim, detailed examination of registry data from countries with a high rate of cementless implantation may provide some useful insights.

REFERENCES

1. National Joint Registry for England and Wales 9th Annual Report. 2012.
2. Epinette JA, Brunschweiler B, Mertl P, et al. Unicompartmental knee arthroplasty modes of failure: Wear is not the main reason for failure: A multicentre study of 418 failed knees. Orthop Traumatol Surg Res 2012;98(Suppl 6):S124–30.
3. Ashraf T, Newman JH, Desai VV, et al. Polyethylene wear in a non-congruous unicompartmental knee replacement: a retrieval analysis. Knee 2004; 11(3):177–81.
4. O'Connor JJ, Goodfellow JW. Theory and practice of meniscal knee replacement: designing against wear. Proc Inst Mech Eng H 1996; 210(3):217–22.
5. Lombardi AV Jr, Berend KR, Walter CA, et al. Is recovery faster for mobile-bearing unicompartmental than total knee arthroplasty? Clin Orthop Relat Res 2009;467(6):1450–7.
6. Brown NM, Sheth NP, Davis K, et al. Total knee arthroplasty has higher postoperative morbidity than unicompartmental knee arthroplasty: a multicenter analysis. J Arthroplasty 2012;27(S8):86–90.
7. Hopper GP, Leach WJ. Participation in sporting activities following knee replacement: total versus unicompartmental. Knee Surg Sports Traumatol Arthrosc 2008;16(10):973–9.
8. Murray DW, Goodfellow JW, O'Connor JJ. The Oxford medial unicompartmental arthroplasty: a ten-year survival study. J Bone Joint Surg Br 1998;80(6):983–9.
9. Steele RG, Hutabarat S, Evans RL, et al. Survivorship of the St Georg Sled medial unicompartmental knee replacement beyond ten years. J Bone Joint Surg Br 2006;88(9):1164–8.
10. Saxler G, Temmen D, Bontemps G. Medium-term results of the AMC-unicompartmental knee arthroplasty. Knee 2004;11(5):349–55.
11. Naudie D, Guerin J, Parker DA, et al. Medial unicompartmental knee arthroplasty with the Miller-Galante prosthesis. J Bone Joint Surg Am 2004; 86(9):1931–5.
12. Price AJ, Svard U. A second decade lifetable survival analysis of the Oxford unicompartmental knee arthroplasty. Clin Orthop Relat Res 2011; 469(1):174–9.
13. Pandit H, Jenkins C, Gill HS, et al. Minimally invasive Oxford phase 3 unicompartmental knee replacement: results of 1000 cases. J Bone Joint Surg Br 2011;93(2):198–204.
14. Australian Orthopaedic Association National Joint Replacement Registry Annual Report. 2011.
15. The Swedish Knee Arthroplasty Register Annual Report. 2012.
16. Curtin B, Malkani A, Lau E, et al. Revision after total knee arthroplasty and unicompartmental knee arthroplasty in the medicare population. J Arthroplasty 2012;27(8):1480–6.
17. Lyons MC, Macdonald SJ, Somerville LE, et al. Unicompartmental versus total knee arthroplasty database analysis: is there a winner? Clin Orthop Relat Res 2012;470(1):84–90.
18. Goodfellow JW, O'Connor JJ, Murray DW. A critique of revision rate as an outcome measure: reinterpretation of knee joint registry data. J Bone Joint Surg Br 2010;92:1628–31.
19. Hamilton WG, Ammeen D, Engh CA Jr, et al. Learning curve with minimally invasive unicompartmental knee arthroplasty. J Arthroplasty 2010; 25(5):735–40.
20. Robertsson O, Knutson K, Lewold S, et al. The routine of surgical management reduces failure after unicompartmental knee arthroplasty. J Bone Joint Surg Br 2001;83(1):45–9.
21. Song MH, Kim BH, Ahn SJ, et al. Early complications after minimally invasive mobile-bearing medial unicompartmental knee arthroplasty. J Arthroplasty 2009;24(8):1281–4.
22. Dervin GF, Carruthers C, Feibel RJ, et al. Initial experience with the Oxford unicompartmental knee arthroplasty. J Arthroplasty 2011;26(2): 192–7.
23. Choy WS, Kim KJ, Lee SK, et al. Mid-term results of oxford medial unicompartmental knee arthroplasty. Clin Orthop Surg 2011;3(3):178–83.
24. Lisowski LA, van den Bekerom MP, Pilot P, et al. Oxford Phase 3 unicompartmental knee arthroplasty: medium-term results of a minimally invasive surgical procedure. Knee Surg Sports Traumatol Arthrosc 2011;19(2):277–84.
25. Foran JR, Brown NM, Della Valle CJ, et al. Long-term survivorship and failure modes of unicompartmental knee arthroplasty. Clin Orthop Relat Res 2012;471(1):102–8.
26. Luscombe KL, Lim J, Jones PW, et al. Minimally invasive Oxford medial unicompartmental knee arthroplasty. A note of caution! Int Orthop 2007;31(3): 321–4.
27. Barrett WP, Scott RD. Revision of failed unicondylar unicompartmental knee arthroplasty. J Bone Joint Surg Am 1987;69(9):1328–35.
28. Seeger JB, Jaeger S, Bitsch RG, et al. The effect of bone lavage on femoral cement penetration and

interface temperature during oxford unicompart-mental knee arthroplasty with cement. J Bone Joint Surg Am 2013;95(1):48–53.

29. Miskovsky C, Whiteside LA, White SE. The ce-mented unicondylar knee arthroplasty. An in vitro comparison of three cement techniques. Clin Or-thop Relat Res 1992;(284):215–20.

30. Kendrick BJ, Longino D, Pandit H, et al. Polyeth-ylene wear in Oxford unicompartmental knee replacement: a retrieval study of 47 bearings. J Bone Joint Surg Br 2010;92(3):367–73.

31. Voss F, Sheinkop MB, Galante JO, et al. Miller-Galante unicompartmental knee arthroplasty at 2- to 5-year follow-up evaluations. J Arthroplasty 1995;10(6):764–71.

32. Tibrewal SB, Grant KA, Goodfellow JW. The radio-lucent line beneath the tibial components of the Oxford meniscal knee. J Bone Joint Surg Br 1984;66(4):523–8.

33. Kendrick BJ, James AR, Pandit H, et al. Histology of the bone-cement interface in retrieved Oxford unicompartmental knee replacements. Knee 2012;19(6):918–22.

34. Gulati A, Chau R, Pandit HG, et al. The incidence of physiological radiolucency following Oxford uni-compartmental knee replacement and its relation-ship to outcome. J Bone Joint Surg Br 2009;91(7):896–902.

35. Kalra S, Smith TO, Berko B, et al. Assessment of radiolucent lines around the Oxford unicompart-mental knee replacement: sensitivity and speci-ficity for loosening. J Bone Joint Surg Br 2011;93(6):777–81.

36. Simpson DJ, Price AJ, Gulati A, et al. Elevated proximal tibial strains following unicompartmental knee replacement–a possible cause of pain. Med Eng Phys 2009;31(7):752–7.

37. Liddle AD, Pandit H, O'Brien S, et al. Cementless fixation in Oxford unicompartmental knee replace-ment: a multicentre study of 1000 knees. Bone Joint J 2013;95(2):181–7.

38. Scott RD, Santore RF. Unicondylar unicompartmen-tal replacement for osteoarthritis of the knee. J Bone Joint Surg Am 1981;63(4):536–44.

39. Forsythe ME, Englund RE, Leighton RK. Unicondy-lar knee arthroplasty: a cementless perspective. Can J Surg 2000;43(6):417–24.

40. Swank M, Stulberg SD, Jiganti J, et al. The natural history of unicompartmental arthroplasty. An eight-year follow-up study with survivorship analysis. Clin Orthop Relat Res 1993;(286):130–42.

41. Magnussen PA, Bartlett RJ. Cementless PCA uni-compartmental joint arthroplasty for osteoarthritis of the knee. A prospective study of 51 cases. J Arthroplasty 1990;5(2):151–8.

42. Blunn GW, Joshi AB, Lilley PA, et al. Polyethylene wear in unicondylar knee prostheses. 106

43. Arastu MH, Vijayaraghavan J, Chissell H, et al. Early failure of a mobile-bearing unicompartmental knee replacement. Knee Surg Sports Traumatol Ar-throsc 2009;17(10):1178–83.

44. Jeer PJ, Keene GC, Gill P. Unicompartmental knee arthroplasty: an intermediate report of survivorship after the introduction of a new system with analysis of failures. Knee 2004;11(5):369–74.

45. Hall MJ, Connell DA, Morris HG. Medium to long-term results of the UNIX uncemented unicom-partmental knee replacement. Knee 2012. pii:S0968-0160(12)00162-7.

46. Epinette JA, Manley MT. Is hydroxyapatite a reli-able fixation option in unicompartmental knee ar-throplasty? A 5- to 13-year experience with the hydroxyapatite-coated unix prosthesis. J Knee Surg 2008;21(4):299–306.

47. Lecuire F, Fayard JP, Simottel JC, et al. Mid-term results of a new cementless hydroxyapatite coated anatomic unicompartmental knee arthroplasty. Eur J Orthop Surg Traumatol 2008;18(4):279–85.

48. Bontemps G, Schlüter-Brust K. 10 year survival after unicompartmental knee arthroplasty: prospective long-term follow-up study. Geneva (Switzerland): ESSKA; 2012.

49. The New Zealand Joint Registry Thirteen Year Report. 2012.

50. Pandit H, Jenkins C, Beard DJ, et al. Cementless Oxford unicompartmental knee replacement shows reduced radiolucency at one year. J Bone Joint Surg Br 2009;91(2):185–9.

51. Pandit H, Liddle AD, Kendrick BJ, et al. Improved fixation in cementless unicompartmental knee replacement: five year results of a randomised controlled trial. J Bone Joint Surg Am, in press.

52. Australian Orthopaedic Association National Joint Replacement Registry Annual Report. 2012.

53. Hooper GJ, Maxwell AR, Wilkinson B, et al. The early radiological results of the uncemented Oxford medial compartment knee replacement. J Bone Joint Surg Br 2012;94(3):334–8.

54. Seeger JB, Haas D, Jager S, et al. Extended sagittal saw cut significantly reduces fracture load in cementless unicompartmental knee arthro-plasty compared to cemented tibia plateaus: an experimental cadaver study. Knee Surg Sports Traumatol Arthrosc 2012;26(6):1087–91.

55. Kim KT, Lee S, Cho KH, et al. Fracture of the medial femoral condyle after unicompartmental knee ar-throplasty. J Arthroplasty 2009;24(7):e21–4.

56. Rudol G, Jackson MP, James SE. Medial tibial plateau fracture complicating unicompartmental knee arthroplasty. J Arthroplasty 2007;22(1):148–50.

57. Van Loon P, de Munnynck B, Bellemans J. Periprosthetic fracture of the tibial plateau after unicompartmental knee arthroplasty. Acta Orthop Belg 2006;72(3):369–74.

58. Clarius M, Haas D, Aldinger PR, et al. Periprosthetic tibial fractures in unicompartmental knee arthroplasty as a function of extended sagittal saw cuts: an experimental study. Knee 2010; 17(1):57–60.

59. Pandit H, Murray DW, Dodd CA, et al. Medial tibial plateau fracture and the Oxford unicompartmental knee. Orthopedics 2007;30(Suppl 5):28–31.

The Clinical Outcome of Patellofemoral Arthroplasty

Jess H. Lonner, MD[a],*, Michael R. Bloomfield, MD[b]

KEYWORDS

- Patellofemoral arthroplasty (replacement) • Knee arthritis • Knee arthroplasty (replacement) results
- Knee arthroplasty (replacement) design • Trochlea

KEY POINTS

- Patellofemoral arthroplasty (PFA) has a long record of use in the treatment of isolated patellofemoral arthritis, with outcomes influenced by patient selection, surgical technique, and trochlear implant design.
- The trochlear components have evolved from inlay-style to onlay-style designs, which have reduced the incidence of patellar instability.
- Inlay-design trochlear prostheses are inset within the native trochlea, flush with the surrounding articular cartilage. The component rotation is therefore influenced by the native trochlear inclination, which tends to be internally rotated relative to the anteroposterior and transepicondylar axes of the femur, accounting for the high incidence of patellar instability with inlay-design components.
- Onlay-design trochlear components are implanted perpendicular to the anteroposterior axis of the femur, resecting the anterior trochlear surface flush with the anterior femoral cortex and positioning the implant irrespective of the native trochlear inclination, which is the number one reason for the significant improvement in patellar tracking with onlay-style trochlear implants.
- Minimizing the risk of patellar instability with onlay-design PFAs has enhanced mid-term and long-term results and leaves progressive tibiofemoral arthritis as the primary failure mechanism beyond 10 to 15 years.
- Revision PFA to an onlay-design is reasonable to consider in the situation of a failed inlay-style trochlear prosthesis, if no tibiofemoral arthritis is present. Otherwise, revision to total knee arthroplasty can yield predictable results.

INTRODUCTION

Epidemiologic studies indicate that isolated patellofemoral arthritis affects nearly 10% of the population over 40 years of age.[1] In one study, women were more than twice as likely as men to have isolated anterior compartment degeneration (24% vs 11%),[2] likely related to subtle dysplasia and malalignment.[3] As the population ages and the burden of arthritis increases,[4] more patients will likely seek treatment for this condition in the upcoming years. In addition, as younger patients in their 30s through 50s continue to present with isolated patellofemoral arthritis, conservative operative treatments like patellofemoral arthroplasty (PFA) will remain important alternatives to total knee arthroplasty (TKA) when nonoperative interventions are ineffective.

J.H. Lonner: Consultant: Zimmer, Blue Belt Technologies, Mako Surgical Corporation, CD Diagnostics, Healthpoint Capital. Royalties: Zimmer, Blue Belt Technologies, CD Diagnostics. Shareholder: Blue Belt Technologies, CD Diagnostics, Healthpoint Capital.
M.R. Bloomfield: No conflicts to disclose.
[a] Rothman Institute, Thomas Jefferson University, 925 Chestnut Street, 5th Floor, Philadelphia, PA 19107, USA;
[b] Rothman Institute, Thomas Jefferson University Hospital, 925 Chestnut Street, 5th Floor, Philadelphia, PA 19107, USA
* Corresponding author.
E-mail addresses: Jess.lonner@rothmaninstitute.com; jesslonner@comcast.net

Most patients with patellofemoral arthritis can be treated symptomatically and with nonoperative modalities (including anti-inflammatory medications, physical therapy, weight reduction, bracing, and injections). However, a small percentage of patients may require surgical intervention if these treatments fail. Surgical options include nonarthroplasty procedures (arthroscopic debridement, tibial tubercle unloading procedures, cartilage restoration, and patellectomy) and partial (patellofemoral) or TKA. Historically, nonarthroplasty surgical treatment has provided mixed and inconsistent results, with success rates of 60% to 70%, especially in patients with advanced arthritis.[5] Although TKA provides reproducible results in patients with isolated patellofemoral arthritis, it may be undesirable for those interested in a more conservative, kinematic-preserving approach, particularly in younger patients. Due to these limitations, PFA continues to emerge as a more mainstream option. This review focuses on the historical and contemporary results of PFA as influenced by advances in prosthetic (specifically trochlear component) design.

Indications for PFA

As with any surgical procedure, a prerequisite for good outcomes with PFA is proper patient selection. Therefore, results of any series of PFA should be interpreted in the context of appropriate indications. The ideal candidate for PFA has isolated, noninflammatory anterior compartment arthritis resulting in pain and functional limitations that are persistent despite reasonable attempts at nonoperative treatments. Patients should have only retropatellar and/or peri-patellar pain that is exacerbated by stairs, sitting with the knee flexed, and standing from a seated position. Symptoms should be reproducible during physical examination with squatting and patellar inhibition testing. An abnormal Q-angle or J-sign indicates significant maltracking and/or dysplasia, particularly with a previous history of patellar dislocations. The presence of these findings may necessitate concomitant realignment surgery with PFA. However, with newer prosthesis designs, moderate maltracking can be corrected with proper orientation of the prosthesis and occasionally a lateral release. Often, patients with patellofemoral arthritis will have significant quadriceps weakness, which should be corrected with preoperative physical therapy to prevent prolonged postoperative pain and functional limitations.

Radiographs should be consistent with isolated patellofemoral arthritis, indicated by joint space narrowing and osteophytes on the lateral and Merchant views (**Fig. 1**). Narrowing within the medial or lateral compartments on weight-bearing views may disqualify that patient from a PFA. The authors also prefer obtaining a preoperative magnetic resonance imaging scan to further evaluate the tibiofemoral compartments for evidence of chondral damage or reactive edema, to guide treatment between PFA and bicompartmental or total knee arthroplasty. Previous arthroscopy photographs are especially valuable in documenting the extent of anterior compartment cartilage loss and the presence or absence of degeneration elsewhere in the knee.

PFA DESIGN CONSIDERATIONS

PFA was first developed over 30 years ago, although it has remained somewhat controversial until recently because of high failure rates seen with early (and even some contemporary) inlay-style trochlear prosthesis designs (**Fig. 2**A). With contemporary onlay-style trochlear implants (see **Fig. 2**B) that replace the entire anterior trochlear surface and are more optimally positioned, high success rates and good functional outcomes are more easily achievable. **Table 1** summarizes key design differences between inlay-style and onlay-style trochlear components.

Inlay Style

Initial attempts at PFA used trochlear components inset into the native trochlea, attempting to position the prosthesis flush with the surrounding trochlear articular cartilage (**Fig. 3**). The resulting design characteristics have proved problematic when coupled with the inherent anatomic variations and inclination of the native trochlea, which make positioning of the component challenging relative to the articular surfaces and biases the component into internal rotation, predisposing to high rates of patellar maltracking, catching, and subluxation.

- The shapes of these components frequently do not match the shape of the trochlea, particularly in the situation of trochlear dysplasia, leading to malpositioning of the prosthesis as it will not sit flush against all surfaces. Several inlay prostheses have large radii of curvature. To avoid impingement of the implant on the anterior cruciate ligament or tibia by a proud inferior aspect of the prosthesis, flexion of these components may be necessary. Flexion of these components results in offset of the proximal aspect of the prosthesis from the anterior femoral cortex,

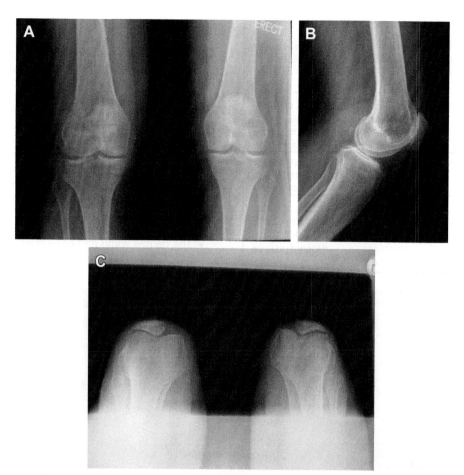

Fig. 1. Preoperative weight-bearing anteroposterior (*A*), lateral (*B*), and sunrise (*C*) radiographs demonstrating advanced patellofemoral arthritis.

causing catching and subluxation of the patella in the initial 15 to 30° of flexion.

- The rotation of the component is determined by the native trochlear orientation. A recent

study by Kamath and colleagues[6] examined trochlear inclination angles in 329 patients with either normal or dysplastic patellofemoral anatomy. Based on magnetic

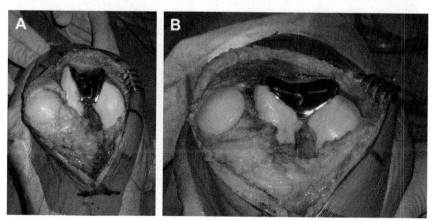

Fig. 2. Intraoperative photos showing components positioned after inlay (*A*) and onlay (*B*) methods of bone preparation.

Table 1
Generalized design characteristics of inlay and onlay designed patellofemoral prostheses

	Inlay	Onlay
Positioning	Inset flush with native trochlea	Replaces entire trochlea, perpendicular to AP axis
Rotation	Determined by native trochlea	Set by surgeon, perpendicular to AP axis
Width	Narrower	Wider
Proximal extension	No further than native trochlear surface	Extends further proximal than native trochlea

resonance imaging scans, both groups had trochlear inclination angles averaging 11.4° and 9.4° of internal rotation, respectively, relative to the anatomic landmarks (anteroposterior and transepicondylar axes). This finding explains the propensity to internally malrotate inlay-style trochlear components, which predisposes to patellar maltracking and subluxation. Like internally rotated femoral components in TKA, internal rotation of the trochlear component in PFA effectively medializes the trochlear groove, increases the Q-angle, and puts tension on the lateral retinaculum, all of which predispose to patellar maltracking and instability.

• The narrow width and often deep constraining sulcus of some inlay-style trochlear

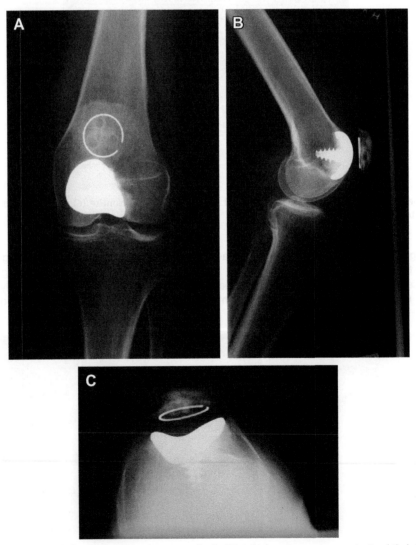

Fig. 3. Inlay design patellofemoral arthroplasty prosthesis. Weight-bearing anteroposterior (A), lateral (B), and sunrise (C) radiographs.

components are more constraining to the patella with little accommodation for patellar tracking, which also increases the potential for patellar maltracking.

- The proximal aspect of the inlay-style trochlear component does not extend proximal to the trochlear articular margin. This proximal aspect often results in the patella not being engaged in the trochlear component when the knee is in full extension, particularly in patients with patella alta. As the knee flexes, the patella transitions onto the trochlear component, which may cause catching and subluxation, particularly if the trochlear component is flexed, offset proximally, and internally rotated.

Onlay Style

Onlay-style trochlear prostheses (**Fig. 4**) replace the entire anterior trochlear surface, alleviating many of the issues described above when having to accept the constraints of native anatomic aberrations common in this population. This design can be applied to all patients, regardless of anatomic variations, and is therefore more versatile and suitable for general use.

- Most onlay prostheses have anatomic radii of curvature, ensuring the prosthesis sits flush with the anterior femoral cortex proximally and the articular cartilage above the intercondylar notch distally.
- The rotation of the trochlear component is determined by the surgeon intraoperatively based on anatomic landmarks, similar to TKA. The component is positioned perpendicular to the anteroposterior axis (Whiteside's line) and parallel to the transepicondylar axis, facilitating patellar tracking and eliminating the effect of native

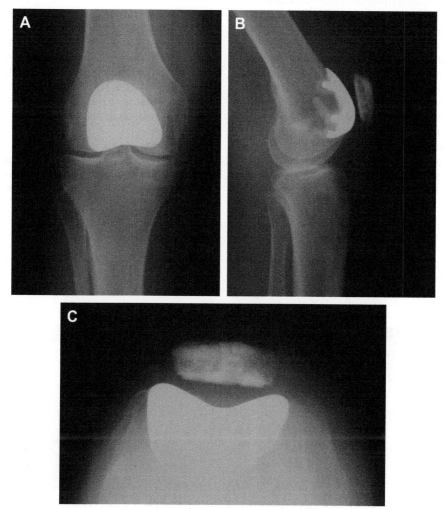

Fig. 4. Onlay design patellofemoral arthroplasty prosthesis. Weight-bearing anteroposterior (*A*), lateral (*B*), and sunrise (*C*) radiographs.

trochlear rotation seen with inlay prostheses (**Fig. 5**).

- Onlay prostheses are wider and less constraining than inlay designs, thus allowing greater excursion of the patella throughout the arc of motion.
- Onlay prostheses often extend further proximal than the native trochlear cartilage and are positioned flush against the anterior femoral cortex, eliminating the catching common to inlay designs and also keeping the patella engaged in the trochlea even in full extension.

RESULTS OF PFA
Primary PFA

Although patient selection and sound surgical technique are important drivers of success in PFA, the results of PFA have shown a disparity in the early and mid-term failures that occur as a result of patellar instability and maltracking, depending on whether an inlay-style or onlay-style component is used.[5] **Tables 2** and **3** contain the cumulative results of published series of inlay-style and onlay-style trochlear prosthesis designs, respectively. Although no studies have directly compared inlay-style and onlay-style trochlear prostheses, the preponderance of the evidence shows lower revision rates and need for secondary surgery to address patellar maltracking, and higher functional success rates and durability with the latter. Although initially poorly understood, high reoperation and revision rates with inlay-style trochlear designs were often attributed to poor patient selection, soft tissue imbalance, and component malposition. In those series, the components were likely positioned flush with some, but not all, articular surfaces (due to morphologic mismatches between surface anatomy and trochlear implant) and internally rotated due to the native trochlear inclination. Again,

although poorly defined in the published series, the disproportionately low rates of satisfactory outcomes can likely be attributed at some level to trochlear component design features, which helps explain the data published in the Australian National Joint Registry, showing that the 5-year cumulative revision rate was greater than 20% for inlay prostheses and less than 10% for onlay designs.[7] Series reviewing the results of inlay-style implants have reported an incidence of patellar maltracking ranging between 17% and 36%.[5,8–10] Other studies that have reviewed the experience with different onlay-style trochlear designs in PFA have found a considerably lower incidence of patellar maltracking, typically less than 1%.[11–14] Several of the older and contemporary inlay-style PFA systems are no longer in use today. If patella tracking is satisfactory after PFA, the primary mode of failure will be progressive tibiofemoral arthritis, irrespective of the type of trochlear prosthesis used.

Late complications of PFA

As opposed to the short-term complications related most frequently to patellar catching and maltracking, late complications requiring revision may occur in the setting of a well-functioning PFA. Revision rates have been shown to be higher in obese patients,[15] likely due to a combination of the factors discussed below.

- Progression of tibiofemoral arthritis is the most common reason for long-term "failure" after successful PFA. In one series, 25% of patients at 15 years required additional surgery for progressive arthritis.[16] Two other series also found radiographic evidence of progressive degeneration in greater than 20% of knees.[11,17] Similarly, Nicol and colleagues[18] found a 12% revision rate for symptomatic tibiofemoral arthritis at a mean of 55 months. These authors also observed that the

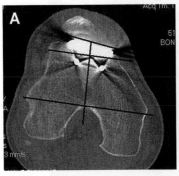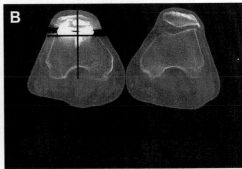

Fig. 5. (A) Axial CT scan of an inlay-style implant demonstrating internal rotation relative to the anteroposterior axis of the distal femur, resulting in lateral patellar catching and subluxation. (B) Axial CT scan of an onlay style trochlear prosthesis showing rotation perpendicular to the AP axis of the femur.

Table 2
Published results of inlay-style patellofemoral arthroplasty prostheses

Series (y)	Implant	No. of PFAs	Age in Years (Range)	Duration of Follow-up in Years (Range)	% of Good/ Excellent Results	% Revised
Blazina et al,[8] 1979	Richards Types I & II	57	39 (19–81)	2 (0.6–3.5)	NA	35
Krajca & Coker,[36] 1996	Richards Types I & II	16	64 (42–84)	5.8 (2–18)	88	6
Arciero & Toomey,[37] 1988	Richards Type II (14); CFS-Wright (11)	25	62 (33–86)	5.3 (3–9)	85	28
De Winter et al,[9] 2001	Richards Type II	26	59 (22–90)	11 (1–20)	76	19
Kooijman et al,[16] 2003	Richards Type II	45	50 (20–77)	17 (15–21)	86	22
van Jonbergen et al,[38] 2010	Richards Type II	185	52 (NA)	13.3 (2–30.6)	NA	25
Cartier et al,[39] 1990	Richards Types II & III	72	65 (23–89)	4 (2–12)	85	7
Cartier et al,[40] 2005	Richards Types II & III	79	60 (36–81)	10 (6–16)	77	25
Argenson et al,[21] 1995	Autocentric	66	57 (19–82)	5.5 (2–10)	84	15
Argenson et al,[19] 2005	Autocentric	66	57 (21–82)	16 y (12–20)	NA	42
van Wagenberg et al,[15] 2009	Autocentric	24	63 (31–81)	4.8 (2–11)	30	29
Tauro et al,[10] 2001	Lubinus	62	66 (50–87)	7.5 (5–10)	45	28
Smith et al,[41] 2002	Lubinus	45	72 (42–86)	4 (0.5–7.5)	69	19
Lonner,[5] 2004	Lubinus	30	38 (34–51)	4 (2–6)	84	33
Merchant,[42] 2004	Low contact stress	15	49 (30–81)	3.8 (2.3–5.5)	93	0
Charalambous et al,[43] 2011	Low contact stress	51	64 (47–84)	2.1 (0.4–5)	33	33
Sisto & Sarin,[44] 2006	Kinematch	25	45 (23–51)	6 (2.6–10)	100	0

Table 3
Published results of onlay-style patellofemoral arthroplasty prostheses

Series (y)	Implant	No. of PFAs	Age in Years (Range)	Duration of Follow-up in Years (Range)	% of Good/ Excellent Results	% Revised
Lonner,[5] 2004	Avon trochlea; Nexgen patella	25	44 (28–59)	0.5 (0.1–1)	96	0
Ackroyd et al,[11] 2007	Avon	109	68 (46–86)	5.2 (5–8)	80	3.6
Starks et al,[12] 2009	Avon	37	66 (30–82)	2 (NA)	86	0
Leadbetter et al,[13] 2009	Avon	79	58 (34–77)	3 (2–6)	84	6.3
Gao et al,[45] 2010	Avon	11	54 (46–74)	2 (0.5–4)	100	0
Odumenya et al,[17] 2010	Avon	50	66 (42–88)	5.3 (2.1–10.2)	NA	4
Mont et al,[14] 2012	Avon	43	29 (27–67)	7 (4–8)	NA	12
Beitzel et al,[46] 2012	Journey PFJ	22	46 (26–67)	2 (NA)	NA	4.5

indication for primary PFA was osteoarthritis in all of the revised patients, whereas none of the patients with trochlear dysplasia as the primary cause were revised. Other authors have also found that patients with primary trochlear dysplasia tend to have better long-term outcomes than those with primary osteoarthritis.[13,19]

- Loosening is an infrequent cause of late revision in most series.[11,20] Kooijman and coworkers found a loosening rate of 2% of prostheses at a mean of 15 years.[16]

- Despite relatively good mid-term clinical results,[21] Argenson and coworkers found in a subsequent follow-up study using the same patient series that the extended survivorship declined significantly, with 58% survivorship at mean 16 years postoperatively.[19] Most of these patients were revised for progression of arthritis (25%) or loosening (14%). In that series, most trochlear components that were revised for aseptic loosening were cementless designs. Cemented components fared substantially better.

PFA with Concomitant Procedures for Tibiofemoral Arthritis

One study has reported results of combined PFA and biologic reconstruction of isolated articular cartilage lesions of the tibiofemoral compartments. Lonner and colleagues[22] performed PFA with simultaneous autologous osteochondral transplantation in 4 knees with isolated full-thickness femoral condylar lesions. Lesion sizes ranged from 10 × 9 mm and 24 × 7 mm, which were reconstructed with up to 3 plugs taken from uninvolved areas of the trochlea that would be resurfaced by the prosthesis. At an average 2.7-year follow-up (range 2–4 years), good clinical results and improved Knee Society scores were reported. No reoperations or complications occurred, and no radiographic evidence of tibiofemoral arthritis was seen. These results are limited by the small sample size and short duration of follow-up.

Modular bicompartmental knee arthroplasty, consisting of both PFA and medial or lateral unicompartmental knee arthroplasty (UKA), has been proposed for the treatment of knee arthritis whereby one of the tibiofemoral compartments is spared and the ligaments are intact.[23,24] Although complications with a monolithic bicompartmental knee arthroplasty have been reported arising from potential femoral component malpositioning/malrotation,[25,26] use of a separate UKA and PFA (modular approach) allows independent placement of the prostheses and optimized sizing and orientation with superior results. Heyse and

colleagues[27] reported on 9 knees in 9 patients treated with medial UKA and PFA. Three procedures were performed in a staged fashion, with a mean of 5 years between UKA and PFA. At a mean follow-up of 12 years (range, 4–17 years), no revision surgeries were necessary, although one asymptomatic patient had substantial progression of lateral arthritis. Knee Society scores increased significantly, as did the range of motion. Mahoney and colleagues[24] reported on their short-term experience with 17 unlinked UKA and PFA, observing mild or no pain and >120° of flexion in all patients. In that series all patients were able to rise unassisted and ascend stairs in a reciprocal manner. There were no cases of incompatibility between the UKA or PFA components. Lonner and colleagues[28] reviewed the initial 28 consecutive modular unlinked bicompartmental UKA/PFAs performed by the authors and found that at a minimum 2-year follow-up (range, 2–4 years), WOMAC, and Knee Society subscores all improved significantly. There were no perioperative complications and no radiographic evidence of loosening, polyethylene wear, or progressive arthritis of the lateral tibiofemoral compartment.

Revision Patellofemoral Arthroplasty

One study investigated the use of the role of revision PFA. Hendrix and colleagues[20] reported 14 failed first-generation inlay-style prostheses that were revised to a second-generation onlay-style PFA implant. The primary failure modes were component malposition, patellar subluxation/catching, polyethylene wear, and overstuffing; no loosening was reported. At a mean 5-year follow-up (range 3–7 years), significant improvements were noted in the Bristol Knee Scores, as well as its pain and function subscores. Five patients had evidence of mild tibiofemoral arthritis at reoperation, which predicted poorer outcome. Two of these 5 patients were revised to TKA by final follow-up. No malposition, loosening, wear, or subluxation was noted in any of the revision PFA prostheses. The authors concluded that revision PFA using an onlay-style trochlear component is a viable option when faced with a failed inlay-style PFA, provided there is no evidence of degeneration elsewhere within the joint. In addition, although the design characteristics of the inlay prosthesis likely contributed to its clinical failure, it also facilitated a relatively easy revision due to the bone-preserving nature of the early design.

As opposed to conversion of UKA to TKA, little has been written about revision of PFA to TKA. Lonner and colleagues[29] reported the results of a series of failed PFAs revised to TKA. Twelve PFA in 10 patients failed at a mean of 4 years postoperatively due to progression of arthritis alone or in combination with patellar maltracking and catching. Significant improvements in the clinical and functional Knee Society scores after revision were noted, with no evidence of wear, maltracking, or failure of the resultant reconstruction at a mean of 3 years. In that series, outcomes of conversion to TKA were similar to those after primary TKA; however, only the trochlear components were revised. Outcomes may not have been as optimal if the patellar components required revision as well.

PFA Versus TKA for Isolated Patellofemoral Arthritis

Several studies have reported successful results of TKA for isolated anterior compartment arthritis, with good midterm results in up to 90% of patients.[30–32] One retrospective study compared outcomes in 45 patients undergoing PFA or TKA at mean of 2.5 years of follow-up.[33] They found similar Knee Society and pain scores, but the PFA group had significantly higher activity scores. However, high-quality comparisons of PFA to other treatments, including TKA, for isolated patellofemoral arthritis have not been reported to date. One ongoing randomized controlled trial is currently evaluating PFA compared with TKA in this scenario and is expected to report results in 2013.[34]

A recent meta-analysis of 28 studies compared complications with PFA and TKA performed for isolated patellofemoral arthritis.[35] The authors found an eightfold higher likelihood of reoperation and revision for all PFA compared with TKA. However, when comparing second-generation onlay prostheses only, no significant differences in reoperation, revision, pain, or mechanical complications were found, indicating a significant effect of implant design. On subgroup analysis, first-generation inlay-style prostheses had over fourfold higher rates of significant complications than second-generation prostheses, likely biasing the overall results. These data indicate that modern onlay-style PFA and TKA likely have similar rates of complications in this patient population.

In conclusion, the significant failure rates and patellar tracking complications that plagued early inlay PFA designs have now been minimized with the modern generation of onlay-style prostheses. PFA outcomes can be optimized with proper patient selection, meticulous surgical technique, and selection of an onlay-style implant that can be positioned perpendicular to the AP axis of the femur. These factors have contributed to a renewed enthusiasm for PFA as a successful treatment option for this challenging clinical problem.

REFERENCES

1. Davies AP, Vince AS, Shepstone L, et al. The radiologic prevalence of patellofemoral osteoarthritis. Clin Orthop Relat Res 2002;(402):206–12.
2. McAlindon TE, Snow S, Cooper C, et al. Radiographic patterns of osteoarthritis of the knee joint in the community: the importance of the patellofemoral joint. Ann Rheum Dis 1992;51(7):844–9.
3. Grelsamer RP, Dejour D, Gould J. The pathophysiology of patellofemoral arthritis. Orthop Clin North Am 2008;39(3):269–74, v.
4. Kurtz S, Ong K, Lau E, et al. Projections of primary and revision hip and knee arthroplasty in the United States from 2005 to 2030. J Bone Joint Surg Am 2007;89(4):780–5.
5. Lonner JH. Patellofemoral arthroplasty: pros, cons, and design considerations. Clin Orthop Relat Res 2004;(428):158–65.
6. Kamath AF, Slattery TR, Levack AE, et al. Trochlear inclination angles in normal and dysplastic knees. J Arthroplasty 2013;28(2):214–9.
7. Australian Oarthopaedic Association National Joint Replacement Registry. Available at: http://dmac. adelaide.edu.au/aoanjrr/publications.jsp. Accessed on January 15, 2013.
8. Blazina ME, Fox JM, Del Pizzo W, et al. Patellofemoral replacement. Clin Orthop Relat Res 1979;(144):98–102.
9. de Winter WE, Feith R, van Loon CJ. The Richards type II patellofemoral arthroplasty: 26 cases followed for 1-20 years. Acta Orthop Scand 2001; 72(5):487–90.
10. Tauro B, Ackroyd CE, Newman JH, et al. The lubinus patellofemoral arthroplasty. A five- to ten-year prospective study. J Bone Joint Surg Br 2001;83(5): 696–701.
11. Ackroyd CE, Newman JH, Evans R, et al. The Avon patellofemoral arthroplasty: five-year survivorship and functional results. J Bone Joint Surg Br 2007; 89(3):310–5.
12. Starks I, Roberts S, White SH. The avon patellofemoral joint replacement: independent assessment of early functional outcomes. J Bone Joint Surg Br 2009;91(12):1579–82.
13. Leadbetter WB, Kolisek FR, Levitt RL, et al. Patellofemoral arthroplasty: a multi-centre study with minimum 2-year follow-up. Int Orthop 2009;33(6): 1597–601.
14. Mont MA, Johnson AJ, Naziri Q, et al. Patellofemoral arthroplasty: 7-year mean follow-up. J Arthroplasty 2012;27(3):358–61.
15. van Wagenberg JM, Speigner B, Gosens T, et al. Midterm clinical results of the autocentric II

patellofemoral prosthesis. Int Orthop 2009;33(6): 1603–8.

16. Kooijman HJ, Driessen AP, van Horn JR. Long-term results of patellofemoral arthroplasty. A report of 56 arthroplasties with 17 years of follow-up. J Bone Joint Surg Br 2003;85(6):836–40.

17. Odumenya M, Costa ML, Parsons N, et al. The Avon patellofemoral joint replacement: five-year results from an independent centre. J Bone Joint Surg Br 2010;92(1):56–60.

18. Nicol SG, Loveridge JM, Weale AE, et al. Arthritis progression after patellofemoral joint replacement. Knee 2006;13(4):290–5.

19. Argenson JN, Flecher X, Parratte S, et al. Patellofemoral arthroplasty: an update. Clin Orthop Relat Res 2005;440:50–3.

20. Hendrix MR, Ackroyd CE, Lonner JH. Revision patellofemoral arthroplasty: three- to seven-year follow-up. J Arthroplasty 2008;23(7):977–83.

21. Argenson JN, Guillaume JM, Aubaniac JM. Is there a place for patellofemoral arthroplasty? Clin Orthop Relat Res 1995;(321):162–7.

22. Lonner JH, Mehta S, Booth RE Jr. Ipsilateral patellofemoral arthroplasty and autogenous osteochondral femoral condylar transplantation. J Arthroplasty 2007;22(8):1130–6.

23. Lonner JH. Modular bicompartmental knee arthroplasty with robotic arm assistance. Am J Orthop (Belle Mead NJ) 2009;38(Suppl 2):28–31.

24. Argenson JN, Parratte S, Bertani A, et al. The new arthritic patient and arthroplasty treatment options. J Bone Joint Surg Am 2009;91(Suppl 5):43–8.

25. Palumbo BT, Henderson ER, Edwards PK, et al. Initial experience of the journey-deuce bicompartmental knee prosthesis: a review of 36 cases. J Arthroplasty 2011;26(Suppl 6):40–5.

26. Muller M, Matziolis G, Falk R, et al. The bicompartmental knee joint prosthesis journey deuce: failure analysis and optimization strategies. Orthopade 2012;41(11):894–904 [in German].

27. Heyse TJ, Khefacha A, Cartier P. UKA in combination with PFR at average 12-year follow-up. Arch Orthop Trauma Surg 2010;130(10):1227–30.

28. John T, Sheth N, Lonner JH. Modular bicompartmental arthroplasty of the knee. Proceedings Knee Society 2010.

29. Lonner JH, Jasko JG, Booth RE Jr. Revision of a failed patellofemoral arthroplasty to a total knee arthroplasty. J Bone Joint Surg Am 2006;88(11): 2337–42.

30. Parvizi J, Stuart MJ, Pagnano MW, et al. Total knee arthroplasty in patients with isolated patellofemoral arthritis. Clin Orthop Relat Res 2001;(392):147–52.

31. Mont MA, Haas S, Mullick T, et al. Total knee arthroplasty for patellofemoral arthritis. J Bone Joint Surg Am 2002;84(11):1977–81.

32. Laskin RS, van Steijn M. Total knee replacement for patients with patellofemoral arthritis. Clin Orthop Relat Res 1999;(367):89–95.

33. Dahm DL, Al-Rayashi W, Dajani K, et al. Patellofemoral arthroplasty versus total knee arthroplasty in patients with isolated patellofemoral osteoarthritis. Am J Orthop (Belle Mead NJ) 2010;39(10):487–91.

34. Odumenya M, McGuinness K, Achten J, et al. The Warwick patellofemoral arthroplasty trial: a randomised clinical trial of total knee arthroplasty versus patellofemoral arthroplasty in patients with severe arthritis of the patellofemoral joint. BMC Musculoskelet Disord 2011;12:265.

35. Dy CJ, Franco N, Ma Y, et al. Complications after patello-femoral versus total knee replacement in the treatment of isolated patello-femoral osteoarthritis. A meta-analysis. Knee Surg Sports Traumatol Arthrosc 2012;20(11):2174–90.

36. Krajca-Radcliffe JB, Coker TP. Patellofemoral arthroplasty. A 2- to 18-year followup study. Clin Orthop Relat Res 1996;(330):143–51.

37. Arciero RA, Toomey HE. Patellofemoral arthroplasty. A three- to nine-year follow-up study. Clin Orthop Relat Res 1988;(236):60–71.

38. van Jonbergen HP, Werkman DM, Barnaart LF, et al. Long-term outcomes of patellofemoral arthroplasty. J Arthroplasty 2010;25(7):1066–71.

39. Cartier P, Sanouiller JL, Grelsamer R. Patellofemoral arthroplasty. 2-12-year follow-up study. J Arthroplasty 1990;5(1):49–55.

40. Cartier P, Sanouiller JL, Khefacha A. Long-term results with the first patellofemoral prosthesis. Clin Orthop Relat Res 2005;(436):47–54.

41. Smith AM, Peckett WR, Butler-Manuel PA, et al. Treatment of patello-femoral arthritis using the lubinus patello-femoral arthroplasty: a retrospective review. Knee 2002;9(1):27–30.

42. Merchant AC. Early results with a total patellofemoral joint replacement arthroplasty prosthesis. J Arthroplasty 2004;19(7):829–36.

43. Charalambous CP, Abiddin Z, Mills SP, et al. The low contact stress patellofemoral replacement: high early failure rate. J Bone Joint Surg Br 2011;93(4): 484–9.

44. Sisto DJ, Sarin VK. Custom patellofemoral arthroplasty of the knee. J Bone Joint Surg Am 2006; 88(7):1475–80.

45. Gao X, Xu ZJ, He RX, et al. A preliminary report of patellofemoral arthroplasty in isolated patellofemoral arthritis. Chin Med J (Engl) 2010;123(21): 3020–3.

46. Beitzel K, Schottle PB, Cotic M, et al. Prospective clinical and radiological two-year results after patellofemoral arthroplasty using an implant with an asymmetric trochlea design. Knee Surg Sports Traumatol Arthrosc 2013;21(2):332–9.

Bicompartmental Knee Arthroplasty: The Clinical Outcomes

Alfred J. Tria Jr, MD*

KEYWORDS

- Bicompartmental arthroplasty • Implants • Patellofemoral joint • Medial tibiofemoral joint

KEY POINTS

- Bicompartmental arthroplasty is a bone-preserving procedure that also preserves both of the cruciate ligaments.
- The two separate implant technique allows the surgeon to concentrate on one area and then the other without compromising either arthroplasty.
- Presently, bicompartmental arthroplasty does not have acceptable long-term results. However, there may still be a place for the procedure with custom-made implants that are positioned more accurately either with navigation control or patient-specific cutting blocks.

INTRODUCTION

Partial knee arthroplasty was developed in the 1950s with such devices as the McKeever and MacIntosh implants.[1–3] Unicondylar (UKA)[4–7] and patellofemoral (PFA) prostheses[8,9] were used in the late 1970s and publications showed acceptable results at midterm follow-up. Some surgeons combined the UKA and PFA when the pathology presented itself at the time of the surgical procedure.[10,11] The results were once again acceptable at midterm follow-up and had the advantage of ligament preservation and improved proprioception. However, long-term follow-up showed a high revision rate.[12] As the total knee arthroplasty (TKA) designs improved, there was less interest in partial knee arthroplasty until Repicci and coworkers offered a smaller incision for UKA.[13,14] Limited incisions for knee arthroplasty became more popular and partial knee arthroplasty became more common.[15–18] The bicompartmental replacements from the early 1970s had some recognized advantages over TKA with preservation of the cruciate ligaments, increased motion, and improved proprioception; however, the two separate implants removed a considerable amount of bone and the operative procedure was complex. A monoblock femoral component was designed to simplify the surgery and limit the amount of resected bone (Journey-Deuce; Smith and Nephew, Memphis, TN).[19] The prosthesis removed less bone and spared all of the ligaments of the knee. A similar prosthesis is now available that is custom designed from a computed tomography of each individual knee (iDuo; Conformis, Burlington, MA).[20]

The separate prostheses for the patellofemoral and the medial tibiofemoral joints have also been improved over the past few years and resect less bone with improved accuracy. The question is whether either of the approaches can produce clinical results that compare with standard UKA or TKA.

CLINICAL REPORTS
Bicompartmental Arthroplasty Using a Single Piece Femoral Component

The author performed 100 of the monoblock designed components and followed the first 40 patients for 5 years.[21] Two operations were

The author is a consultant for Smith and Nephew Orthopedics, Memphis, TN, USA.
Robert Wood Johnson Medical School, New Brunswick, NJ, USA
* The Orthopaedic Center of New Jersey, 1527 State Highway 27, Suite 1300, Somerset, NJ 08873.
E-mail address: Atriajrmd@aol.com

Orthop Clin N Am 44 (2013) 281–286
http://dx.doi.org/10.1016/j.ocl.2013.03.003
0030-5898/13/$ – see front matter © 2013 Elsevier Inc. All rights reserved.

bilateral procedures. The patients were chosen for the operation based on the preoperative office interview, physical examination, and radiographic evaluation.

The patients were asked to indicate the location of their pain and the prevalence. If the pain was medial tibiofemoral with associated medial patellofemoral symptoms, the patient was considered a good candidate. The indications were very similar to those used for UKA but allowed more symptoms relating to the patellofemoral joint. Global knee pain that was equally distributed in all areas of the knee was a definite contraindication despite any of the physical examination and radiographic findings to the contrary.

The physical examination included medial tibiofemoral and patellofemoral tenderness. The clinical deformity did not exceed 10 degrees of varus or flexion contracture. When the varus deformity corrected to neutral with valgus stress, the knee was a more ideal one for the replacement. However, it was not absolutely necessary for the knee to correct completely. The cruciate ligaments were clinically intact. Some degree of anterior laxity was accepted but grade four instability was not included. Inflammatory arthritis and knees with previous ligament reconstructions or osteotomies were excluded.

The standing anteroposterior radiograph showed an anatomic varus deformity that was less than 10 degrees with minimal translocation of the tibia beneath the femur. Patellofemoral arthritic changes of any extent were acceptable. Mild lateral osteoarthritic changes were considered acceptable. If there were changes in the lateral compartment, there should be no significant symptoms of pain or tenderness on physical examination.

The operative procedure was performed using a curvilinear medial incision with an associated similar medial arthrotomy. No attempt was made

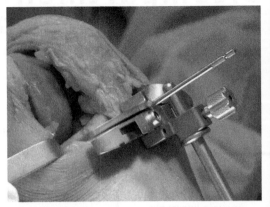

Fig. 1. The extramedullary tibial guide references the medial tibial plateau surface.

to specifically limit the incision; however, the smallest possible exposure was chosen that permitted adequate joint visualization and implant positioning. Most of the procedures included a 1- to 2-cm incision into the quadriceps tendon as part of the medial arthrotomy.

The tibial plateau was addressed first and an extramedullary guide was used to cut the surface 2 to 4 mm below the lowest point (**Fig. 1**). The space was then evaluated using a spacer block with the 8-mm insert (**Fig. 2**). The gap at 90 degrees of flexion was compared with the gap in extension to plan the distal femoral resection. An intramedullary instrumentation system was used to make the femoral cuts. The anteroposterior axis was used for referencing proper external rotation. The first femoral guide sized the femur from anterior to posterior and set the anterior femoral resection depth and rotation (**Fig. 3**). The distal femoral resection was performed by setting the depth on the medial side of the femur and referencing a point on the lateral side of the previously anterior cut surface where the edge of the prosthesis would meet the lateral aspect of the femoral cortex (**Fig. 4**). After

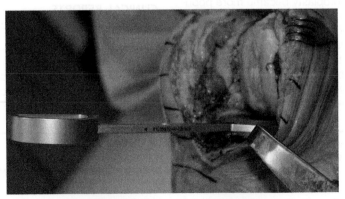

Fig. 2. The spacer block is placed into the flexion gap and used as a reference for the extension gap.

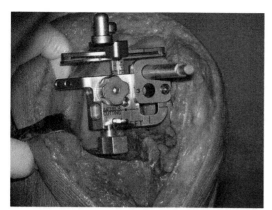

Fig. 3. The first femoral guide references the posterior medial femoral condyle and sets the depth and rotation for the anterior cut.

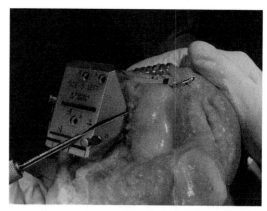

Fig. 5. The femoral finishing block references the width of the medial femoral condyle and the lateral femoral cortex.

the distal medial resection was completed, the space in full extension was compared with the space in flexion and minor adjustments made before proceeding. The finishing block for the femur was set on the cut surface and adjusted with reference to the medial femoral condyle and the lateral femoral cortex (**Fig. 5**). It was often difficult to match the femur with a femoral component size that would allow the medial femoral runner to sit exactly in the center of the tibial tray and also extend across the anterior surface to the lateral cortex.

The tibial tray size was chosen by covering the entire surface with cortical support without overhang in either the sagittal or coronal planes (**Fig. 6**).

The patellar surface was resected in a manner similar to the technique used for TKA and the thickness was 1 to 2 mm thinner than the original patella. The trial components were inserted and the range of motion, tracking of the patella,

tracking of the medial femoral condyle on the tibial polyethylene insert, and the laxity in full extension and 90 degrees of flexion were all evaluated. Two milliliters of laxity in full extension and at 90 degrees of flexion was considered to be ideal. The components were all cemented (**Fig. 7**). Surgical drains were used and the closure was performed in the standard fashion.

The patients started physical therapy and weight-bearing ambulation on the day of surgery. A low-molecular-weight heparin anticoagulation was used within 24 hours after surgery and was continued for 12 to 14 days. Routine Doppler ultrasound surveillance was used for all patients. The hospital stay was 3 days, and then the patients were discharged to a rehabilitation facility or to home. Outpatient physical therapy was continued for approximately 4 weeks.

The average age of the patients was 70 with a range from 49 to 89. The average weight was

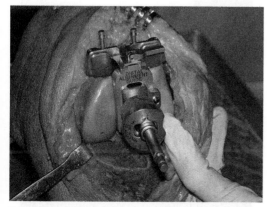

Fig. 4. The distal femoral cut references the medial femoral condyle for the depth of resection and the lateral femoral cortex for the proper angulation.

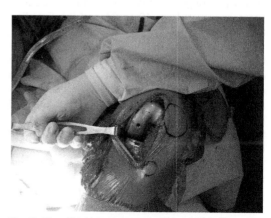

Fig. 6. The tibial tray is centered on the tibial cut surface resting on the cortical bone without overhang.

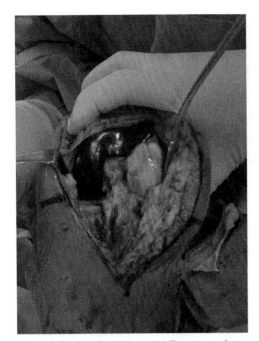

Fig. 7. The final components are all cemented.

185 lb (84 kg) with a range from 114 (52 kg) to 262 lb (119 kg). The average body mass index was 30 (range, 20–42). The average operative time (including surgery and anesthesia) was 114 minutes. The average tourniquet time was 68 minutes. There were no pulmonary emboli, proximal thigh deep venous thromboses, myocardial infarctions, infections, or mortalities. The average length of stay was 3 days (range, 1–6 days). The average preoperative flexion was 122 degrees (range, 115–130). The postoperative flexion at 2 to 4 weeks after surgery was 102 degrees and increased to 120 degrees at the last recorded office visit. The average preoperative anatomic axis was 3 degrees of varus and the average postoperative axis was 2 degrees of valgus. The Knee Society score improved from 49 to 84 and the Function Score from 57 to 81.

One patient expired after the first year of follow-up. One patient developed a subluxing patella in deep flexion at 6 weeks after the surgery. The components were not malaligned or internally rotated and there was no disruption of the medial retinacular closure. The patient was returned to the operating room for a lateral release and went on to have a good result.

Five knees had global pain (12%) and four have been revised to a standard TKA with a good result. At the time of the revisions, the prostheses did not seem to have any specific indicating factors for the failure. The fifth patients was lost to follow-up and considered to be a revision.

Ten patients (24%) have persistent anterior knee pain. Two tibial trays fractured in the coronal plane (**Fig. 8**). Both underwent revision to a TKA. One tray settled anteriorly at 20 months after surgery with a reverse in the tibial slope (**Fig. 9**). The patient's pain is presently tolerable without revision.

There are two other reports in the literature concerning the monoblock femoral design. Palumbo and colleagues[22] reviewed 36 cases in 32 patients with shorter follow-up of 21 months. There were 19 women and 13 men with an average age of 66. Four patients underwent staged bilateral procedures separated by a mean of 6 months. The operative time averaged 87 minutes and the mean length of stay was 2 days (range, 1–5). The mean Knee Society Score for function was 65.4. Seventeen knees had an excellent or good result (48%). A total of 53% of the patients said they would not repeat the surgery. Fourteen percent were converted to a TKA. The average follow-up was less than 2 years and there was no comparison group: however, five knees underwent conversion to TKA because of persistent medial tibial pain. All five of the tibial trays were loose and one was fractured.

Morrison and colleagues[23] reported on a prospective cohort of patients who underwent either a bicompartmental arthroplasty or a TKA. The cohort assignment was determined by the patients after a discussion of the two approaches. There were 21 bicompartmental knees in 20 patients

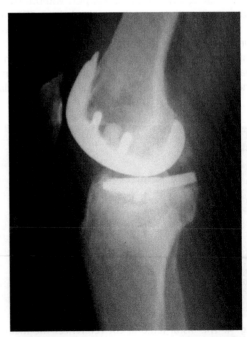

Fig. 8. Lateral radiograph showing the fracture of the tibial tray.

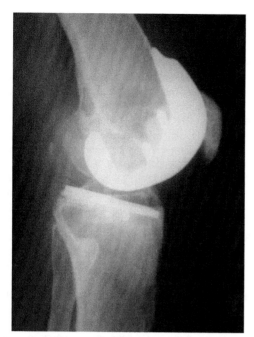

Fig. 9. Lateral radiograph showing the collapse of the tibial tray anteriorly with reverse slope.

(14 women and 6 men) and 33 TKAs in 31 patients (25 women and 6 men). The bicompartmental patients achieved better improvement in stiffness, pain, and physical function at 3 months after surgery. However, the bicompartmental cohort experienced higher overall complications with three revisions for pain, one patellar subluxation, and one patellar fracture. The TKA complications included one patellar tendon tendinitis, one deep venous thrombosis, and no revisions. The patients were not randomly assigned and the follow-up was short (2 years) but the difference in the revision rate was significant.

Bicompartmental Arthroplasty Using Two Separate Implants

The patellofemoral and medial compartments can be replaced using two completely separate implants. Argenson and coworkers[11] reported a review of patellofemoral arthroplasty in association with medial compartment UKA. A total of 183 operations were performed between 1972 and 1990. The surgeries were begun as patellofemoral replacements, and in 104 of the cases the medial compartment had enough arthritic changes to warrant UKA. The average age of the patients was 57 and the mean Knee Society Score was 94 (range, 53–100) but the results concentrated on the cases with isolated patellofemoral arthroplasties.

Parratte and coworkers[12] published a 5- to 23-year follow-up of bicompartmental replacements using two separate implants. There were 71 patients with 77 knees. The average age was 60, with 43 women and 28 men. The survivorship of the prostheses at 17 years was 54%. A total of 28 knees underwent revision. Twenty of the 27 aseptic loosenings involved the patellofemoral arthroplasty. The authors concluded that the revisions were caused by "early generation of implant and limited instrumentation."

Heyse and coworkers[24] published a report on nine cases (eight women and one man) of the combined procedures with an average of 12 years of follow-up. The Knee Society scores improved from 68 to 87. The patients were questioned concerning the level of satisfaction: six of nine were very satisfied and three were just satisfied. There were no revisions.

Lonner[25] has looked at the combined procedures and has tried to improve the surgical approach with updated instruments and robotic assistance. The surgical procedure is demanding but does lead to greater accuracy.

DISCUSSION

Bicompartmental arthroplasty is a bone-preserving procedure that also preserves both of the cruciate ligaments. Some of the early postoperative results are good and the Knee Society scores are close to the scores for TKA but not quite the same. The single-piece femoral design is difficult to implant and forces the surgeon to compromise the position of the implant in the coronal plane to resurface the trochlea and the medial compartment. This leads to transposition of the component and may explain the high incidence of patellofemoral symptoms. Three different authors have failed to show acceptable results even in the first 2 years after the surgery. The custom-designed femoral component may allow for the matching of the two areas but there are no long-term publications as of this time.

The two separate implant technique allows the surgeon to concentrate on one area and then the other without compromising either arthroplasty. The approach takes time, resects more bone than the single-piece femur, and has not shown a distinct advantage in the few papers that have been published. Heyse's paper was encouraging but only involved nine cases. Parrate's report showed good early results but 54% had failed by 17 years. It may not be possible to attain good results beyond the first decade after surgery but that remains to be seen.

Presently, bicompartmental arthroplasty does not have acceptable long-term results. However, there may still be a place for the procedure with custom-made implants that are positioned more accurately either with navigation control or patient-specific cutting blocks.

REFERENCES

1. McKeever DC. Tibial plateau prosthesis. Clin Orthop Relat Res 1960;18:86–95.
2. MacIntosh DL. Hemiarthroplasty of the knee using a space occupying prosthesis for painful varus and valgus deformities. J Bone Joint Surg Am 1958; 40:1431.
3. MacIntosh DL. Arthroplasty of the knee in rheumatoid arthritis. J Bone Joint Surg Br 1966;48:179.
4. Marmor L. Marmor modular knee in unicompartmental disease. Minimum four-year follow-up. J Bone Joint Surg Am 1979;61:347–53.
5. Berger RA, Nedeff DD, Barden RN, et al. Unicompartmental knee arthroplasty. Clin Orthop Relat Res 1999;367:50–60.
6. Gesell MW, Tria AJ Jr. MIS unicondylar knee arthroplasty: surgical approach and early results. Clin Orthop Relat Res 2004;(428):53–60.
7. Goodfellow JW, Kershaw CJ, Benson MK, et al. The Oxford knee for unicompartmental osteoarthritis. The first 103 cases. J Bone Joint Surg Br 1988;70: 692–701.
8. Krajca-Radcliffe JB, Coker TP. Patellofemoral arthroplasty. A 2 to 18 year follow up study. Clin Orthop 1996;330:143–51.
9. Argenson JN, Flecher X, Parratte S, et al. Patellofemoral arthroplasty: an update. Clin Orthop 2005; 440:50–3.
10. Cartier P, Sanouiller JL, Grelsamer R. Patellofemoral arthroplasty: 2–12 year follow-up study. J Arthroplasty 1990;5(1):49–55.
11. Argenson JN, Guillaume JM, Aubaniac JM. Is there a place for patellofemoral? Arthroplasty? Clin Orthop Relat Res 1995;321:162–7.
12. Parratte S, Pauly V, Aubaniac JM, et al. Survival of bicompartmental total knee arthroplasty at 5 to 23 years. Clin Orthop 2010;468:64–72.
13. Repicci JA, Eberle RW. Minimally invasive surgical technique for unicondylar knee arthroplasty. J South Orthop Assoc 1999;8(1):20–2.
14. Romanowski MR, Repicci JA. Minimally invasive unicondylar arthroplasty: eight year follow up. J Knee Surg 2002;15(1):17–22.
15. Price AJ, Webb J, Topf H, et al, The Oxford Hip and Knee Group. Rapid recovery after Oxford Unicompartmental Arthroplasty through a short incision. J Arthroplasty 2001;16:970–6.
16. Emerson RH. Higgins. Unicompartmental knee arthroplasty with the Oxford prosthesis in patients with medial compartment arthritis. J Bone Joint Surg Am 2008;90(1):118–22.
17. Berger RA, Meneghini RM, Jacobs JJ, et al. Results of unicompartmental knee arthroplasty at a minimum of ten years of follow up. J Bone Joint Surg Am 2005; 87(5):999–1006.
18. Pandit H, Jenkins C, Gill JS, et al. Minimally invasive Oxford phase 3 unicompartmental knee replacement: results of 1000 cases. J Bone Joint Surg Br 2011;93(2):198–204.
19. Rolston L, Bresch J, Engh G, et al. Bicompartmental knee arthroplasty: a bone sparing, ligament-sparing, and minimally invasive alternative for active patients. Orthopedics 2007;30(Suppl 8):70–3.
20. Koeck FX, Perlick L, Luring C, et al. Leg axis correction with ConforMIS iForma (interpositional device) in unicompartmental arthritis of the knee. Int Orthop 2009;33(4):955–60.
21. Shin MS, Karthik VK, Tria AJ. Bicompartmental knee arthroplasty. In: Scott WN, editor. Insall and Scott surgery of the knee. Philadelphia: Elsevier, Churchill Livingstone; 2012. p. 1021–5.
22. Palumbo BT, Henderson ER, Edwards PK, et al. Initial experience of the Journey-Deuce bicompartmental knee prosthesis. A review of 36 cases. J Arthroplasty 2011;26(Suppl 6):40–5.
23. Morrison TA, Nyce JD, Macaulay WB, et al. Early adverse results with bicompartmental knee arthroplasty. A prospective cohort comparison to total knee arthroplasty. J Arthroplasty 2011;26(Suppl 6): 35–9.
24. Heyse TJ, Khefacha A, Cartier P. UKA in combination with PFR at average 12 year follow up. Arch Orthop Trauma Surg 2010;130(10):1227–30.
25. Lonner JH. Modular bicompartmental knee arthroplasty with robotic arm assistance. Am J Orthop 2009;38(Suppl 2):28–31.

Results and Outcomes of Unicompartmental Knee Arthroplasty

Matthieu Ollivier, MD, Sebastien Parratte, MD, PhD,
Jean-noël Argenson, MD, PhD*

KEYWORDS

- Unicompartmental knee arthroplasty • Fluoroscopy • Total knee arthroplasty
- Unicompartimental knee arthroplasty • Outcomes measurement • Results

KEY POINTS

- Over the past decade, progress in the UKA ancillary and technique had increased the results of the procedure in terms of survivorship and satisfaction even for young patients.
- To access functional outcomes of UKA, different dimensions must be taken into consideration. Some refer to objective elements, such radiographic outcomes, kinematics or survivorship.
- Some are more subjective and individual parameters of our patients should be evaluated by specific scoring systems, including both patient's and surgeon's experience of the UKA.

INTRODUCTION

Management of osteoarthritis of the femorotibial compartments in young subjects is controversial.[1] In cases of medical treatment failure, surgery can be required to relieve pain and restore function.[1] Available surgical possibilities include conservative surgical treatments with limited arthroscopic débridement or valgus high tibial osteotomy, which is effective in certain precise indications.[1–4] When conservative treatments are no longer efficient, prosthetic replacement must be considered: unicompartmental knee arthroplasty (UKA) or total knee arthroplasty (TKA).[1–4] The population of subjects ages less than 60 years includes active patients whose management must take particular needs into consideration: functional recuperation, resumption of sports activities, and the lifespan of the implants are 3 of the specific problems added to limiting extension of osteoarthritis to the neighboring compartments.[1,3] Over the past decade, progress in the ancillary instrumentation used to implant these unicompartment prostheses associated with better patient selection has accelerated functional recuperation and increased the satisfactory clinical results based on the classical scores and satisfactory implant survival, even if the wear rates seem higher in this age group.[2,5,6] The study of implant survival has, however, thus far been insufficient to demonstrate the value of an intervention, particularly in a population that is young and active, whose quality of life can be strongly related to the condition of the knee.[7,8] To access the functional outcomes of UKA, different dimension must be taken into consideration. The aim of this article is to provide up-to-date information concerning the different tools of function evaluation after UKA, including (1) clinical and radiographic analysis, (2) knee kinematics evaluation, (3) survivorship of implant (medial or lateral after primary arthritis, osteonecrosis, or trauma), and (4) subjective results based on patient-rated outcomes questionnaires, including knee-related quality-of-life or general knee-related quality-of-life questionnaires.

Institute for Locomotion, Center for Arthritis Surgery, Sainte-Marguerite Hospital, Aix-Marseille University, 270 Boulevard de Sainte-Marguerite, 13009 Marseille, France
* Corresponding author.
E-mail address: Jean-noel.ARGENSON@ap-hm.fr

Orthop Clin N Am 44 (2013) 287–300
http://dx.doi.org/10.1016/j.ocl.2013.03.004
0030-5898/13/$ – see front matter © 2013 Elsevier Inc. All rights reserved.

OBJECTIVE EVALUATION OF UNICOMPARTMENTAL KNEE ARTHROPLASTY

Clinical Evaluation

The clinical evaluation is classical and based on the evaluation of the pain, range of motion, the stability of the knee, and the function of the patient. The Knee Society Score was classically used to compile these results.[9] This evaluation most of the time was not sufficient for patients with a UKA due to the high demand and the lack of subjective evaluation. Furthermore, younger patients operated on with a UKA[10,11] place a high demand on their knee when performing sport activities. The new Knee Society Score[12] includes items concerning the subjective feeling of patients not only during daily living and standard activities but also during advanced and recreational activities. The validation of this new Knee Society Score for UKA is currently under process and will be an effective tool to better address patient expectations.

Radiologic Evaluation

Classically, radiographic evaluation (**Figs. 1–3**) has been based on long-leg radiographs and on anteroposterior (AP), lateral, and skyline radiographs of the knee to obtain measurement of preoperative

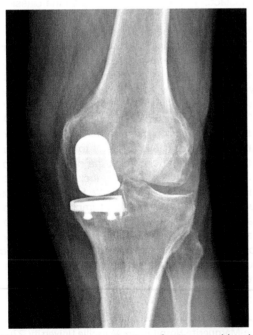

Fig. 1. Radiographic evaluation of a 65-year-old male patient suffering from medial knee pain without signs of inflammation and progressive nontraumatic frontal instability, at 10 years of medial unicompartimental (*left*) knee replacement. Frontal view.

and postoperative hip-knee-ankle angles and to classify lower limb alignment (described by Kennedy and White[13]). The lower limb alignment is considered correct when the mechanical axis passes through either the medial part of the medial tibial plateau (zone 2) or the central part of the tibia (zone C) (**Fig. 4**). During this evaluation, alignment and position of the components must be assessed on screened AP and lateral radiographs and the presence, extent, or progression of femoral or tibial radiolucencies (**Figs. 5** and **6**) according to the Knee Society roentgenographic score is recorded.[14] Progression of osteoarthritis has to be evaluated in the uninvolved compartment on the AP radiographs and in the patellofemoral joint on skyline views according to Berger 4-point scale.[15] According to this scale, grade 1 radiologic change is defined as no measurable loss of joint space but with changes, such as osteophyte formation. Grade 2 changes are defined as up to 25% loss of joint space, grade 3 up to 50%, and grade 4 as more than 50%.

Knee Kinematics After Unicompartmental Knee Arthroplasty

Fluoroscopy has been described as an effective tool[16,17] to evaluate in vivo motions of knee replacement. This peculiar device may help surgeons understand range of motion after UKA, by giving dynamic information during flexion-extension movement or during gait (**Figs. 7–10**).

Some fluoroscopic analyses, focused on the kinematics of posterior cruciate–retaining and posterior stabilized total knee replacements, determined that a paradoxic anterior slide occurs during gait and deep flexion in subjects with total knee replacement.[18,19] From these studies, it has been hypothesized that the anterior cruciate ligament plays an important role in knee kinematics. Argenson and colleagues[18] reported, in 2002, the results of their series of 70 medial UKA and 3 lateral UKA kinematics in knees in which the anterior cruciate ligament was intact at the time of the surgery. All the knee arthroplasties were judged clinically successful with a Hospital for Special Surgery score of greater than 90 points, with no ligamentous laxity or pain. Under fluoroscopic surveillance, each subject was asked to perform successive weight-bearing deep knee bends to maximum flexion. Subjects with a medial unicompartmental knee replacement had only minimal motion during flexion, and kinematic patterns varied among the subjects. The average AP contact position was 0.0 mm at full extension, −2.1 mm at 30° of knee flexion, −2.1 mm at 60° of knee flexion, and −0.8 mm at 90° of knee flexion. Seven of the

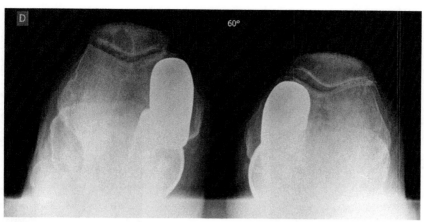

Fig. 2. Radiographic evaluation of a 65-year-old male patient suffering from medial knee pain without signs of inflammation and progressive nontraumatic frontal instability, at 10 years of medial unicompartimental (*left*) knee replacement. Skyline view.

17 subjects had normal posterior femoral rollback of the medial condyle from full extension to 90° of knee flexion. At full extension, 8 of the 17 subjects had a too anterior contact of the medial condyle. In other hand, patients with a lateral unicompartmental knee replacement had posterior femoral rollback. The average AP contact position between implants for these subjects was −1.95 mm at full extension, −5.1 mm at 30° of knee flexion, −6.7 mm at 60° of knee flexion, −6.0 mm at 75°

of knee flexion, and −4.5 mm at 90° of knee flexion. There was increased rollback of the lateral condyle in the posterior direction from full extension to 60° of knee flexion. From 60° to 75° of knee flexion, minimal motion of the lateral condyle was detected on the average, and from 75° to 90° of knee flexion, an average of 1.5 mm of anterior motion was detected. With both medial and lateral UKA, there were variable kinematic patterns, with an anterior slide with increasing knee flexion (especially with

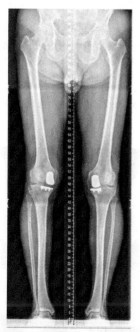

Fig. 3. Radiographic evaluation of a 65-year-old male patient, suffering from medial knee pain without signs of inflammation and progressive nontraumatic frontal instability, at 10 years of medial unicompartimental (*left*) knee replacement. Long-axis evaluation.

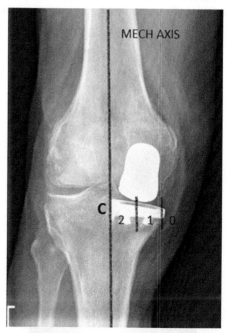

Fig. 4. Lower limb alignment, as described by Kennedy and White.[13] The lower limb alignment is considered correct when the mechanical axis passes through either the medial part of the medial tibial plateau (zone 2) or the central part of the tibia (zone C).

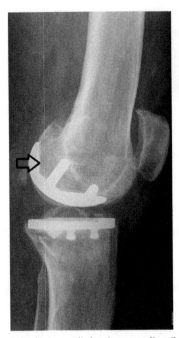

Fig. 5. Nonevolutive radioluminescent line 5 years after UKA for a 52-year-old patient.

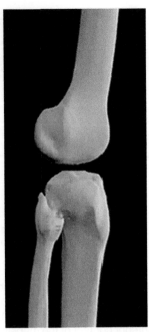

Fig. 7. Kinematic evaluation of a 60-year-old woman with limited range of motion at 2 years after UKA. Mapping of the controlateral knee.

medial UKA) occurring at either 30° or 60° of knee flexion. The results of this study suggested that progressive laxity of the anterior cruciate ligament may occur over time. In this study, it seemed that 8 subjects with medial UKA had an anterior contact position at full extension, which may lead to the hypothesis that the anterior cruciate ligament was not functioning properly, because the anterior cruciate ligament was unable to provide an anterior constraint force with the necessary magnitude to thrust the femur in the anterior direction at full extension. This suggests inconsistent function of the anterior cruciate ligament after UKA and may account, at least in part, for the premature polyethylene wear occasionally seen after UKA.[20–22]

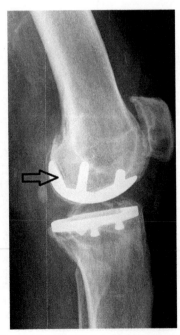

Fig. 6. Nonevolutive radioluminescent line at 6 years after UKA for a 52-year-old patient.

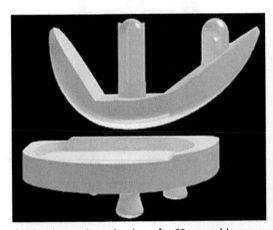

Fig. 8. Kinematic evaluation of a 60-year-old woman with limited range of motion at 2 years after UKA. 3-D reconstruction of the UKA (Lateral View).

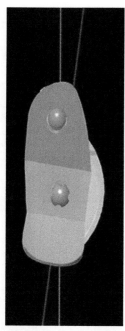

Fig. 9. Kinematic evaluation of a 60-year-old woman with limited range of motion at 2 years after UKA. 3-D reconstruction of the UKA (Top view).

Implant Survival

Survivorship of UKA is classically based on the evaluation of the number of complete or partial revision. Because the indications are different with high tibial osteotomy or TKA, the survivorship of these 3 procedures cannot be directly compared.[1,2,4,23] Reliable function and good survival have been reported for TKA in younger patients,[24–30] and this type of treatment has also been advocated for unicompartmental osteoarthritis. Recently, Morgan and colleagues[27] reported a 96% 12-year survival in a series of 63 young patients (mean age 50.7 years) treated with TKA for osteoarthritis. Mont and colleagues[23] also reported only 1 failure because of polyethylene wear in a series of 31 knees in patients under 50 treated with a TKA for osteoarthritis, with a mean follow-up of 86 months. According to Hanssen and colleagues,[1] despite the good clinical results, TKA should continue to be considered with caution for young patients because of the issues related to the eventual need for a revision. In a study by Pennington and colleagues,[5] 2 of 45 UKAs (4.5%) were revised for polyethylene wear in patients under 60. Price and colleagues,[6] in a multicenter study of the Oxford UKA, compared 512 patients older or equal to 60 and 53 patients younger than 60 and showed that this implant functions well and is durable in patients younger than 60, although the survival was lower for this group (91% at 10 years in the <60 group vs 96% in the >60 group).

In another recent report, 93% of patients successfully returned to regular sporting and physical activities after a UKA, but the patients were older, with a mean age of 64.[31]

Medial UKA

Fixed-bearing UKA Several studies compared the results between fixed-bearing and mobile-bearing UKA.[31,32] Although mobile-bearing congruent polyethylene may be an alternative to fixed bearing,[33] the risk of dislocation remains higher than in fixed-bearing UKAs in the young patient group.[6,19,30,34] It has been demonstrated in a biomechanical study that running and jumping produce surface loads that exceed the limits of polyethylene resistance.[30] To recommend specific activities after a UKA, factors, such as wear, joint load, and the type of prosthesis, must be taken into account for each patient.[8,30,31,35] Based on the authors' results and previous reports, decreasing wear seems the main factor in improving long-term results of UKA.[5,30,36] The diagnosis of polyethylene wear was made clinically and radiologically. Two major symptoms were observed with polyethylene wear (**Fig. 11**), medial knee pain without signs of inflammation and progressive nontraumatic frontal instability. There was no clinical or biologic sign of infection. Physical examination is important to confirm the development of frontal instability in these patients. When these symptoms occurred, the authors' performed weight-bearing and varus and valgus stress radiographs to confirm wear and to look for osteolysis. When there was no evidence of infection, loosening or osteolysis exchange of the polyethylene insert was undertaken and the wear was mainly found on the posterior aspect (see **Fig. 3**; **Figs. 12** and **13**).

In 2011, the authors and colleagues presented the results in term of survivorship of fixed-bearing UKA versus mobile-bearing UKA in young patients.[32] The authors retrospectively reviewed 75 patients (79 knees) with a fixed-bearing UKA and 72 patients (77 knees) with a mobile-bearing UKA operated on between 1989 and 1992. The mean age of patients was 63 years; gender and body mass index (26 kg/m^2) were comparable in the 2 groups. Knee Society function and radiographic scores were determined and survival determined. The minimum follow-up was 15 years (mean 17.2 ± 4.8 years; range, 15–21.2 years). Radiographically, the number of overcorrections and the number of radiolucencies were statistically higher in the mobile-bearing group (69% vs 24%) but at final follow-up, considering revision for any reason, 12 of 77 (15%) UKAs were revised (for

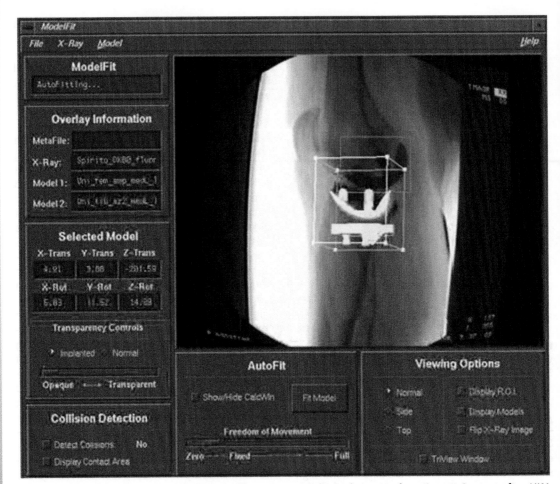

Fig. 10. Kinematic evaluation of a 60-year-old woman with limited range of motion at 2 years after UKA. Computer-assisted method of kinematic analysis: model fitting.

aseptic loosening, dislocation, and arthritis progression) in the mobile-bearing group and 10 of 79 (12%) in the fixed-bearing group (for wear and arthritis progression). This difference did not reach the significance level.

Mobile-bearing UKA Mobile-bearing UKA, using a specific design, Oxford Partial Knee System (Biomet, Warsaw, Indiana), has shown a recent increase in use. The challenges with mobile-bearing design include technical issues of ligament balancing with the potential risk of bearing dislocation. Several studies have suggested excellent long-term survivorship. Murray and colleagues[37] reported 98% cumulative prosthetic survivorship at 10-year follow-up. Svärd and coworkers[38,39] retrospectively evaluated 124 mobile-bearing UKA, with a cumulative survivorship of 95%. They noted that balancing the flexion and extension gaps was challenging. Price and colleagues,[39] using the same implant, found a 15-year survivorship of up to 92%. They noted, however, a high

frequency of complete radiolucent lines around the tibial component in half of the tibial components. Other studies, however, suggest contradictory results with similar mobile-bearing implants. Lewold and colleagues,[40] in evaluating the Swedish Knee Arthroplasty register, found 90% survivorship at 5-year follow-up, using the same Oxford implant. Vorlat and colleagues[41] reported an 84% survival of 149 consecutive Oxford partial knees at 5.5 years. In a US Investigative Device Exemption study, 125 Oxford UKAs were followed at 8 sites.[42] This was a prospective multicenter study and found at 7 years that there was only an 80.6% survivorship, and the clinical success rate was only 74.2%. There are 3 comparison studies evaluating fixed-bearing and mobile-bearing designs. Confalonieri and colleagues[43] found no statistical difference in outcome. Gleeson and colleagues[44] found 3 bearing dislocations in the mobile-bearing group and 4 additional revisions. In the fixed-bearing group, there were only 3 revisions. They found that the Oxfords had a high

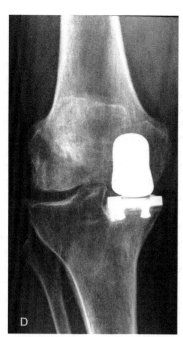

Fig. 11. Frontal view showing an important amount of polyethylene wear 20 years after UKA for a 75-year-old male patient.

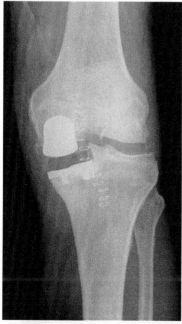

Fig. 12. Frontal view: Polyethylene exchange for a 65-year-old male patient, suffering from medial knee pain without signs and progressive frontal instability, at 10 years after UKA.

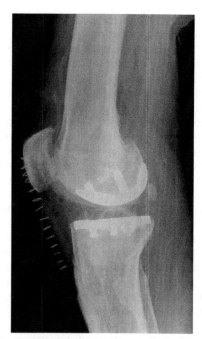

Fig. 13. Lateral View: Polyethylene exchange for a 65-year-old male patient, suffering from medial knee pain without signs and progressive frontal instability, at 10 years after UKA.

reoperation rate and the St. Georg Sled (Waldemar Link, Hamburg, Germany) device achieved better pain relief. The functional results of both implants were similar. These comparative studies show no consensus between mobile bearing and fixed bearing in regards to function, success, or recovery, and a mobile-bearing design has the potential complication of bearing dislocation.

Lateral UKA
Midterm and long-term studies suggest reasonable outcome at 10 years, with survivorship greater than 95% of UKA performed for medial osteoarthritis or osteonecrosis,[45] but few long-term follow-up data are available for lateral UKA.[46–48] The investigators of 1 small series of UKA in the lateral compartment reported only 1 failure out of 19 patients at 89 months of follow-up.[49] Recently, 2 other series reported high functional scores without revision at 5.2 years for 1 and at 12.4 years for another.[46,48] Both the anatomic and biomechanical characteristics are different in each of the knee femorotibial compartments, and similar surgical treatment may not provide reproducible results when applied to a different compartment.[45,47] Furthermore, UKA in the lateral compartment has been described as technically more challenging and 10 times less performed than medial UKA, thus representing fewer than 1% of all knee arthroplasty

procedures.[50] These facts may explain the few data available concerning outcomes of lateral UKA.[46] In 2008, the authors presented results of a consecutive series of 39 lateral UKA.[51,52] The data demonstrate lateral UKA can provide reasonable clinical and radiographic results, with survivorship at 10 and 16 years comparable to the survivorship obtained for medial UKA (**Figs. 14–18**). Recent studies reported a low failure rate, whereas the results of older series were more controversial.[45–47,51] Gunther and colleagues[46] reported a 21% failure rate using the mobile-bearing Oxford unicompartmental prosthesis in the lateral compartment, with a 10% rate of bearing dislocation. This difference with the commonly reported high-functioning long-term outcomes using the same implant for the medial compartment may be explained by the amount of femoral translation of the lateral condyle whereas the medial one remains fairly stationary.[47] When studying the in vivo kinematics of patients implanted with either a medial or lateral UKA, the authors showed an important posterior femoral translation of the lateral condyle during flexion compared with the medial one.[18] According to these results and as a result of the biomechanical properties of the lateral compartment, fixed-bearing implants seem more appropriate.[18] Sah and Scott[48]

reported no revision at 5 years in a group of 49 knees implanted with lateral UKA. The rate of radiolucencies observed in the authors' series (10% of nonprogressive tibial radiolucencies) was comparable with those observed in previous series of lateral UKA at the same follow-up.[48,53] Because both the anatomic and the biomechanical characteristics are different in each of the knee's femorotibial compartments, some surgical considerations may be outlined for the lateral compartment.[18,54,55] The rule of undercorrection of the deformity should be strictly applied on lateral UKA[53] to avoid medial OA progression. Furthermore, the positioning of the femoral component should accommodate the femoral divergence of the lateral condyle when the knee is flexed to avoid impingement with the tibial spines when brought into extension.[54] The mediolateral positioning of the femoral component should also avoid the excessive lateral placement in extension, which may lead to an overload of the lateral part of the tibial plateau when the knee is flexed to 30°.[54] Additionally, internal rotation of the tibial component when performing lateral UKA accommodates the typical screw-home mechanism occurring during knee flexion, and this should be included when performing the sagittal tibial cut.[5,55]

Frontal view   **Lateral View**

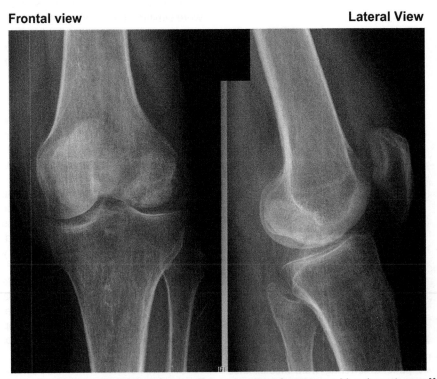

Fig. 14. Radiographic (preoperative and postoperative) evaluation of a 55-year-old male patient suffering from an osteonecrosis of the femoral (*lateral*) condyle. Frontal and lateral view.

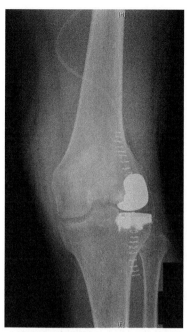

Fig. 15. Radiographic (preoperative and postoperative) evaluation of a 55-year-old male patient suffering from an osteonecrosis of the femoral (*lateral*) condyle. Frontal view after knee resurfacing.

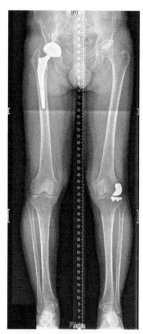

Fig. 17. Radiographic (preoperative and postoperative) evaluation of a 55-year-old male patient suffering from an osteonecrosis of the femoral (*lateral*) condyle. Long-axis evaluation after knee resurfacing.

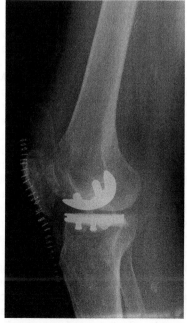

Fig. 16. Radiographic (preoperative and postoperative) evaluation of a 55-year-old male patient suffering from an osteonecrosis of the femoral (*lateral*) condyle. Lateral view after knee resurfacing.

Unicompartmental knee arthroplasty for osteonecrosis

Osteonecrosis of the knee classically includes 2 distinct entities: spontaneous osteonecrosis or secondary osteonecrosis.[56–62] Spontaneous osteonecrosis occurs most often in patients older than 55, unilaterally, and in 1 compartment of the knee.[56,57,59,60] Secondary osteonecrosis could appear after corticosteroid therapy, renal and systemic disease, or barotrauma, and occurs most often in younger patients with bilateral multicompartmental disease.[56,60] For both types of osteonecrosis, the natural evolution without treatment is arthritis.[56,61,62] Four stages of the radiographic evolution of the lesion have been described, according to Mont and colleagues.[59] In the first stage, the knee maintains a normal aspect. In the second stage, cystic or osteosclerotic lesions are observed with normal contour, whereas subchondral collapse is observed in stage 3. In stage 4, a narrowing of the joint is observed.[56] For stages 1, 2, and 3, core decompression,[63,64] arthroscopic débridement, or high tibial osteotomy has been used with success. Stage 4 is associated with severe clinical symptoms, and TKA[65,66] or UKA[67–70] has been advocated. To date, there are few data analyzing the clinical and radiologic outcomes after modern UKA for spontaneous and secondary osteonecrosis of the knee and these outcomes

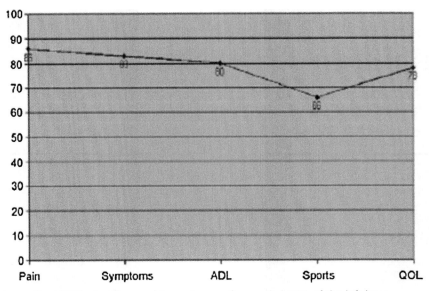

Fig. 18. Postoperative KOOS of a 65-year-old man 1 year after medial UKA of the left knee.

should be clarified. The utility of UKA in secondary osteonecrosis should be clarified, because this entity typically involves the metaphyseal region and both compartments.[56] Furthermore, the place of UKA for secondary osteonecrosis that more often involves the metaphyseal regions and both compartments should be determined.[56] The authors presented, in 2007,[44] a series of 31 UKAs performed after osteonecrosis of the knee; according to the Ahlbäck classification, 2 patients (6%) were grade 1, 14 (45%) were grade 2, and 15 (49%) were grade 3. The causes of the osteonecrosis were spontaneous in 21 knees (67%) and secondary in 10 knees (33%), including steroidinduced osteonecrosis in 7 and barotraumatic osteonecrosis in professional scuba divers in 3. All patients in cases of steroid-induced osteonecrosis have had long-term steroid therapy, in 4 cases for a systematic lupus erythematosus and in 3 cases after a renal transplantation.

In a retrospective study, the author and colleagues[45] analyzed the results of UKA for osteonecrosis using a modern implant and strict inclusion criteria, first regarding the limitation of the osteonecrosis to 1 compartment of the knee even for the cases of secondary osteonecrosis and second regarding the status of patellofemoral articulation and the anterior cruciate ligament. The 12-year survival rate was 96.7% ± 3% with revision for any reason or radiographic loosening as the endpoint. No intraoperative complications occurred. One knee underwent revision for aseptic loosening at 30 months. The knee was revised with a cemented TKA with good clinical and radiographic results at the latest follow-up. These data suggest the UKA is reliable in osteonecrosis (see **Figs. 14–17**) for alleviating pain and improving function, restoring proper lower limb mechanical axis, and achieving durable survivorship.

SUBJECTIVE EVALUATION OF UNICOMPARTMENTAL KNEE ARTHROPLASTY: KNEE SCORING SYSTEMS

Outcome scoring is vital in the accurate evaluation of interventions around the knee. There has been a paradigm shift in the determinants of success over the past 2 decades, from those based on physical examination and radiographic variables to a more patient-centered assessment of outcome. Modern knee surgery has allowed patients' expectations and activity levels to increase but it remains difficult to accurately assess outcome. Evidence in the current literature confirms that few scoring systems have satisfactory levels of reliability and validity.[71] What is clear is that those systems that use a high degree of patient involvement, such as the Knee Injury and Osteoarthritis Outcome Score (KOOS),[8] Oxford Knee Score,[72] and International Knee Documentation Committee[72] scores, are performing better as a patient-based assessment tool.[7] Several scoring systems largely concentrate on pathology and knee-specific, patient-based systems.[71] The use of generic instruments to complement these is, however, encouraged.[71,73] They have a greater potential to measure side effects or unforeseen effects of treatment. The Western Ontario and McMaster Universities Osteoarthritis Index (WOMAC),[74,75] in particular, remains valid, reliable, and responsive.

Significant advances have been made in prosthetic design and function. This has changed the emphasis from one of the alleviation of disabling pain and a limited return of functional activity as the primary endpoint to a more generalized improvement in quality of life and knee function. Expectations vary greatly between patients and the mismatch of experience versus expectation after knee replacement is a potent cause of patient dissatisfaction. Scoring systems in turn have evolved to accommodate more active patients at both ends of the age spectrum.[71,74–78] As a result of earlier surgical intervention, patients now expect not only pain relief but also correction of any deformity added to an early return to physical and recreational activities. Currently, there is no single best outcome measure for total knee replacement. There are, however, several reliable, responsive, and validated systems.

The WOMAC is one of the disease-specific scores most frequently used.[72] The WOMAC[74,75] underwent vigorous psychometric validation before its introduction and requires licensed use from the copyright holders. This may be obtained free online for educational and clinical use (www.womac.org). It is ubiquitous, easy to use, and evaluates 3 domains: pain (5 questions), stiffness (2 questions), and physical function (17 questions), each weighted on a similar computation. The WOMAC is sensitive to change and has shown greater efficiency than most of other instruments in the assessment of osteoarthritis.[77]

The KOOS[8] questionnaire had been developed in the 1990s as an instrument to assess a patient's opinion about a knee and associated problems. It includes WOMAC in its complete and original format and other questions grouped in a self assessed-questionnaire. The results of KOOS are presented in 5 subscales: pain, other symptoms, activities of daily living, function in sport, and recreation and knee-related quality of life. The previous week is the time period considered when answering the questions. Standardized answer options are given (5 Likert boxes) and each question is assigned a score from 0 to 4. A normalized score (100 indicating no symptoms and 0 indicating extreme symptoms) is calculated for each subscale (see **Fig. 18**). Since the first publication in 1998, the psychometric properties of the KOOS have been assessed in more than 20 individual studies from all over the world. Furthermore, KOOS has been evaluated and compared with other instruments in several reviews.[79–81]

The 12-item Oxford Knee Score, published in 1998,[68] contains 12 questions scored from 0 to 4, with 4 the best outcome. The scoring system ranges from 0 to 48, with 48 representing the most favorable outcome. In contrast with the patient-assessed and equally weighted Oxford Knee Score, the American Knee Society Score is a surgeon-assessed weighted score developed through consensus by the Knee Society in 1989.[9] It comprises 2 parts. The first addresses pain, stability, and range of movement. The second part examines function, with particular reference to walking distance and stair climbing. Maximum scores of 100 are possible in each section. The American Knee Society Score has been validated and is responsive and reproducible. It suffers, however, from high interobserver and intraobserver variation when assessments are performed by less-experienced doctors and nurses.[82]

To improve the measurement of patient outcomes, the new Knee Society scoring system, with both preoperative and postoperative versions that include both patient and surgeon sections, have been developed (www.kneesociety.org).[12,83] In the preoperative instrument, patients supply demographic information and complete questions relating to their symptoms (pain measures), knee function, satisfaction with their current functional activities, and expectations of the results of the TKA. A surgeon completes information on functional status and objective information on the alignment, instability, and range of motion of the knee. In addition to questions about standard activities, such as walking on an uneven surface or climbing a flight of stairs, the instrument also asks about discretionary activities that are important to the patient. These include both recreational and workout activities. The postoperative version asks patients to compare their initial expectations with current reality for pain relief, activities of daily living, and discretionary (leisure, recreational, and sports) activities. The score has been validated and published for TKA[12] and is under validation and publication process for UKA.[83]

SUMMARY

Precise outcome evaluation is mandatory to improve analysis of the results of knee replacement procedures. Patients' expectations toward surgery and activity levels increased with the change of patient population and improvement of the surgical results. It is difficult, however, to accurately assess outcomes because objective evaluation of the patient function performed by a surgeon only remains highly inaccurate. For these reasons, new methods of objective evaluation after UKA have been developed, including fluoroscopic analysis devices. These devices can give objective information about range of motion and prosthesis function during daily activities.

Using a knee replacement scoring system can bring first, objective data filled by a surgeon, and then, subjective data as experienced by a patient. The mismatch of experience versus expectation after knee replacement is a potent cause of patient dissatisfaction. Therefore, knee scoring systems have evolved to accommodate more active patients at both ends of the age spectrum. The next generation of knee scoring system should include the new IKS score, have been developed to include all of these dimensions (patient's and surgeon's experience) to clearly evaluate outcomes of knee replacement procedures.

REFERENCES

1. Hanssen AD, Stuart MJ, Scott RD, et al. Surgical options for the middle-aged patient with osteoarthritis of the knee joint. Instr Course Lect 2001;50: 499–511.
2. Argenson JN, Chevrol-Benkeddache Y, Aubaniac JM. Modern unicompartmental knee arthroplasty with cement: a three to ten-year follow-up study. J Bone Joint Surg Am 2002;84:2235–9.
3. Dennis MG, Di Cesare PE. Surgical management of the middle age arthritic knee. Bull Hosp Jt Dis 2003;61:172–8.
4. Flecher X, Parratte S, Aubaniac JM, et al. A 12-28 year follow-up study of closing wedge high tibial osteotomy. Clin Orthop 2006;452:91–6.
5. Pennington DW, Swienckowski JJ, Lutes WB, et al. Unicompartmental knee arthroplasty in patients sixty years of age or younger. J Bone Joint Surg Am 2003;85:1968–73.
6. Price AJ, Dodd CA, Svard UG, et al. Oxford medial unicompartmental knee arthroplasty in patients younger and older than 60 years of age. J Bone Joint Surg Br 2005;87(11):1488–92.
7. Ornetti P, Parratte S, Gossec L, et al. Cross-cultural adaptation and validation of the French version of the Knee injury and Osteoarthritis Outcome Score (KOOS) in knee osteoarthritis patients. Osteoarthr Cartil 2008;16(4):423–8.
8. Roos EM, Lohmander LS. The Knee injury and Osteoarthritis Outcome Score (KOOS): from joint injury. Health Qual Life Outcomes 2003;1(1):64.
9. Insall JN, Dorr LD, Scott RD, et al. Rationale of the Knee Society clinical rating system. Clin Orthop 1989;248:13–4.
10. Parratte S, Argenson JN, Pearce O, et al. Medial unicompartmental knee replacement in the under-50s. J Bone Joint Surg Br 2009;91:351–6.
11. Felts E, Parratte S, Pauly V, et al. Function and quality of life following medial unicompartmental knee arthroplasty in patients 60 years of age or younger. Orthop Traumatol Surg Res 2010;96: 861–7.
12. Noble PC, Scuderi GR, Brekke AC, et al. Development of a new Knee Society scoring system. Clin Orthop Relat Res 2012;470:20–32.
13. Kennedy WR, White RP. Unicompartmental arthroplasty of the knee: postoperative alignment and its influence on overall results. Clin Orthop 1987; 221:278–85.
14. Berger RA, Meneghini RM, Sheinkop MB. The progression of patellofemoral arthrosis after medial unicompartmental replacement: results at 11 to 15 years. Clin Orthop 2004;428:92–9.
15. Lafortune MA, Cavanagh PR, Sommer HJ 3rd, et al. Three-dimensional kinematics of the human knee during walking. J Biomech 1992;25:347–57.
16. Dennis DA, Komistek RD, Hoff WA, et al. In vivo knee kinematics derived using an inverse perspective technique. Clin Orthop Relat Res 1996;331:107–17.
17. Dennis D, Komistek RD, Hoff WA, et al. In vivo anteroposterior femorotibial translation: a multicenter analysis. Clin Orthop 1998;356:47–57.
18. Argenson JN, Komistek RD, Aubaniac JM, et al. In vivo determination of knee kinematics for subjects implanted with a unicompartmental arthroplasty. J Arthroplasty 2002;17:1049–54.
19. Blunn GW, Walker PS, Joshi A, et al. The dominance of cyclic sliding in producing wear in total knee replacements. Clin Orthop 1991;273:253–60.
20. Deschamps G, Lapeyre B. Rupture of the anterior cruciate ligament: a frequently unrecognized cause of failure of unicompartmental knee prostheses. Rev Chir Orthop Reparatrice Appar Mot 1987; 73:544–51.
21. Moller JT, Weeth RE, Keller JO, et al. Unicompartmental arthroplasty of the knee. Cadaver study of the importance of the anterior cruciate ligament. Acta Orthop Scand 1985;56:120–3.
22. Palmer SH, Morrison PJ, Ross AC. Early catastrophic tibial component wear after unicompartmental knee arthroplasty. Clin Orthop 1998;350: 143–8.
23. Mont MA, Lee CW, Sheldon M, et al. Total knee arthroplasty in patients ≤50 years old. J Arthroplasty 2002;17:538–43.
24. Hofmann AA, Heithoff SM, Camargo M. Cementless total knee arthroplasty in patients 50 years or younger. Clin Orthop 2002;404:102–7.
25. Lonner JH, Hershmann S, Mont M, et al. Total knee arthroplasty in patients 40 years of age and younger with osteoarthritis. Clin Orthop 2000;380: 85–90.
26. Flecher X, Argenson JN, Aubaniac JM. Hip and knee replacement and sport. Ann Readapt Med Phys 2004;47:382–8.
27. Morgan M, Brooks S, Nelson RA. Total knee arthroplasty in young active patients using a highly congruent fully mobile prosthesis. J Arthroplasty 2007;22:525–30.

28. Weale AE, Newman JH. Unicompartmental arthroplasty and high tibial osteotomy for osteoarthrosis of the knee: a comparative study with a 12- to 17-year follow-up period. Clin Orthop 1994;302:134–7.

29. Duffy GP, Trousdale RT, Stuart MJ. Total knee arthroplasty in patients 55 years old or younger: 10- to 17-year results. Clin Orthop 1998;356:22–7.

30. Argenson JN, Parratte S. The unicompartmental knee: design and technical considerations in minimizing wear. Clin Orthop 2006;452:137–42.

31. Fisher N, Agarwal M, Reuben SF, et al. Sporting and physical activity following Oxford medial unicompartmental knee arthroplasty. Knee 2006;13:296–300.

32. Parratte S, Pauly V, Aubaniac JM, et al. No long-term difference between fixed and mobile medial unicompartmental arthroplasty. Clin Orthop Relat Res 2012;470:61–8.

33. Price AJ, Short A, Kellett C, et al. Ten-year in vivo wear measurement of a fully congruent mobile bearing unicompartmental knee arthroplasty. J Bone Joint Surg Br 2005;87:1493–7.

34. Walton NP, Jahromi I, Lewis PL, et al. Patient-perceived outcomes and return to sport and work: TKA versus mini-incision unicompartmental knee arthroplasty. J Knee Surg 2006;19:112–6.

35. Steele RG, Hutabarat S, Evans RL, et al. Survivorship of the St Georg Sled medial unicompartmental knee replacement beyond ten years. J Bone Joint Surg Br 2006;88:1164–8.

36. Deshmukh RV, Scott RD. Unicompartmental knee arthroplasty for younger patients: an alternative view. Clin Orthop 2002;404:108–12.

37. Murray D, Goodfellow J, O'Connor J. The Oxford medial unicompartmental arthroplasty. J Bone Joint Surg Br 1998;80:983.

38. Svärd U, Price A. Oxford medial unicompartmental knee arthroplasty. J Bone Joint Surg Br 2001;83:191.

39. Price A, Wait J, Svärd U. Long-term clinical results of the medial Oxford unicompartmental knee arthroplasty. Clin Orthop Relat Res 2005;(435):171.

40. Lewold S, Goodman S, Knutson K, et al. Oxford meniscal bearing knee versus the Marmor knee in unicompartmental arthroplasty for arthrosis. J Arthroplasty 1995;10:722.

41. Vorlat P, Putzeys G, Cottenie D, et al. The Oxford unicompartmental knee prosthesis: an independent 10-year survival analysis. Knee Surg Sports Traumatol Arthrosc 2005;14:40.

42. US IDE. FDA pre market approach. Summary of safety and effectiveness. P010014. 2004. FDA website.

43. Confalonieri N, Manzotti A, Pullen C. Comparison of a mobile with a fixed tibial bearing unicompartmental knee prosthesis: a prospective randomized trial using a dedicated outcome score. Knee 2004;11:357.

44. Gleeson R, Evans C, Ackroyd J, et al. Fixed or mobile bearing unicompartmental knee replacement? A comparative cohort study. Knee 2004;11(5):379–84.

45. Parratte S, Argenson JN, Dumas J, et al. Unicompartmental knee arthroplasty for avascular osteonecrosis. Clin Orthop Relat Res 2007;464:37–42.

46. Ashraf T, Newman JH, Evans RL, et al. Lateral unicompartmental knee replacement survivorship and clinical experience over 21 years. J Bone Joint Surg Br 2002;84:1126–30.

47. Gunther T, Murray D, Miller R. Lateral unicompartmental knee arthroplasty with Oxford meniscal knee. Knee 1996;3:33–9.

48. Sah AP, Scott RD. Lateral unicompartmental knee arthroplasty through a medial approach. Study with an average five-year follow-up. J Bone Joint Surg Am 2007;89:1948–54.

49. Marmor L. Lateral compartment arthroplasty of the knee. Clin Orthop Relat Res 1984;186:115–21.

50. Scott RD. Lateral unicompartmental replacement: a road less traveled. Orthopedics 2005;28:983–4 J Arthroplasty 2002;17:1049–54.

51. Argenson JN, Parratte S, Bertani A, et al. Long-term results with a lateral unicondylar replacement. Clin Orthop Relat Res 2008;466:2686–93.

52. Engh GA. The lateral unicompartmental replacement: a road less traveled. Orthopedics 2006;29:825–6.

53. Ohdera T, Tokunaga J, Kobayashi A. Unicompartmental knee arthroplasty for lateral gonarthrosis: midterm results. J Arthroplasty 2001;16:196–200.

54. Cartier P, Sanouiller JL, Grelsamer RP. Unicompartmental knee arthroplasty surgery. 10-year minimum follow-up period. J Arthroplasty 1996;11:782–8.

55. Weidow J. Lateral osteoarthritis of the knee. Etiology based on morphological, anatomical, kinematic and kinetic observations. Acta Orthop Suppl 2006;77:3–44.

56. Aglietti P, Insall JN, Buzzi R, et al. Idiopathic osteonecrosis of the knee: aetiology, prognosis and treatment. J Bone Joint Surg Br 1983;65:588–97.

57. Ahlback S, Bauer GC, Bohne WH. Spontaneous osteonecrosis of the knee. Arthritis Rheum 1968;11:705–33.

58. Ecker ML. Spontaneous osteonecrosis of the distal femur. Instr Course Lect 2001;50:495–8.

59. Mont MA, Baumgarten KM, Rifai A, et al. Atraumatic osteonecrosis of the knee. J Bone Joint Surg Am 2000;82:1279–90.

60. Myers TG, Cui Q, Kuskowski M, et al. Outcomes of total and unicompartmental knee arthroplasty for secondary and spontaneous osteonecrosis of the knee. J Bone Joint Surg Am 2006;88(Suppl):76–82.

61. Marmor L. Unicompartmental arthroplasty for osteonecrosis of the knee joint. Clin Orthop Relat Res 1993;294:247–53.

62. Muheim G, Bohne WH. Prognosis in spontaneous osteonecrosis of the knee. J Bone Joint Surg Br 1970;52:605–12.

63. Carro LP, Cimiano JG, Del Alamo GG, et al. Core decompression and arthroscopic bone grafting for avascular necrosis of the knee. Arthroscopy 1996;12:323–6.

64. Mont MA, Tomek IM, Hungerford DS. Core decompression for avascular necrosis of the distal femur: long term followup. Clin Orthop Relat Res 1997; 334:124–30.

65. Bergman NR, Rand JA. Total knee arthroplasty in osteonecrosis. Clin Orthop Relat Res 1991;273: 77–82.

66. Lotke PA, Battish R, Nelson CL. Treatment of osteonecrosis of the knee. Instr Course Lect 2001;50: 483–8.

67. Mont MA, Rifai A, Baumgarten KM, et al. Total knee arthroplasty for osteonecrosis. J Bone Joint Surg Am 2002;84:599–603.

68. Atsui K, Tateishi H, Futani H, et al. Ceramic unicompartmental knee arthroplasty for spontaneous osteonecrosis of the knee joint. Bull Hosp Jt Dis 1997;56:233–6.

69. Lotke PA, Abend JA, Ecker ML. The treatment of osteonecrosis of the medial femoral condyle. Clin Orthop Relat Res 1982;171:109–16.

70. Soucacos PN, Xenakis TH, Beris AE, et al. Idiopathic Osteonecrosis of the medial femoral condyle: classification and treatment. Clin Orthop Relat Res 1997;341:82–9.

71. Paxton EW, Fithian DC, Stone ML, et al. The reliability and validity of knee-specific and general health instruments in assessing acute patellar dislocation outcomes. Am J Sports Med 2003; 31(4):487–92.

72. Dawson J, Fitzpatrick R, Murray D, et al. Questionnaire on the perceptions of patients about total knee replacement. J Bone Joint Surg Br 1998;80: 63–9.

73. Garratt AM, Brealey S, Gillespie WJ. Patient-assessed health instruments for the knee: a structured review. Rheumatology (Oxford) 2004;43(11): 1414–23.

74. Collins NJ, Misra D, Felson DT, et al. Measures of knee function: International Knee Documentation Committee (IKDC) Subjective Knee Evaluation Form, Knee Injury and Osteoarthritis Outcome Score (KOOS), Knee Injury and Osteoarthritis Outcome Score Physical Function Short Form (KOOS-PS), Knee Outcome Survey Activities of Daily Living Scale (KOS-ADL), Lysholm Knee Scoring Scale, Oxford Knee Score (OKS), Western Ontario and McMaster Universities Osteoarthritis Index (WOMAC), Activity Rating Scale (ARS), and Tegner Activity Score (TAS). Arthritis Care Res 2011;63(Suppl 11):S208–28.

75. Whitehouse SL, Crawford RW, Learmonth ID. Validation for the reduced Western Ontario and McMaster Universities Osteoarthritis Index function scale. J Orthop Surg 2008;16(1):50–3.

76. Hefti F, Muller W, Jakob RP, et al. Evaluation of knee ligament injuries with the IKDC form. Knee Surg Sports Traumatol Arthrosc 1993;1(3–4):226–34.

77. Davies AP. Rating systems for total knee replacement. Knee 2002;9(4):261–6.

78. Patt JC, Mauerhan DR. Outcomes research in total joint replacement: a critical review and commentary. Am J Orthop (Belle Mead NJ) 2005;34(4): 167–72.

79. Tanner SM, Dainty KN, Marx RG, et al. Knee-specific quality-of-life instruments: which ones measure symptoms and disabilities most important to patients? Am J Sports Med 2007;35(9):1450–8.

80. Hambly K, Griva K. IKDC or KOOS? Which measures symptoms and disabilities most important to postoperative articular cartilage repair patients? Am J Sports Med 2008;36(9):1695–704.

81. Wright RW. Knee injury outcomes measures. J Am Acad Orthop Surg 2009;17:31–9.

82. Liow RY, Walker K, Wajid MA, et al. The reliability of the American Knee Society Score. Acta Orthop Scand 2000;71(6):603–8.

83. Argenson JN, Berend KR, Parratte S, et al. The Validation of the New Knee Society Score for Unicompartmental Knee Arthroplasty. Presented at the open meeting of the Knee Society, AAOS. Chicago, March 23, 2013.

TRAUMA

Preface
Trauma

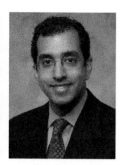

Saqib Rehman, MD
Editor

In just the last few years, there has been a remarkable transition in the way orthopedic surgeons obtain point-of-care information. Online journals and textbooks as well as mobile devices and tablets have taken off as the "go-to" means of obtaining information for many of us. Information "on-the-go" demands that the journals have readily accessible information on topics of current interest to orthopedic surgeons. As the *Orthopedic Clinics in North America* moves to this new format, I'll be doing my best to shape the content of the Trauma section to meet today's needs of you, our readers. In this issue, we have 2 excellent reviews on topics that I am sure you will find useful when the time comes.

Treating pelvic trauma in pregnancy is an uncommon event, but like most things in trauma, the surgeon better figure out what to do quickly to best serve our patients. Drs Amorosa, Helfet, and colleagues draw on their experience managing both traumatic pelvic fractures in pregnant patients as well as pubic symphyseal disruption of pregnancy

to provide a comprehensive review of the management of these challenging conditions.

Proximal humeral fractures remain difficult cases to manage, whether treated nonoperatively, or with osteosynthesis or arthroplasty methods. For those of us who do shoulder arthroplasty only occasionally, it can be a humbling experience to try and recover satisfactory function for our patients. Drs Wiesel, Nagda, and Williams review their technical pearls and tips for obtaining improved results with shoulder arthroplasty for these injuries.

Saqib Rehman, MD
Associate Professor of Orthopaedic Surgery
Director of Orthopaedic Trauma
Department of Orthopaedic Surgery
Temple University Hospital
3401 North Broad Street
Philadelphia, PA 19140, USA

E-mail address:
Saqib.Rehman@tuhs.temple.edu

Orthop Clin N Am 44 (2013) xv
http://dx.doi.org/10.1016/j.ocl.2013.05.003
0030-5898/13/$ – see front matter © 2013 Published by Elsevier Inc.

Management of Pelvic Injuries in Pregnancy

Louis F. Amorosa, MD[a],*,
Jennifer Harms Amorosa, MD, MAT[b],
David S. Wellman, MD[c], Dean G. Lorich, MD[c],
David L. Helfet, MD[c]

KEYWORDS

- Pelvic fracture • Acetabular fracture • Pregnancy • Pubic symphysis rupture • Pelvic instability

KEY POINTS

- Pelvic trauma in pregnant women represents a life-threatening condition to both the mother and child. In the acute setting, the mother's life takes precedence over that of the unborn child.
- Acute pubic symphysis rupture caused by pregnancy is rare and can usually be managed nonoperatively. However, with diastasis of greater than 4 cm, open pubic symphysis rupture, and continued pelvic malreduction in a pelvic binder, operative intervention should be considered.
- Chronic pelvic instability related to parturition is a common syndrome and can almost always be managed nonoperatively.
- In most cases, history of pelvic ring injury or pubic symphysis rupture is not a contraindication to vaginal delivery. However, women with a history of pelvic trauma do have a higher incidence of cesarean section as a result of multiple factors.

PELVIC RING TRAUMA IN THE PREGNANT WOMAN

Epidemiology of Trauma in Pregnancy

After primary obstetric causes, trauma is the leading cause of maternal death during pregnancy.[1] Trauma occurs in approximately 7% of all pregnancies[2] and is most often in conjunction with motor vehicle accidents (MVAs).[3,4] Similar to the trauma-related mortality in nonpregnant women, the maternal mortality from trauma is approximately 10%, with the highest risk of maternal death occurring in the third trimester.[5–7] Fetal death rates are significantly higher and have been reported to be as high as 50% to 65% in cases of severe trauma.[8–10]

Fetal Morbidity and Mortality

Maternal death from trauma is associated both with fetal death and a high injury severity score.[3,9,11] If the fetus survives the initial traumatic event, it is still at a higher risk of low birth weight, premature delivery, and permanent neurocognitive dysfunction than a pregnancy not affected by a traumatic event.[12] Multiple case reports and series have identified associations between maternal trauma during pregnancy and cerebral palsy or developmental delay in the child.[13–16] This brain injury is believed to be caused by a hypoxic insult to the developing fetal brain either from maternal hypotension or placental embolus at the time of the traumatic event.[14]

The fetus is at greater risk of death caused by trauma than the mother. Fetal demise can be caused by direct trauma, preterm labor, maternal-fetal hemorrhage, placental abruption, or uterine rupture.[4] Before 12 weeks of gestation, the fetus is contained entirely within the bony pelvis and is protected from direct trauma. However, after

[a] Department of Orthopaedic Surgery, New York Medical College, 19 Bradhurst Ave, Suite 1300, Hawthorne, NY 10532, USA; [b] Department of Obstetrics and Gynecology, Columbia University Medical Center, 622 W 168th Street, New York, NY 10032, USA; [c] Division of Orthopaedic Trauma, Hospital for Special Surgery, 535 East 70th Street, New York, NY 10021, USA
* Corresponding author.
E-mail address: lou53nd@gmail.com

Orthop Clin N Am 44 (2013) 301–315
http://dx.doi.org/10.1016/j.ocl.2013.03.005
0030-5898/13/$ – see front matter © 2013 Elsevier Inc. All rights reserved.

12 weeks' gestation, direct injury to the fetus can occur through the same mechanism as the pelvic fracture. Placental abruption is the most common complication of blunt trauma in pregnancy[17] and is responsible for fetal death in 40% to 60% of trauma-related deaths versus 1% to 5% in non-traumatic causes of fetal death.[9] It is theorized that the force of the traumatic event causes the elastic uterine lining to separate from the inelastic placenta,[18] interrupting the gas exchange that occurs across the placental interface. If a complete placental abruption occurs, the fetus, if viable, must be delivered rapidly in order not to deprive the fetus of oxygenated blood. Even minor trauma can increase the risk of preterm labor, placental abruption, and fetal demise, especially if the abdomen or pelvis is involved.[19,20]

Prevention Strategies

Because most severe trauma in pregnant women is caused by MVAs, the best evidence-based strategy to prevent related maternal and fetal morbidity and mortality is the use of safety belts. Approximately one-half of all fetal fatalities caused by MVAs are estimated to be preventable if seat belts are worn properly.[21] The use of seat belts has been shown to reduce the rate of preterm labor and fetal demise in pregnant women involved in MVAs.[21,22] Safety belts should have both a shoulder harness and lap belt. The lap belt should sit across the pelvic brim, not the gravid uterus, and the shoulder harness should rest between the breasts.[7,8]

Epidemiology of Pelvic and Acetabular Fractures in Pregnancy

Few evidence-based studies have examined the outcomes of pregnant women who sustain pelvic fractures, because such cases are rare; however, 1 large population-based study found that pregnant women who sustain pelvic fractures were at high risk for placental abruption and fetal demise.[12] A systematic review of the literature that reported on 101 total cases of pelvic or acetabular fractures in pregnant women found that although no single institution had significant experience with this combined patient-injury demographic, maternal and fetal death were more likely to occur with MVAs and pedestrians struck by a motor vehicle than with a fall. Mortality was not affected by fracture classification (simple or complex), type (pelvic or acetabular), pregnancy trimester, or study era.[11] In this review, the fetal mortality was 35% and the maternal mortality was 9%, which is similar to mortality from high-energy trauma in general. In a 24-year study

from a major European trauma center of 4196 patients with blunt polytrauma, only 7 of the patients who sustained a pelvic fracture were pregnant (0.17% incidence in the overall population of patients with polytrauma).[23] The mean injury severity score of these 7 women was 29.9. Five of 7 mothers survived their injuries; however, only 3 of 7 fetuses survived, and 4 were found to be deceased at the scene of the accident. In 2 of the 3 mothers in whom the fetus survived, treatment was modified based on the viability of the fetus. In all 3 cases in which the fetus survived, the mother went on to uneventful delivery of the child without any long-term effects related to the mother's injury. Almog and colleagues[24] found that over a 15-year period, only 15 of 1345 patients who were treated at a trauma center for a pelvic or acetabular fracture were pregnant (1.1%). One woman died of her injuries and there were 4 cases of fetal death. Four of the 15 women underwent operative fixation of their fractures, and the rest were treated nonoperatively.

Acetabular fractures are considered part of the spectrum of injuries to the pelvic ring. Most studies that have reported on acetabular fractures in pregnant women are case reports; however, Porter and colleagues[25] reported a case series of 8 pregnant women with acetabular fractures (of a total of 518 patients) who presented to a level I trauma center over a 6-year period. Gestational age in this group ranged from 5 to 26 weeks at the time of injury. All of the patients went on to deliver at at least 36 weeks with normal Apgar scores at delivery. Long-term follow-up on the children was not reported.

Evaluation and Treatment

Initial assessment

The most unique aspect of pregnancy-related trauma is that the trauma team must simultaneously address 2 patients: the mother and the fetus. Therefore, the treatment team should include not only the standard trauma team members but also a maternal-fetal medicine specialist. The priority in a pregnant trauma patient is timely treatment and resuscitation of the mother, because this leads to better outcomes for the fetus.[7] Standard protocol of advanced trauma life support should be adhered to by addressing airway, breathing, circulation, disability, and exposure. All female trauma patients of childbearing age should have a rapid urine pregnancy test, because sometimes neither the patient nor the trauma team may be aware of an early pregnancy. Pelvic fractures caused by high-energy mechanisms are an indicator of severe polytrauma, and there is a high incidence of associated injuries, including head, thoracic, abdominal, and spinal injuries, some of which are immediately more life-threatening than the pelvic fracture itself.[26]

Sources of blood loss, if not obvious on physical examination, should be discovered via chest radiograph, pelvic radiograph, and focused assessment with sonography in trauma (FAST) survey. A Foley catheter should be placed to monitor adequacy of resuscitation. The presence of blood at the vaginal introitus in a pregnant trauma patient should prompt the trauma and obstetric team to rule out placenta previa, placental abruption, or labor. Nonobstetric causes include urethral or bladder injury; if a nonobstetric cause is suspected, the patient should be evaluated by a urologist before Foley catheter placement.[27] Blood at the vagina or rectum in the presence of a high-energy pelvic fracture may also indicate an open pelvic fracture, a diagnosis that carries a mortality of near 50% and requires operative debridement and stabilization once the patient is hemodynamically stable.[28]

Fetal considerations in the acute setting

In any pregnant women beyond the threshold of viability, continuous fetal heart rate monitoring and a maternal tocometer to monitor for uterine contractions should be used in the acute setting.[8] Depending on the center, fetuses are typically considered viable at 24 weeks' gestational age; however, fetuses born at less than 30 weeks are at a significantly increased risk of cerebral palsy.[29] In obtunded or intubated patients for whom no history is available, the location of the uterine fundus allows for a close estimate of gestational age, and in early pregnancies, the standard FAST scan may be diagnostic.[8] On secondary survey, a pelvic examination should be performed by an obstetrician, who should look for bleeding, signs of labor, and cervical length or dilation. In the setting of a pelvic fracture, such an examination may need to be performed under sedation or general anesthesia because of pain or instability.[7] In addition, a Kleihauer-Betke (KB) blood test, which detects fetal hemoglobin in maternal circulation, can aid in detecting occult maternal-fetal hemorrhage.[30] It is unnecessary in obvious cases of severe trauma and maternal-fetal hemorrhage,[31] but a positive KB test should prompt the treatment team to administer Rh immunoglobulin in all Rh-negative women.[8]

Emergent reduction of the pelvis in the pregnant patient

If an open-book pelvic fracture (anteroposterior compression type) is diagnosed on examination or radiograph, and the patient is hemodynamically unstable, a pelvic sheet or binder should be placed to tamponade presumed bleeding from disrupted pelvic vessels. The pelvis can be close reduced by internally rotating the legs and compressing on the iliac wings when applying the sheet or binder. Internally rotating the legs and holding them together by taping the knees with cushioning between them is an assistive maneuver to hold the reduction. Military antishock trousers (MAST), although effective in keeping the pelvis reduced and creating a tamponade, are no longer recommended for treatment, because they limit access to the abdomen and cannot be used for any significant period out of concern for MAST-induced lower extremity compartment syndrome.[32]

There are several unique aspects to closed reduction of the pregnant patient's pelvis. The gravid uterus acts as a compressive device on the inferior vena cava (IVC) when the pregnant patient is supine, which inhibits venous return and decreases cardiac output. Close reducing an open-book pelvic fracture with a sheet or a binder may worsen this problem by increasing the compression of the gravid uterus on the IVC, further decreasing venous return to the heart and cardiac output. Certain measures may help to mitigate this problem once the pelvic binder or sheet is placed.[18] If the patient is too unstable to be placed into the full left lateral decubitus position or if there is a concurrent spinal injury preventing safe left lateral decubitus positioning, a roll or wedge may be placed under the right side of the backboard in spinal immobilized patients, or the bed rotated with the right side up.[8] This left lateral tilt position mechanically allows the uterus to fall to the left, relieving some pressure on the compressed IVC and improving venous return to the heart and improving cardiac output by as much as 30%.[31] There is little clinical evidence to support what degree of tilt to use[33]; however, the general recommendation is that 15° of left lateral tilt is acceptable.[34] Another maneuver that may help take pressure off the IVC is for an experienced obstetrician to manually shift the gravid uterus to the left of the abdomen.[7]

Resuscitation measures specific to a pregnant woman

Many physiologic changes during pregnancy occur and must be considered during resuscitation (**Box 1, Table 1**). After 20 weeks of gestation, the pregnant woman's plasma volume is significantly increased and up to 1500 mL of blood loss can occur before hemodynamic instability becomes apparent.[10] About 50% more fluid than usual may be required before improvement in hemodynamic status is observed.[7] The treatment team should be aware of certain normal

Box 1
Physiologic changes affecting diagnosis and treatment of the pregnant patient with an orthopedic injury

First Trimester

Major organogenesis (radiosensitive)

Central nervous system development (most sensitive period)

Increased risk of teratogenesis

Increased white blood cell count may be normal

Increased erythrocyte sedimentation rate may be normal

Hypercoagulable state

Increased risk of spontaneous abortion related to general anesthesia

Second Trimester

Fetal central nervous system relatively radioresistant

Hypotension possible with supine positioning caused by aortocaval compression (as a result of increased uterus size)

Increased white blood cell count may be normal

Increased erythrocyte sedimentation rate may be physiologically normal

Hypercoagulable state

Increased risk of spontaneous abortion related to general anesthesia

Increased risk of seat belt–related injury to the fetus

Third Trimester

Maternal plasma expands by 40% to 50% (dilutional anemia)

Pregnancy-related osteoporosis possible

Increased risk of seat belt–related injury to the fetus

Increased white blood cell count may be physiologically normal

Increased erythrocyte sedimentation rate may be physiologically normal

Data from Flik K, Kloen P, Toro JB, et al. Orthopaedic trauma in the pregnant patient. J Am Acad Orthop Surg 2006;14:175–82.

laboratory values in pregnant women; for instance, the normal arterial Pco_2 (partial pressure of carbon dioxide) level is less than a nonpregnant patient, and if a pregnant patient's value is in the normal nonpregnant range, hypoxia is present.[8] If the mother's blood type is not known, all blood products administered acutely should be Rh-negative to prevent a fetal transfusion reaction and Rh immunoglobulin should be administered. Moreover, a secondary coagulopathy or acute hypoxic event can occur as a result of amniotic fluid embolus.[23]

Continued hemodynamic instability in setting of an unstable pelvic fracture

If closed reduction of the pelvis and fluid resuscitation measures have failed to restore hemodynamic stability, there are 2 options to consider. Most often pelvic fractures result in venous plexus bleeding, which cannot be repaired surgically or embolized with angiography. In these cases, an open laparotomy with retroperitoneal packing and rapid external fixation of the pelvis can be performed to tamponade bleeding and has been shown to have lower mortality and less transfusion requirements than angiography.[35] At the time of laparotomy, any obstetric issues can be concurrently addressed. If an arterial source of bleeding is suspected, angiography may be the more appropriate choice over laparotomy. The decision of whether to proceed first to laparotomy or angiography depends primarily on the clinical situation and institutional resources available.

Emergent cesarean section

If the fetus is viable and massive placental abruption resulting in nonreassuring fetal status or uterine rupture has occurred, the fetus should be rapidly delivered via cesarean section with a pediatric intensivist team ready to treat the neonate on delivery. In the setting of massive maternal hemorrhage and coagulopathy, hysterectomy may also need to be performed. In situations in which the mother has expired, a perimortem cesarean section should be performed emergently to save the life of a viable fetus.[36] If cardiopulmonary resuscitation (CPR) is being performed for cardiac arrest, the treatment team must also immediately consider cesarean delivery. Perimortem cesarean section should be performed within 4 to 5 minutes of maternal cardiac arrest to increase the chances of both maternal and fetal survivability[37]; a review of the literature found that beyond 4 minutes of maternal CPR time, there is a low probability of fetal survival and a high probability of severe neurologic dysfunction if the fetus does survive.[38] Perimortem cesarean section allows for better maternal perfusion with chest compressions once the mother's abdomen is relieved of the gravid uterus.[7]

Table 1
Important physiologic changes during pregnancy

Parameter	Change	Implication
Maternal blood volume	Increased	Attenuated initial response to hemorrhage
Cardiac output	Increased	Increased metabolic demands
Uterine size	Enlarged	Potential for supine hypotension from aortocaval compression
Functional lung residual volume	Decreased	Hypoxemia from atelectasis
Gastrointestinal motility	Decreased	Greater risk for aspiration
Minute ventilation	Increased	Compensated respiratory alkalosis

Data from Flik K, Kloen P, Toro JB, et al. Orthopaedic trauma in the pregnant patient. J Am Acad Orthop Surg 2006;14:175–82.

Surgical considerations unique to the pregnant female

Surgical indications for pelvic and acetabular fractures are the same in pregnant women as in the general population. If surgery is indicated and the fetus remains viable through the acute stages of the trauma and resuscitation period, modifications to the standard surgical treatment of pelvic and acetabular fractures may be necessary to accommodate the fetus (**Fig. 1**). If the fetus is not viable then surgical considerations are more straightforward and follow the standard of care for any pelvic or acetabular fracture once the patient is stabilized.

If the fetus is viable, modifications to the standard treatment include using external fixation only as the

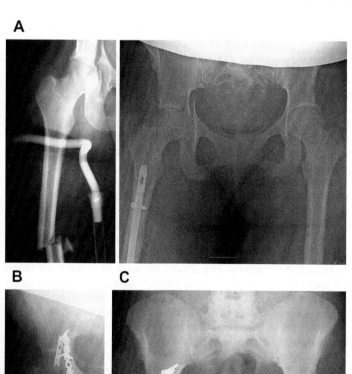

A

B   **C**

Fig. 1. (*A*) Injury radiographs showing a right transverse/posterior wall acetabular fracture and ipsilateral femur fracture in a 26-week pregnant female. After undergoing retrograde nailing of her femur, she was transferred to our institution for further management of her injuries. (*B*) The patient underwent operative fixation of her acetabular fracture through the Kocher-Langenbeck approach in the left lateral decubitus position in conjunction with close obstetric and anesthesia consultation and using minimal fluoroscopic assistance. (*C*) The patient went on to deliver a healthy baby vaginally at full term at 38 weeks. Follow-up radiographs at 38 months after the accident show preservation of the joint space and no evidence of post-traumatic arthritis. (*From* Kloen P, Flik K, Helfet DL. Operative treatment of acetabular fracture during pregnancy: a case report. Arch Orthop Trauma Surg 2005;125:209–12; with permission.)

definitive treatment, assuming that the reduction and stability are adequate. This strategy avoids further insult to the surrounding uterine environment.[8] Other options include using temporary skeletal traction with elective delivery of the fetus at a more advanced gestational age, followed by definitive operative treatment of the fracture.[11] If possible, delivery should be delayed to at least 28 weeks' gestational age to decrease the risks of immature lung development and intraventricular hemorrhage. Little benefit is seen by delaying delivery past 34 weeks of gestation.[39] If a fetus is to be delivered before 34 weeks' gestational age, antenatal steroids should be administered to aid in fetal lung maturity.[40] In addition, if the fetus is less than 32 weeks' gestational age, magnesium sulfate should be administered to help decrease rates of cerebral palsy.[41] Postponing delivery for fetal benefit must be weighed against the risks of waiting to perform operative treatment of the mother. After 3 weeks after injury, it becomes more challenging to obtain an adequate reduction during pelvic and acetabular fracture surgery[42]; additional risks are related to long-term immobilization and bed rest, including aspiration, pulmonary embolus, and pressure ulcers. The risk of prolonged bed rest immobilization and the prognosis for posttraumatic deformity, early arthritis, and likelihood of needing future deformity correction surgery or arthroplasty should be discussed with the patient and family if delayed open reduction and internal fixation (ORIF) or nonoperative management is chosen. Alternatively, if the fetus is near term or full term, surgical fixation of the pubic symphysis can be performed at the same time as cesarean section via the same Pfannenstiel incision.[24] In certain acetabular fracture patterns in which an anterior ilioinguinal approach is normally used, such as a transverse acetabular fracture, a posterior Kocher-Langenbeck incision may be used instead to stay on the outside of the pelvis and further away from the surrounding uterine environment.[24] Although the goal of surgery is anatomic reduction of the pelvis or acetabulum, in pregnant patients, the aim may be a less than anatomic reduction to limit the length of the case, potential blood loss, and amount of radiation to the fetus. If less than an anatomic reduction is considered, the patient or her family should be counseled preoperatively about the increased risk of malunion, future progression to posttraumatic arthritis, and need for early arthroplasty.[23,24]

Positioning in the pregnant patient

During surgery, the supine position should be avoided in the second and third trimesters in combination with general anesthesia, because it reduces cardiac output and can cause maternal hypotension and hypoxia to the placenta and fetus as a result of compression of the gravid uterus on the IVC.[43] The left lateral decubitus position is ideal, because it takes the weight of the gravid uterus off the IVC and allows for better venous return and cardiac output. With respect to specific fracture patterns, alternatives to standard positioning may be elected. For instance, in a left posterior wall acetabular fracture, which is usually surgically fixed in the right lateral decubitus position, it would be safer to have the patient completely prone to take the weight of the uterus off the IVC. When the prone position is used, the abdomen and gravid uterus need to be carefully padded and free.[25]

Intraoperative fetal monitoring in pelvic and acetabular surgery

There is significant controversy about the use of intraoperative fetal heart monitoring.[44] The decision of whether or not to use it should be made on an individual basis in consultation with the obstetrics and anesthesia teams.[43] If continuous fetal monitoring is used, an obstetrics team should be available in case emergent delivery is warranted. In case of emergency or signs of fetal distress, fetal monitoring equipment should be used when possible and an obstetrician available.[24]

Anesthesia risks in the pregnant patient

An anesthesiologist experienced in obstetric anesthesia should be used. Modern general anesthesia in a pregnant woman is safe.[45] Regional anesthesia reduces the risk of aspiration as well as the amount of systemic chemicals from general anesthesia to the mother and fetus; however, there is a risk of sympathetic blockade and hypotension, with resultant fetal hypoxia, more likely to occur with spinal than epidural anesthesia.[46] Frequent blood pressure monitoring and in most cases an arterial line should be used to monitor for blood pressure fluctuations.[46] In addition to the safety of the mother, the anesthesia team must consider risk of teratogenicity, fetal hypoxia, and preterm labor.[44] Although most anesthetic agents are teratogenic in high doses in animal studies, they are considered safe in clinical practice. It is essential to avoid maternal hypotension, hypoxia, or major changes in physiologic acid-base levels of normal pregnancy to prevent fetal hypoxia. There is an increased risk of preterm labor postoperatively with abdominopelvic surgery.[47] However, the risk of this complication is low, and prophylactic tocolytic therapy to inhibit contractions is generally not recommended because of its significant maternal side effects and unproved efficacy.[44]

Radiation risks to the fetus

Pregnant patients undergoing trauma surgery are often concerned about the risk of radiation exposure on the developing fetus. So great are these fears that many women electively chose to terminate their pregnancy based on perceived risk of exposure.[48,49] Patients should be counseled that most of these fears are unfounded.[50,51] If the patient and family have questions or concerns regarding radiation exposure to the developing fetus, a radiation safety evaluation should be conducted to assess the amount of exposure and risk to the fetus so that the patient can make informed decisions.[52]

Although studies of Japanese atomic bomb survivors have shown a dose-related correlation between prenatal exposure to ionizing radiation and teratogenesis, the doses required exceed any single diagnostic study.[51,53] There is no association between fetal anomalies or demise with radiation doses of less than 5 rad (5 mGy) according to the American College of Obstetricians and Gynecologists and other radiation safety organizations.[51,54] Major organ development occurs in the third to eighth week of gestation, and organ malformations can also be affected by high doses of radiation in this period. However, the risk of teratogenesis is greatest at 10 to 17 weeks of gestation (8–15 weeks after conception), a time of critical human brain development.[55] Although carcinogenic risk, especially childhood leukemia, has been shown to be increased with as little as 1 to 2 rad of radiation exposure, the absolute risk of increase with this amount of exposure is extremely low, on the order of 1 in 10,000.[51]

The risks of modern low-dose imaging techniques must be weighed against the risks of not having necessary and timely information to save the mother's life and that of the fetus, as well as the risk of poor long-term function from a malunited pelvic ring or acetabulum. However, certain modifications can be made when considering radiation reduction exposure to the developing fetus. In acute trauma situations, all standard imaging studies should be obtained, which include anteroposterior view of the pelvis, lateral view of the cervical spine, and chest radiograph. Although some trauma centers have replaced the standard trauma radiographic series with a pan-scan, that is, a screening computed tomography (CT) scan of the entire body in polytrauma situations, this should be bypassed in known or suspected pregnancies (**Table 2**).

The essential orthopedic radiographic studies are pelvic inlet and outlet views to characterize the fracture pattern in pelvic fractures or Judet views of the pelvis if there is an acetabular fracture.

Table 2 Fetal radiation exposure (approximate) during common radiographic studies		
Radiographic Study	Rad	No. of Studies to Reach Cumulative 5 Rad
Cervical spine	0.002	2500
Chest (2 views)	0.00007	71,429
Pelvis	0.040	125
Hip (single view)	0.213	23
CT head (10 slices)	<0.050	>100
CT chest (10 slices)	<0.100	>50
CT abdomen (10 slices)	2.600	1
CT lumbar spine (5 slices)	3.500	1
Ventilation-perfusion scan	0.215	23

Data from Flik K, Kloen P, Toro JB, et al. Orthopaedic trauma in the pregnant patient. J Am Acad Orthop Surg 2006;14:175–82.

Although a CT scan is now the standard for examining for posterior pelvic ring involvement, sacral dysmorphism, or intra-acetabular fracture fragments, fracture pattern and morphology of the pelvis can almost always be diagnosed with plain radiographs alone. A pelvic CT scan (which conveys greater than the recommended maximum 5 rad amount to the fetus) should be bypassed to avoid high-dose radiation to the fetus.[25] When a pelvic CT scan is deemed necessary by the treatment team, modifications of slice width and number have been described, which images only the areas of most interest to decrease the amount of radiation to the fetus.[24]

An alternative to pelvic CT scan is magnetic resonance imaging (MRI). MRI/magnetic resonance venography (MRV) can be performed on preoperative patients with pelvic and acetabular fracture to diagnose pelvic vein thrombosis, and although not as specific as CT scan for assessing bone, it is usually adequate to assess for fracture pattern, intra-articular fragments, and sacral morphology.[43] Furthermore, MRI has not been shown to have any deleterious effects on the developing fetus.[56]

Intraoperatively, lead shielding of the uterus should be used if it does not interfere with imaging, and collimation of the image intensifier should be used to reduce exposure. Fluoroscopy should be used sparingly, and a more open approach than usual may be necessary to avoid relying heavily on intraoperative imaging. Furthermore, only the minimal amount of intraoperative fluoroscopy should be used to obtain the necessary intraoperative reduction. A carefully planned preoperative template should help the surgeon better understand the fracture and reduce the length of surgery and amount of intraoperative fluoroscopy.[43]

Prophylaxis considerations for deep venous thrombosis and pulmonary embolism in pregnant women

The hypercoagulable states of pregnancy and trauma combined put the patient at high risk for developing deep venous thrombosis (DVT), so these patients should be placed on preventative doses of subcutaneous heparin or low-molecular-weight heparin once hemodynamically stabilized.[34] These medications do not cross the placental barrier and are safe to use in pregnancy; warfarin is contraindicated in pregnancy because it crosses the placenta and enters fetal circulation. Mechanical prophylaxis with intermittent pneumatic compression devices should also be used. Preoperatively, screening Doppler ultrasonography should also be performed. Although an IVC filter is commonly used in patients with polytrauma with pelvic fractures, placement of the filter requires further radiation exposure and therefore is not indicated as a preventative measure. However, if a large-vein DVT is diagnosed by Doppler ultrasonography or MRV, an IVC filter may be indicated, because the risk of a fatal pulmonary embolus outweighs the risk of radiation to the fetus from IVC filter placement.

Summary

Pelvic fractures in pregnancy are life-threatening to both the mother and fetus. The priority of the trauma team should always be to the mother, because prompt treatment gives both the mother and the fetus the best chance for a favorable outcome. A multidisciplinary team approach should be used to address what are often complex and challenging cases and should involve input from general trauma surgery, orthopedics, obstetrics, pediatrics, obstetric anesthesia, and radiology as well as the patient and her family whenever possible. Modifications to the standard treatment of pelvic and acetabular fractures in pregnant women are often necessary with regards to anesthesia, radiation exposure, and surgery.

ACUTE PUBIC SYMPHYSIS RUPTURE CAUSED BY PREGNANCY
Epidemiology of Acute Pubic Symphysis Rupture Caused by Pregnancy

The incidence of acute pubic symphysis rupture caused by pregnancy is rare and estimates vary greatly from between 1 in 600 to 800[57,58] to 1 in 30,000.[59] Multiple risk factors and associations have been suggested, including a large fetal birth weight, prolonged labor, epidural anesthesia, previous nulliparity (first child), a shoulder dystocia associated with a large birth weight, forceps delivery, and maternal developmental dysplasia of the hip.[60] Even when any of these conditions is present, the patient has a low risk of suffering from a pubic symphysis rupture during or after labor.

Pathogenesis of Acute Pubic Symphysis Rupture in Pregnancy

Mechanistically, the reason that the pubic symphysis ruptures is simple: the fetus descends rapidly into the birth canal during stage 2 of labor, and the head drives into the true pelvis.[57] Most women physiologically respond appropriately to this; however, in rare cases, the pelvis cannot adjust quickly enough and the pelvic ring begins to fail at its weakest point: the symphysis.

Some primate pelvii, namely those of rodents, do require significant diastasis of the pubic symphysis to allow passage of the head during delivery. However, in normal human pregnancies, slight increases in symphysis width are physiologic and subtle.[61] Early radiographic studies showed the symphysis to stretch cephalad-caudad an average of 7 mm and medial-lateral by 3 mm.[62] Later ultrasonographic studies have largely corroborated these findings: during labor, the average width of the pubic symphysis measures only 5.8 mm.[63] Physiologic pelvic ligamentous laxity and pubic symphyseal widening begin to reverse after delivery and normally return to normal by 12 weeks after birth.

The Role of Hormones

The pubic symphysis and pelvic ligaments undergo changes during pregnancy. Pregnant women have increased ligamentous laxity not just in the pelvis but throughout the body. This change is believed to be caused by changes in estradiol, progesterone, and relaxin levels; however, studies have failed to show a correlation between specific hormonal levels and amount of joint laxity in pregnant women.[64,65]

Diagnosis of Pubic Symphysis Rupture

Frank pubic symphysis disruption caused by parturition is pathologic. Reported injuries associated with pubic symphysis rupture include massive hemorrhage, hemodynamic instability,[59] sacroiliac (SI) dislocation,[66] sacral fracture, lumbosacral plexopathy,[67,68] bladder injury, and death.[59] As opposed to physiologic symphyseal widening, frank pubic symphysis rupture is usually accompanied by the sudden onset of severe tearing pain and a sensation of separation directly over the symphysis at the time of delivery or shortly thereafter. An audible click or snap may be heard. Examination may reveal a palpable gap at the symphysis as well as abnormal mobility, with lateral to medial compression of the iliac wings or greater trochanters. One or both SI joints may be tender to palpation. Less acute signs of diastasis include pain and difficulty with weight bearing, and a waddling or wide-based gait, and the patient may have a positive Patrick test if testable, with pain at the SI joint with flexion, abduction, and external rotation of the hip.[66] If any of these signs are present, diagnostic radiographs should be performed. If the patient has severe tenderness to palpation posteriorly or radiographic findings suggestive of associated widening of the SI joint or sacral fracture in addition to pubic symphysis diastasis, a CT scan of the pelvis should be obtained to better define the extent of the injury and any posterior ring involvement.[66]

Treatment

If a diagnosis of symphyseal rupture is suspected clinically or radiographically and the patient is hemodynamically unstable, the most important orthopedic intervention is to control and tamponade internal pelvic hemorrhage with provisional closed reduction of the pelvic ring. This procedure can be performed by internally rotating the legs and placing a sheet or binder around the greater trochanters. Other hemodynamic stabilization or resuscitative measures should be performed as needed. Once the patient is hemodynamically stabilized, further imaging studies should be obtained to guide definitive treatment. Nonoperative treatment with a pelvic binder is the initial treatment of choice, followed by early mobilization with a walker and pain control. This procedure is usually effective at keeping the symphysis reduced. Close follow-up radiographs should be obtained to make sure the pelvis stays reduced and symmetric in the binder.[57]

Surgical intervention is warranted in situations of open pubic symphysis rupture secondary to severe vaginal tearing, significant malreduction of the pelvis, or diastasis with the pelvic binder in place, or if 1 or both SI joints are displaced. Previous investigators[68] have suggested that a symphysis diastasis of 4 cm or more warrants surgical intervention, although the patient's pain level, disability, and preferences should be considered. Open pubic symphysis rupture with severe vaginal tearing should be irrigated and debrided followed by surgical fixation of the pelvis.[69] Surgical options include pubic symphysis ORIF or external fixation of the pelvis followed by reduction and percutaneous iliosacral screws if the SI joints are not indirectly reduced after addressing the symphysis.[66]

CHRONIC PUBIC SYMPHYSIS INSTABILITY RELATED TO PREGNANCY

Pelvic pain during pregnancy is a common syndrome and occurs in 20% to 50% of all pregnancies. Up to 25% of these women develop chronic postpartum pain.[63,70] Pregnancy-associated pelvic pain typically occurs in distinct anatomic locations: the unilateral or bilateral SI joint(s), the pubic symphysis, or in all 3, which is referred to as the pelvic girdle syndrome.[70] Anatomically, the pelvic joints include the symphysis anteriorly and the two SI joints posteriorly on either side of the sacrum. Similarly to any acute pelvic ring injury, if pain exists in 1 of these joints, there is likely associated disease in at least 1 of the other joints, even if asymptomatic.[66] Pelvic stretching and instability after delivery, which localizes with pain to the pubic symphysis or 1 or both SI joints, is likely on a continuum with symphyseal rupture and is caused by the same pathologic mechanism.

Pelvic pain during pregnancy is often multifactorial and has been attributed to a combination of instability, hormonal changes, trauma, and degenerative disease.[63] It is not always related to the pubic symphysis or SI joints and can originate in the low back, hip, or internal organs. Risk factors include history of low back pain, previous trauma to the back or pelvis, multiparity, prepregnancy obesity, and smoking, as well as psychosocial factors such as stress and low job satisfaction.[70]

Diagnosis

The diagnosis of pathologic pregnancy-related pubic symphysis instability related to pregnancy may be subtle clinically. Originally described by Chamberlain in 1930 as a means of diagnosing SI joint instability, single-leg stance radiographs of the pelvis can also be used to diagnose pubic symphysis instability.[71–73] Also called flamingo views, these are performed by having the patient stand on 1 leg and taking an anteroposterior radiograph of the pelvis. The vertical translation of 1 pubic ramus to the other is measured on both radiographs and the 2 measurements are summed to arrive at the amount of total translation. A total translation of 5 mm is considered positive.[71,72]

If radiographs are not diagnostic, more advanced imaging studies can be used to look for other diseases. MRI can diagnose soft tissue abnormalities in the anatomic region of the symphysis, including hernia, fascial defect, or osteitis pubis. MRI can be used to assess the posterior pelvic ring, including the SI joints, for disruption or sacral stress fracture. A bone scan can also be used to diagnose pelvic stress fractures and osteitis pubis.

Treatment of Chronic Pubic Symphysis Pain and Instability Related to Pregnancy

The initial treatment of pubic symphysis instability involves the use of a pelvic corset for comfort and physical therapy, with an emphasis on exercises to strengthen the pelvic muscles.[74] Nonoperative treatment emphasizing muscle strengthening has been shown to be effective in diastasis up to 22 mm.[75]

When considering nonoperative treatment, it is important to differentiate postpartum symphyseal pain from radiographic instability. Although initial treatment of both is the same, namely symptomatic pain relief and corset for comfort, if there is radiographic evidence of diastasis, the patient should be followed more closely with repeat radiographs after a trial of mobilization and physical therapy 6 to 10 weeks after presentation.

Operative treatment of pubic symphysis instability should be considered only in cases of extremely recalcitrant pain with radiographic evidence of instability. Shuler and Gruen[76] reported a case of nearly complete symptom resolution after ORIF of the pubic symphysis and percutaneous fixation of the bilateral SI joints. Similarly, Rommens[77] reported on 3 patients with recalcitrant pubic symphysis pain and radiographic evidence of instability at 3 to 8.5 months post partum who underwent pubic symphysis ORIF and had good relief of their symptoms. One also underwent fixation of the SI joint. All 3 patients had good relief of their symptoms and had their implants removed.

ABILITY TO HAVE A NORMAL VAGINAL DELIVERY AFTER PELVIC TRAUMA

Although there are many injury-associated obstetric indications for cesarean section, a history of previous pelvic fracture or pregnancy-associated pubic symphysis rupture is not by itself an indication for cesarean section (**Fig. 2**).[78,79] If a pelvic fracture occurred during the current pregnancy, factors to consider when determining mode of delivery include the current gestational age relative to the gestational age at which the injury occurred, whether the pelvic fracture is healed, if it is widely displaced, or if there is displaced bone that could impinge on the fetus or bladder during delivery. Healing normally occurs between 8 and 12 weeks after injury, so if the injury occurred early in the pregnancy, it is possible for the patient to deliver vaginally. Conversely, if the fracture is not healed or the pubic rami are displaced, cesarean section should be considered.[11] In addition, a pelvic malunion with a significant lateral compression component may be a contraindication to vaginal

delivery if it decreases the circumference of the true pelvis, making it more difficult for the fetus to descend into the birth canal and raising the risk of dystocia.[80] In a series of pregnant patients with pelvic fractures, of the 9 women with viable fetuses, 7 delivered vaginally and 2 by cesarean section.[24] In a systematic review of 101 cases of pelvic fractures in pregnant women, 43% of cases went on to deliver a live baby vaginally, whereas 16% delivered a live baby via cesarean section. In the remaining 41 cases, the fetus and/or mother did not survive or the mother was lost to follow-up before delivery.[11]

In addition, multiple studies have shown that previous history of pelvic fracture does not preclude a trial of labor and vaginal delivery and is not dependent on whether the patient was treated operatively or nonoperatively or the type of fixation used. For example, in a retrospective review of 34 pregnant women with a history of pelvic fracture, 28 delivered vaginally without complication, and in only 1 case was cesarean section performed out of consideration of the previous pelvic fracture.[81] The evidence does suggest that there is a higher incidence of cesarean section after a pelvic fracture, especially in those patients with greater initial displacement of more than 5 mm.[82]

In a retrospective review of 26 women who delivered infants after a previous healed pelvic fracture, 16 (62%) had cesarean sections, a rate more than double the national average.[83] The decision for cesarean section was based in part on previous history of pelvic fracture in 8 of 16 (50%) cases. In the 10 patients (38%) delivered vaginally, 4 had pelvic fixation in place. Of the patients' obstetricians surveyed in the study, 26% did not believe that a previous pelvic fracture should be a contraindication to vaginal delivery, but most had no previous experience in treating pregnant women with a history of pelvic fracture. Similarly, Vallier and colleagues[84] performed a retrospective review to see whether or not previous pelvic fracture inhibited the ability to have a vaginal delivery in the future. There were 29 patients available for review, with a high percentage of patients (13 of 29, 45%) who subsequently had cesarean sections compared with the rate for the entire hospital (27.3%, $P = .002$). Two patients were lost to follow-up and their postinjury obstetric history was unknown. The remaining 14 patients had vaginal deliveries, 6 of whom had undergone previous operative treatment of their pelvic fracture, and 3 of whom had retained pubic symphyseal plates. There were no complications to vaginal delivery in any of these patients. In cases of cesarean section, 54% of patients (7 of 13) had the cesarean

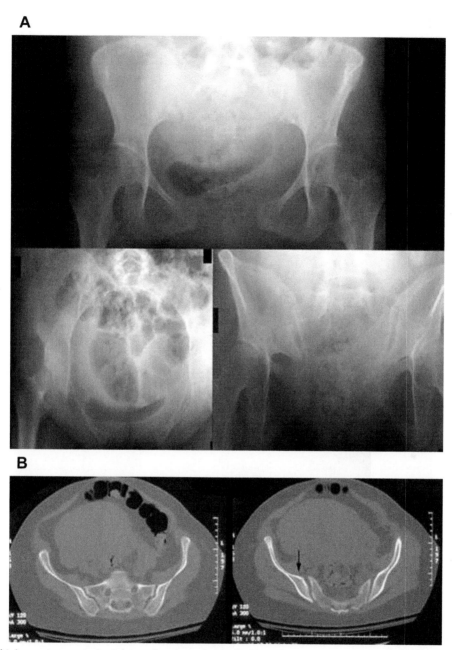

Fig. 2. (*A*) Injury anteroposterior, inlet, and outlet radiographs films of a woman on postpartum day 3 showing pubic symphysis rupture with diastasis of 9.5 cm and widened bilateral SI joints. (*B*) CT scan showed right and left SI widening of 8 and 9 mm, respectively, along with bilateral SI displacement, indicating complete disruption of the joints. (*C*) Postoperative anteroposterior, inlet, and outlet radiographs after ORIF of the pubic symphysis and bilateral SI percutaneous fixation. The woman went on to deliver another child vaginally with all implants in place 15 months postoperatively. (*D*) The SI screws loosened and were removed at 2 years postoperatively because of pain posteriorly, which resolved by 2 months after removal. (*From* Hierholzer C, Ali A, Toro-Arbelaez JB, et al. Traumatic disruption of pubis symphysis with accompanying posterior pelvic injury after natural childbirth. Am J Orthop (Belle Mead NJ) 2007;36:E167–70; with permission. Copyright © 2007 Quadrant HealthCom Inc. All rights reserved.)

section for reasons related to the previous pelvic fracture, 3 of which were decided by the patient and 4 of which were decided by the obstetrician. Misconceptions by both the patient and the treating physicians as well as risk-averse medicolegal decision making may contribute to the high rate of cesarean delivery in patients with a previous pelvic fracture.[82,83]

C

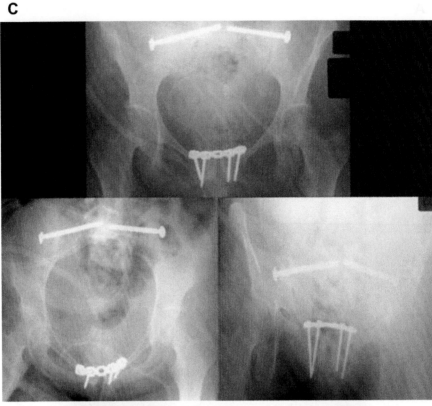

D

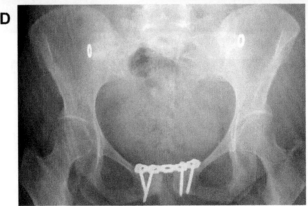

Fig. 2. (*continued*)

We recommend that if a pregnant patient has a healed pelvic fracture with no significant residual pelvic malunion and all implants are appropriately placed within the bony pelvis and not protruding significantly into the pelvis, a trial of vaginal delivery should be attempted if no other primary obstetric contraindications exist. The limited available evidence suggests that plates traversing the pubic symphysis or screws traversing the SI joint do not need to be removed before vaginal delivery, and there has been no report in the literature of symphyseal plates or SI screws breaking with vaginal delivery.[66,84] In a normal vaginal delivery, the pubic symphysis measures 5.8 mm during labor based on ultrasonographic studies, a slight amount, unlikely to cause plate or screw failure.[63] Even if a pubic symphyseal plate or SI screw were to break within the bony pelvis, no clinical relevance would be expected from this. Pregnant patients with a previous history of pelvic fracture should be counseled that vaginal delivery is safe if no other contraindications exist.

SUMMARY

Pelvic fractures in pregnant women are usually high-energy injuries associated with risk of mortality to both mother and fetus. The mother's life always takes precedence. Pubic symphysis rupture and chronic pubic symphysis and pelvic instability related to pregnancy are challenging problems that can almost always be successfully treated nonoperatively. A previous pelvic fracture is not a contraindication by itself to vaginal delivery. A team approach is necessary to dealing with the pregnant trauma patient.

REFERENCES

1. Fildes J, Reed L, Jones N, et al. Trauma: the leading cause of maternal death. J Trauma 1992;32:643–5.
2. Peckham CH, King RW. A study of intercurrent conditions observed during pregnancy. Am J Obstet Gynecol 1963;87:609–24.
3. El-Kady D, Gilbert WM, Anderson J, et al. Trauma during pregnancy: an analysis of maternal and fetal outcomes in a large population. Am J Obstet Gynecol 2004;190:1661–8.
4. Cheng HT, Wang YC, Lo HC, et al. Trauma during pregnancy: a population-based analysis of maternal outcome. World J Surg 2012;36(12):2767–75.
5. Timberlake GA, McSwain NE Jr. Trauma in pregnancy. A 10-year perspective. Am Surg 1989;55:151–3.
6. Esposito TJ, Gens DR, Smith LG, et al. Trauma during pregnancy. A review of 79 cases. Arch Surg 1991;126:1073–8.
7. Chames MC, Pearlman MD. Trauma during pregnancy: outcomes and clinical management. Clin Obstet Gynecol 2008;51:398–408.
8. Mattox KL, Goetzl L. Trauma in pregnancy. Crit Care Med 2005;33:S385–9.
9. Ali J, Yeo A, Gana TJ, et al. Predictors of fetal mortality in pregnant trauma patients. J Trauma 1997;42:782–5.
10. Kissinger DP, Rozycki GS, Morris JA Jr, et al. Trauma in pregnancy. Predicting pregnancy outcome. Arch Surg 1991;126:1079–86.
11. Leggon RE, Wood GC, Indeck MC. Pelvic fractures in pregnancy: factors influencing maternal and fetal outcomes. J Trauma 2002;53:796–804.
12. El Kady D, Gilbert WM, Xing G, et al. Association of maternal fractures with adverse perinatal outcomes. Am J Obstet Gynecol 2006;195:711–6.
13. Baethmann M, Kahn T, Lenard HG, et al. Fetal CNS damage after exposure to maternal trauma during pregnancy. Acta Paediatr 1996;85:1331–8.
14. Hayes B, Ryan S, Stephenson JB, et al. Cerebral palsy after maternal trauma in pregnancy. Dev Med Child Neurol 2007;49:700–6.
15. Gilles MT, Blair E, Watson L, et al. Trauma in pregnancy and cerebral palsy: is there a link? Med J Aust 1996;164:500–1.
16. Murdoch Eaton DG, Ahmed Y, Dubowitz LM. Maternal trauma and cerebral lesions in preterm infants. Case reports. Br J Obstet Gynaecol 1991;98:1292–4.
17. Pearlman MD, Tintinalli JE, Lorenz RP. A prospective controlled study of outcome after trauma during pregnancy. Am J Obstet Gynecol 1990;162:1502–7 [discussion: 7–10].
18. Pearlman MD, Tintinalli JE, Lorenz RP. Blunt trauma during pregnancy. N Engl J Med 1990;323:1609–13.
19. Crosby WM, Snyder RG, Snow CC, et al. Impact injuries in pregnancy. I. Experimental studies. Am J Obstet Gynecol 1968;101:100–10.
20. Pearlman MD. Motor vehicle crashes, pregnancy loss and preterm labor. Int J Gynaecol Obstet 1997;57:127–32.
21. Klinich KD, Flannagan CA, Rupp JD, et al. Fetal outcome in motor-vehicle crashes: effects of crash characteristics and maternal restraint. Am J Obstet Gynecol 2008;198:450.e1–9.
22. Wolf ME, Alexander BH, Rivara FP, et al. A retrospective cohort study of seatbelt use and pregnancy outcome after a motor vehicle crash. J Trauma 1993;34:116–9.
23. Pape HC, Pohlemann T, Gansslen A, et al. Pelvic fractures in pregnant multiple trauma patients. J Orthop Trauma 2000;14:238–44.
24. Almog G, Liebergall M, Tsafrir A, et al. Management of pelvic fractures during pregnancy. Am J Orthop (Belle Mead NJ) 2007;36:E153–9.
25. Porter SE, Russell GV, Qin Z, et al. Operative fixation of acetabular fractures in the pregnant patient. J Orthop Trauma 2008;22:508–16.
26. Papadopoulos IN, Kanakaris N, Bonovas S, et al. Auditing 655 fatalities with pelvic fractures by autopsy as a basis to evaluate trauma care. J Am Coll Surg 2006;203:30–43.
27. Perry MO, Husmann DA. Urethral injuries in female subjects following pelvic fractures. J Urol 1992;147:139–43.
28. Dente CJ, Feliciano DV, Rozycki GS, et al. The outcome of open pelvic fractures in the modern era. Am J Surg 2005;190:830–5.
29. Kaempf JW, Tomlinson MW, Campbell B, et al. Counseling pregnant women who may deliver extremely premature infants: medical care guidelines, family choices, and neonatal outcomes. Pediatrics 2009;123:1509–15.
30. Muench MV, Baschat AA, Reddy UM, et al. Kleihauer-Betke testing is important in all cases of maternal trauma. J Trauma 2004;57:1094–8.

31. Shah AJ, Kilcline BA. Trauma in pregnancy. Emerg Med Clin North Am 2003;21:615–29.

32. Aprahamian C, Gessert G, Bandyk DF, et al. MAST-associated compartment syndrome (MACS): a review. J Trauma 1989;29:549–55.

33. Cluver C, Novikova N, Hofmeyr GJ, et al. Maternal position during caesarean section for preventing maternal and neonatal complications. Cochrane Database Syst Rev 2010;(6):CD007623.

34. Flik K, Kloen P, Toro JB, et al. Orthopaedic trauma in the pregnant patient. J Am Acad Orthop Surg 2006;14:175–82.

35. Osborn PM, Smith WR, Moore EE, et al. Direct retroperitoneal pelvic packing versus pelvic angiography: a comparison of two management protocols for haemodynamically unstable pelvic fractures. Injury 2009;40:54–60.

36. Lavin JP Jr, Polsky SS. Abdominal trauma during pregnancy. Clin Perinatol 1983;10:423–38.

37. Katz VL. Perimortem cesarean delivery: its role in maternal mortality. Semin Perinatol 2012;36:68–72.

38. Katz VL, Dotters DJ, Droegemueller W. Perimortem cesarean delivery. Obstet Gynecol 1986;68:571–6.

39. Goldenberg RL, Nelson KG, Davis RO, et al. Delay in delivery: influence of gestational age and the duration of delay on perinatal outcome. Obstet Gynecol 1984;64:480–4.

40. Effect of corticosteroids for fetal maturation on perinatal outcomes. NIH Consensus Development Panel on the Effect of Corticosteroids for Fetal Maturation on Perinatal Outcomes. JAMA 1995; 273:413–8.

41. American College of Obstetricians and Gynecologists, Committee on Practice B-O. ACOG practice bulletin no. 127: management of preterm labor. Obstet Gynecol 2012;119:1308–17.

42. Letournel E, Judet E. Fractures of the acetabulum. 2nd edition. New York: Springer-Verlag; 1993.

43. Kloen P, Flik K, Helfet DL. Operative treatment of acetabular fracture during pregnancy: a case report. Arch Orthop Trauma Surg 2005;125:209–12.

44. Van De Velde M, De Buck F. Anesthesia for non-obstetric surgery in the pregnant patient. Minerva Anestesiol 2007;73:235–40.

45. Kuczkowski KM. The safety of anaesthetics in pregnant women. Expert Opin Drug Saf 2006;5: 251–64.

46. Steinberg ES, Santos AC. Surgical anesthesia during pregnancy. Int Anesthesiol Clin 1990;28:58–66.

47. Mazze RI, Kallen B. Reproductive outcome after anesthesia and operation during pregnancy: a registry study of 5405 cases. Am J Obstet Gynecol 1989;161:1178–85.

48. Trichopoulos D, Zavitsanos X, Koutis C, et al. The victims of Chernobyl in Greece: induced abortions after the accident. Br Med J (Clin Res Ed) 1987; 295:1100.

49. Cohen-Kerem R, Nulman I, Abramow-Newerly M, et al. Diagnostic radiation in pregnancy: perception versus true risks. J Obstet Gynaecol Can 2006;28: 43–8.

50. Bentur Y, Horlatsch N, Koren G. Exposure to ionizing radiation during pregnancy: perception of teratogenic risk and outcome. Teratology 1991;43: 109–12.

51. Toppenberg KS, Hill DA, Miller DP. Safety of radiographic imaging during pregnancy. Am Fam Physician 1999;59:1813–8, 20.

52. Mann FA, Nathens A, Langer SG, et al. Communicating with the family: the risks of medical radiation to conceptuses in victims of major blunt-force torso trauma. J Trauma 2000;48:354–7.

53. Otake M, Schull WJ. In utero exposure to A-bomb radiation and mental retardation; a reassessment. Br J Radiol 1984;57:409–14.

54. ACOG Committee on Obstetric Practice. ACOG Committee Opinion. Number 299, September 2004 (replaces No. 158, September 1995). Guidelines for diagnostic imaging during pregnancy. Obstet Gynecol 2004;104:647–51.

55. Yamazaki JN, Schull WJ. Perinatal loss and neurological abnormalities among children of the atomic bomb. Nagasaki and Hiroshima revisited, 1949 to 1989. JAMA 1990;264:605–9.

56. Clements H, Duncan KR, Fielding K, et al. Infants exposed to MRI in utero have a normal paediatric assessment at 9 months of age. Br J Radiol 2000; 73:190–4.

57. Taylor RN, Sonson RD. Separation of the pubic symphysis. An underrecognized peripartum complication. J Reprod Med 1986;31:203–6.

58. Scriven MW, Jones DA, McKnight L. The importance of pubic pain following childbirth: a clinical and ultrasonographic study of diastasis of the pubic symphysis. J R Soc Med 1995;88:28–30.

59. Reis RA, Baer JL, Arens RA, et al. Traumatic separation of the symphysis pubis during spontaneous labor: with a clinical and x-ray study of the normal symphysis pubis during pregnancy and the puerperium. Surg Gynecol Obstet 1932;55:336–54.

60. Saugstad LF. Persistent pelvic pain and pelvic joint instability. Eur J Obstet Gynecol Reprod Biol 1991; 41:197–201.

61. Putschar WG. The structure of the human symphysis pubis with special consideration of parturition and its sequelae. Am J Phys Anthropol 1976;45: 589–94.

62. Farbrot E. The relationship of the effect and pain of pregnancy to the anatomy of the pelvis. Acta Radiol 1952;38:403–19.

63. Bjorklund K, Lindgren PG, Bergstrom S, et al. Sonographic assessment of symphyseal joint distention intra partum. Acta Obstet Gynecol Scand 1997;76:227–32.

64. Marnach ML, Ramin KD, Ramsey PS, et al. Characterization of the relationship between joint laxity and maternal hormones in pregnancy. Obstet Gynecol 2003;101:331–5.

65. Schauberger CW, Rooney BL, Goldsmith L, et al. Peripheral joint laxity increases in pregnancy but does not correlate with serum relaxin levels. Am J Obstet Gynecol 1996;174:667–71.

66. Hierholzer C, Ali A, Toro-Arbelaez JB, et al. Traumatic disruption of pubis symphysis with accompanying posterior pelvic injury after natural childbirth. Am J Orthop (Belle Mead NJ) 2007;36: E167–70.

67. Urist M. Obstetric fracture-dislocation of the pelvis. Report of a case with injury to the lumbosacral trunk and first sacral nerve root. JAMA 1953; 152(2):127–9.

68. Kharrazi FD, Rodgers WB, Kennedy JG, et al. Parturition-induced pelvic dislocation: a report of four cases. J Orthop Trauma 1997;11:277–81 [discussion: 81–2].

69. Blum M, Orovano N. Open rupture of the symphysis pubis during spontaneous delivery. Acta Obstet Gynecol Scand 1976;55:77–9.

70. Albert HB, Godskesen M, Korsholm L, et al. Risk factors in developing pregnancy-related pelvic girdle pain. Acta Obstet Gynecol Scand 2006;85: 539–44.

71. Garras DN, Carothers JT, Olson SA. Single-leg-stance (flamingo) radiographs to assess pelvic instability: how much motion is normal? J Bone Joint Surg Am 2008;90:2114–8.

72. Siegel J, Templeman DC, Tornetta P 3rd. Single-leg-stance radiographs in the diagnosis of pelvic instability. J Bone Joint Surg Am 2008;90:2119–25.

73. Chamberlain W. The symphysis pubis in the roentgen examination of the sacro-iliac joint. Am J Roentgenol 1930;24:621–5.

74. Depledge J, McNair PJ, Keal-Smith C, et al. Management of symphysis pubis dysfunction during pregnancy using exercise and pelvic support belts. Phys Ther 2005;85:1290–300.

75. Shim JH, Oh DW. Case report: physiotherapy strategies for a woman with symphysis pubis diastasis occurring during labour. Physiotherapy 2012;98:89–91.

76. Shuler TE, Gruen GS. Chronic postpartum pelvic pain treated by surgical stabilization. Orthopedics 1996;19:687–9.

77. Rommens PM. Internal fixation in postpartum symphysis pubis rupture: report of three cases. J Orthop Trauma 1997;11:273–6.

78. ACOG educational bulletin. Obstetric aspects of trauma management. Number 251, September 1998 (replaces Number 151, January 1991, and Number 161, November 1991). American College of Obstetricians and Gynecologists. Int J Gynaecol Obstet 1999;64:87–94.

79. Culligan P, Hill S, Heit M. Rupture of the symphysis pubis during vaginal delivery followed by two subsequent uneventful pregnancies. Obstet Gynecol 2002;100:1114–7.

80. Voegelin A, McCall ML. Some acquired bony abnormalities influencing the conduct of labor: with reports of recent cases. Am J Obstet Gynecol 1944; 48:361–70.

81. Madsen LV, Jensen J, Christensen ST. Parturition and pelvic fracture. Follow-up of 34 obstetric patients with a history of pelvic fracture. Acta Obstet Gynecol Scand 1983;62:617–20.

82. Copeland CE, Bosse MJ, McCarthy ML, et al. Effect of trauma and pelvic fracture on female genitourinary, sexual, and reproductive function. J Orthop Trauma 1997;11:73–81.

83. Cannada LK, Barr J. Pelvic fractures in women of childbearing age. Clin Orthop Relat Res 2010; 468:1781–9.

84. Vallier HA, Cureton BA, Schubeck D. Pregnancy outcomes after pelvic ring injury. J Orthop Trauma 2012;26:302–7.

Technical Pitfalls of Shoulder Hemiarthroplasty for Fracture Management

Brent B. Wiesel, MD[a],*, Sameer Nagda, MD[b],
Gerald R. Williams, MD[c]

KEYWORDS

- Proximal humerus fractures • Hemiarthroplasty • Tuberosity malunion

KEY POINTS

- The majority of proximal humerus fractures can be managed non operatively.
- Four part fractures and 3 part fracture/dislocations in elderly patients often require management with prosthetic arthroplasty.
- While reverse shoulder arthroplasty is gaining popularity for the management of fractures in patients over the age of 70, hemiarthroplasty remains a valuable tool in the management of these fractures.
- Restoration of the patients' correct humeral head height and version and healing of the greater and lesser tuberosities in an anatomic position are crucial for regaining function after this procedure.

INTRODUCTION

Proximal humerus fractures represent 4% to 5% of all fractures and 50% of all humerus fractures, increase in incidence with age, are more common in females, and are a leading cause of visits to the emergency room or admission to the hospital.[1] According to Neer,[2] 80% of all proximal humerus fractures are nondisplaced and can be managed nonoperatively. However, recent data from a regional trauma center indicates that the incidence of displaced fractures may be higher than originally described by Neer.[3] In his original description, Neer classified displaced fractures as 2-, 3-, and 4-part fractures or fracture dislocations, as discussed in more detail herein. Hemiarthroplasty was indicated for most 4-part fractures and fracture dislocations as well as selected 3-part fractures and fracture dislocations. As techniques for internal fixation have improved, many 3-part and 4-part fractures in young active patients are currently being treated with osteosynthesis rather than arthroplasty.[4] Moreover, inconsistent results from hemiarthroplasty, particularly in patients older than 70 years, has led to the increased use of reverse total shoulder arthroplasty.[5]

Hemiarthroplasty is still a viable alternative in many patients with proximal humerus fractures. As has been emphasized in the past, successful hemiarthroplasty is predicated on anatomic placement of the prosthesis with anatomic healing of the tuberosities. This approach requires optimization of specific patients, implants, and surgical factors. The purposes of this article are to briefly review certain patient factors (anatomy, classification, diagnosis, and indications), discuss important implant-related factors, and highlight key surgical factors so that pitfalls may be minimized and the goals of anatomic reconstruction realized more frequently.

[a] Department of Orthopaedic Surgery – G PHC, Medstar Georgetown University Hospital, Georgetown University School of Medicine, 3800 Reservoir Road, Northwest, Washington, DC 20007, USA; [b] Anderson Orthopaedic Clinic, Georgetown University School of Medicine, Inova Mount Vernon Hospital, 2501 Parkers Lane, Suite 200, Alexandria, VA 22306, USA; [c] Rothman Institute at Thomas Jefferson University, 925 Chestnut Street, Philadelphia, PA 19107, USA
* Corresponding author.
E-mail address: brent.wiesel@gmail.com

Orthop Clin N Am 44 (2013) 317–329
http://dx.doi.org/10.1016/j.ocl.2013.03.006
0030-5898/13/$ – see front matter © 2013 Elsevier Inc. All rights reserved.

ANATOMY AND CLASSIFICATION

The proximal humerus can be separated into 4 parts: the humeral head, the greater tuberosity, the lesser tuberosity, and the shaft.[6] The humeral head is retroverted in relation to the shaft and the humeral epicondyle by 20° to 35° with an average of 30°.[7] The neck shaft angle is extremely variable but averages 135°. The center of the humeral head is most often offset posteriorly and medially with regard to the center of the humeral shaft.[8] However, given the comminution that is usually present, the importance of recreating humeral head offset is unclear. The most superior aspect of the head is situated approximately 5 to 8 mm above the top of the greater tuberosity[9] and approximately 5.6 cm superior to the most superior extent of the pectoralis major insertion.[10] The bicipital groove separates the greater and lesser tuberosity and is, on average, angled approximately 30° more retroverted than the humeral head with respect to the epicondylar axis.[11]

Understanding the muscle attachments on each fragment will aid in fixation of the fragments to the humeral prosthesis. The infraspinatus, supraspinatus, and teres minor attach to the greater tuberosity. As a result, this fragment is most likely to displace posteriorly and superiorly. The lesser tuberosity is most often displaced medially owing to the pull of the subscapularis. Similarly, the shaft is often displaced medially because of the strong pull of the pectoralis major tendon.

There are 3 common classification systems for proximal humerus fractures: the Neer classification,[12] the AO classification,[13] and the Hertel classification.[14] Although reliability of these classification systems has been questioned,[15] the most commonly used system is Neer's, which is a modification of the system originally introduced by Codman. It is based on displacement of the 4 previously described anatomic segments whereby displacement is defined on plain radiographs as 1 cm or 45°. The Neer classification describes 2-, 3-, and 4-part displacement with or without dislocation along with certain special situations such as head-splitting fractures and head-impression fractures.

INDICATIONS, CONTRAINDICATIONS, AND ALTERNATIVES

Indications for hemiarthroplasty include classic (ie, not valgus impacted) 4-part fractures and fracture dislocations as well as selected 3-part fractures and dislocations, and certain special situations including head-split fractures and impression fractures (**Fig. 1**). The more displaced the fragment, the more likely it is to have a negative impact on the blood supply to the humeral head. Displaced 4-part fractures have the highest likelihood of developing avascular necrosis. Studies report this to be between 20% and 30%.[16] In younger patients (eg, younger than 60 years) with 4-part displacement, adequate bone quality, and an intact rotator cuff, open reduction and internal fixation is indicated if an anatomic or near anatomic stable reduction and adequate fixation can be obtained. In addition, patients older than 70 with 4-part displacement, particularly if they have multiple medical comorbidities or are too sedentary or noncompliant to complete postoperative rehabilitation, may be candidates for reverse arthroplasty. Three-part fractures in older individuals with osteoporotic bone, 3-part fracture dislocations, and fractures involving a split or compression of 40% or more of the humeral head may also be considered for hemiarthroplasty. In general, however, open reduction and internal fixation is possible and id preferred for the vast majority of 3-part fractures.

Contraindications to hemiarthroplasty include patients who are medically unable to tolerate surgery and patients with limited or no use of the involved arm because of prior neurologic injury.

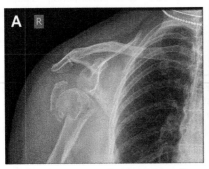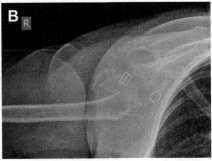

Fig. 1. Anteroposterior (AP) (*A*) and axillary (*B*) radiographs of a 74-year-old woman who sustained a 4-part proximal humerus fracture following a fall.

Patients with active infection are also poor candidates for implantation of a prosthesis. In addition, patients with a known prior rotator cuff tear are not likely to do well with a hemiarthroplasty. These patients will likely have a better outcome with reverse shoulder arthroplasty.

HISTORY

Evaluation of a patient with a proximal humerus fracture should begin with the mechanism of injury. High-energy injuries increase the suspicion for other concurrent injuries. Low-energy injuries raise suspicion of poor bone quality. An evaluation of the medical history for possible risk factors that resulted in injury or that may affect surgical management or postoperative outcome should be performed. For example, a patient with a history of stroke with contralateral weakness may be more reliant on the fractured extremity.

An evaluation of the patient's living situation is also important. The surgical extremity will be protected in a sling for up to 6 weeks postoperatively. In addition, overall function will be limited for an extended period of time beyond that. Evaluation of the patient's home responsibilities (ie, caring for other family members) and available help to assist the patient are critical for a smooth postoperative course. Patients may benefit from temporarily living with other family members, or from having a home health aide or nurse. Alternatively, patients may require discharge to a skilled nursing or rehabilitation facility from the hospital. Inattention to these details may result in noncompliance with postoperative rehabilitation, and activity restrictions and could jeopardize a successful outcome.

Prior shoulder and arm function should be assessed. Any prior shoulder pain needs to be investigated. A history of symptoms suggestive of rotator cuff disease should be thoroughly discussed. Any prior imaging of the shoulder should be assessed and prior surgeries reviewed. Unrecognized prior shoulder abnormality, especially involving the rotator cuff, may have a negative impact on hemiarthroplasty.

Appropriate patient expectation is also critical in optimizing the patient's postoperative satisfaction. In most cases, the patient's shoulder was normal before the fracture and they may expect it to be normal after treatment. It is important to set reasonable patient expectations before surgical intervention. On average, patients undergoing hemiarthroplasty for proximal humerus fractures will take a year to reach a plateau in recovery, and can expect a shoulder with no or mild pain and elevation of 90° to 120°.[17] Their role in maximizing the result should be emphasized. Failure to set appropriate expectations before surgery can result in decreased patient satisfaction.

PHYSICAL EXAMINATION

Physical examination of the involved shoulder is often limited because of pain. However, several key physical findings can affect surgical planning and overall outcome, and should therefore be elicited. Inspection of the shoulder area for open wounds or skin breakdown that may increase the risk of local cellulitis should be performed. Moreover, the level of swelling and bruising in the arm may require delay of the procedure for several days. An evaluation of the vascular status is mandatory, especially with displaced 4-part fractures. In particular, significant medialization of the shaft can place the patient at increased risk for vascular injury.[18] Assessment of the distal pulses bilaterally should be performed. Any decrease in the pulse on the involved side should be further evaluated. Complete laceration of the axillary artery is rare, and is usually obvious and limb threatening. However, collateral periscapular circulation between the third part of the subclavian artery and the third part of the axillary artery will likely keep the extremity perfused, despite complete occlusion of the axillary artery.[19] This situation most commonly occurs with intimal tearing near the origin of the anterior and posterior humeral circumflex arteries. Although this injury is not usually limb threatening, it often results in long-term cold intolerance and pain. The only clue to its existence may be a slight asymmetry in the strength of the pulse. When this is present, confirmation of axillary artery patency of either extremity with ultrasonography or arteriography is suggested.

Neurologic status should also be assessed. Visser and colleagues[20] demonstrated a 67% incidence of nerve injury following proximal humerus fracture. Axillary nerve function should be assessed by documenting the motor firing of the deltoid muscle. Evaluating the sensation over the lateral arm is not an accurate gauge of axillary nerve function. Presence of an axillary nerve injury, especially if the head is anteriorly dislocated, may affect the timing and type of surgical intervention. Distal motor function should also be evaluated to assess for brachial plexus injury. A thorough examination of the cervical spine must be performed to assess for possible concurrent injury. An inadequately performed or documented neurologic examination is a potential pitfall that can affect overall outcome, possibly resulting in litigation.

IMAGING

Radiographic evaluation of the fracture should include a trauma series as defined by Neer: an anteroposterior view in the scapular plane, a y-view, and an axillary view.[12] These radiographs are often done in an emergency room setting, and frequently are inadequate. Pain may limit the ability to attain a standard axillary view. A Velpeaux view can usually be performed in lieu of the axillary view, with much less pain.[21] If these 3 views are all optimal, advanced imaging may not be necessary. However, if any of the views is inadequate, especially the axillary view, a computed tomography scan should be obtained to rule out posterior dislocation of the head and to characterize all fracture lines, tuberosity displacement, and comminution. Three-dimensional reconstruction can be especially helpful, particularly if the glenoid image is subtracted. Understanding the location of the tuberosity fracture lines in particular will allow preoperative planning to exploit existing fracture lines during exposure, rather than creating new ones. The intertubercular fracture line is most commonly located approximately 1 cm posterior to the bicipital groove.

IMPLANT FACTORS

The past decade has seen a significant increase in implant options. Most implant manufactures offer a fracture-specific shoulder implant with multiple head sizes to match patient anatomy. Fracture-specific shoulder stems have been designed with features that are intended to assist the surgeon with anatomic placement of the stem, and optimal reduction and fixation of the tuberosities. These features include fenestrations for bone grafting, implant coatings that induce bone ingrowth, strategically placed holes for suture fixation, size and shape alterations to enhance canal fit for cementless use or tuberosity reduction, and intramedullary or extramedullary jigs for temporary fixation to allow for provisional assessment of stem placement. In addition, some systems provide radiopaque trial heads to aid in assessment of adequacy of reduction, particularly greater tuberosity to head height. The surgeon should be familiar with the specific design features of the stem being used and the rationale behind the specific design characteristics so that any potential advantages can be maximized.

Several recently introduced systems allow for a well-fixed hemiarthroplasty to be converted to a reverse shoulder arthroplasty without removing the entire stem. In most reported series of reverse arthroplasties, revisions of prior shoulder prostheses represent a substantial percentage of the cases, and revision of failed hemiarthroplasties for fracture are among the most common revisions.[22] Therefore, use of a stem that can be converted to a reverse component clearly represents an advantage. Ultimately, the utility of this feature depends on placement of the initial implant. If the hemiarthroplasty has been placed anatomically, most systems allow some correction of version and inclination, either above the humerus or within it. However, some hemiarthroplasties may be so poorly placed that they must be removed. All other factors being equal, use of a convertible stem is advantageous.

Finally, the surgeon should be prepared for any circumstances that may be encountered, such as potential placement of an anatomic glenoid component, fixation of an unrecognized glenoid fracture, or placement of a reverse prosthesis primarily. In the latter instance, having a convertible system that can be used as either an anatomic hemiarthroplasty or a reverse arthroplasty may be advantageous.

SURGICAL TECHNIQUE

The patient is placed in the beach chair position with the head of the bed elevated 30° to 40°, and the operative arm draped so that is it freely mobile (**Fig. 2**). It is important that the surgeon is able to adduct and extend the arm toward the floor to gain access to the humeral shaft. This setting is best accomplished by using either a commercially available beach chair positioner, which secures the head and allows a portion of the back of the bed to be removed, or a standard table with the patient positioned as far toward the edge as is safely possible with the shoulder and arm unsupported. A Mayfield headrest can be used to secure the head and improve access to the top of the shoulder. With either positioning scenario, a bolster should be placed along the ribs on the operative side to prevent inadvertent lateral movement of the patient during the case.

Intraoperative radiographic evaluation is strongly encouraged in all fracture cases. In most instances, intraoperative fluoroscopy is adequate. However, if image quality is poor or acquisition or interpretation is difficult for any reason, portable plain radiography should be available. Preoperative images should be available in the operating room. In addition, the C-arm should be positioned before the patient is prepped and draped to verify that adequate images can be obtained. The C-arm can be positioned parallel to the table, above the head on the operative side or perpendicular to the table from the opposite side. The latter configuration has the advantage of keeping the C-arm

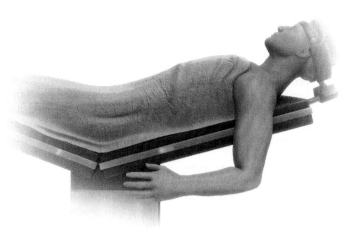

Fig. 2. The patient is placed in the beach chair position with the operative arm freely mobile. (*Courtesy of* DePuy Orthopaedics, Inc, Warsaw, IN; with permission.)

out of the way, but may be difficult when using a standard table.

An 8- to 10-cm incision is made extending inferiorly and laterally from the tip of the coracoid process toward the deltoid tuberosity. The cephalic vein is identified and retracted laterally with the deltoid muscle. Once through the deltopectoral interval, the surgeon will encounter substantial hematoma, which should be evacuated. At least initially, the pectoralis major insertion is preserved so that it can be used to confirm accurate head placement if necessary. In most cases, release of any of the pectoralis major is not required for adequate exposure. A self-retaining retractor is used to retract the pectoralis medially and the deltoid and cephalic vein laterally.

The conjoined tendon of the coracobrachialis and short head of the biceps is identified, and the clavipectoral fascia is incised just lateral to this tendon. This incision is carried superiorly to the coracoacromial ligament and inferiorly to the upper border of the pectoralis major insertion. There is no need to incise the coracoacromial ligament, and there may be some advantage to preserving it as a restraint to future anterosuperior subluxation.[23] The surgeon's finger is then swept medially, deep to the conjoined tendon, from superiorly to inferiorly, to identify the axillary nerve as it passes superficial to the subscapularis muscle belly toward the quadrilateral space. In general, the musculocutaneous nerve passes through the conjoined tendon approximately 5 to 6 cm distal to the tip of the coracoid, and is not within the immediate surgical field. However, this relationship is variable, and the nerve can be as close as 1 to 2 cm distal to the tip of the coracoid.[24] If the musculocutaneous nerve is palpated in this latter position, retraction of the conjoined tendon should be minimized.

The bicipital sheath is then identified and incised. In the setting of an acute fracture there is often a significant amount of hematoma and hemorrhagic bursal tissue, which can make identification of the biceps sheath difficult. The sheath can be most easily identified at the inferior portion of the deltopectoral interval just superior to the pectoralis major. Because the pectoralis major tendon inserts on the lateral lip of the bicipital groove, palpation immediately deep to the pectoralis major insertion will identify the biceps tendon. The biceps can then be followed proximal to the pectoralis major insertion. Once the sheath is identified and opened, the biceps tendon should be traced superiorly to the transverse humeral ligament, which is preserved. This action identifies the bicipital groove proximally and should assist the surgeon in identifying the greater tuberosity fracture line, which is usually located approximately 1 cm posterior to the bicipital groove. This fracture line is widened and, at the superior aspect of the fracture, the soft-tissue is split parallel to the anterior border of the supraspinatus all the way to the glenoid. The biceps is then tenodesed to the upper border of the pectoralis major distally and released just proximal to this tenodesis site. The joint is accessed through the greater tuberosity fracture line and the split created at the anterior border of the supraspinatus. The biceps is then resected by releasing the intra-articular portion from the supraglenoid tubercle and pulling it through the transverse humeral ligament distally.

The humeral metaphysis should now consist of an anterior fragment that includes the bicipital groove and lesser tuberosity and a posterior fragment that includes the greater tuberosity. Either of these fragments may be comminuted. Therefore, care should be exercised in manipulating them.

A heavy, nonabsorbable suture is placed through the bone-tendon junction of each of these fragments at the most lateral extent on each, adjacent to the major intertubercular fracture line (**Fig. 3**). This action will assist in protecting the remaining bone during retraction. The anterior fragment is pulled anteriorly and the posterior fragment is pulled posteriorly, taking care to preserve as much of the periosteal connection between the fragments and the shaft as possible.

Next the humeral head is excised. In many cases of classic 4-part fractures, the head will be easily identifiable and removable. In some cases, however, there may be some residual soft-tissue attachments that must be released to remove the head. In addition, a portion of the head often remains with one or both of the tuberosity fragments. It is important to resect all portions of the head from both tuberosity fragments so that residual head does not interfere with tuberosity reduction. The humeral head size is measured to aid in prosthetic head selection (**Fig. 4**).

The humeral shaft is then delivered into the wound by dropping the arm toward the floor so that the humerus is adducted, slightly extended, and modestly externally rotated. Excessive external rotation is not required and may be detrimental. A small incision is made at the labral-capsule junction anteriorly and posteriorly,

and blunt Homan retractors are placed to retract the tuberosity fragments. Excessive retraction should be avoided so that as much as possible of the remaining periosteal sleeve connecting the tuberosities to the shaft can be preserved. With the head removed, the shaft displaced inferiorly, and the tuberosities retracted, the glenoid is easily visualized. Any glenoid-based abnormality (ie, fracture or arthritis) should be addressed. Discussion of specific techniques for the management of concomitant glenoid-based abnormalities is beyond the scope of this article.

The specific steps for bone preparation, prosthetic placement, and tuberosity reduction and fixation are, to some extent, dependent on the prosthetic used. Successful results can be obtained with any implant, and the surgeon should be thoroughly familiar with the implant he or she is using. The remainder of this section is based on the technique used by the senior author (G.R.W.) using a specific system (Global Unite, DePuy Orthopaedics, Inc, Warsaw, IN).

The shaft is sequentially reamed using hand reamers until there is good circumferential contact between the reamer and the shaft. Care should be exercised to avoid overreaming, as the cortex of the humeral shaft is often thin. The goal is to take the reamer up to the endosteal surface without creating endosteal perforation or notching. A trial component is constructed with a diaphyseal portion the same size as the reamer and a matching size 0 epiphyseal component. Each epiphyseal component comes in 0, −5, and +5 sizes. Using a 0 component initially allows for subsequent lengthening or shortening by 5 mm, depending on the quality of the reduction confirmed radiographically. The two components are connected to one another and the trial is loaded onto the inserter. The trial stem is then inserted into the humerus.

There are 3 major goals for this trialing process: (1) to determine whether enough stability exists for cementless fixation, (2) to set and mark humeral component version, and (3) to evaluate tuberosity reduction and stem height. Unless there is substantial calcar comminution, stability is usually adequate for cementless fixation, which is determined by testing rotational stability after the trial is seated with the trial inserter handle. Excessive impaction with a mallet should be avoided to prevent splitting the shaft. Version can be set by using the alignment rod in the inserter handle and aligning it with the forearm. Options exist for 0°, 10°, 20°, and 30°. In most cases, 30° is acceptable (**Fig. 5**). With the trial seated in appropriate version, the inserter is removed, the shaft is marked where the anterior fin contacts it (usually at the anterior

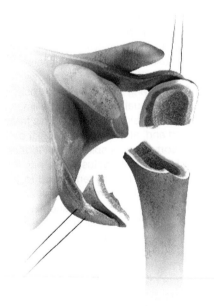

Fig. 3. The tuberosity fragments are controlled by placing heavy, nonabsorbable sutures through the bone-tendon junction. (*Courtesy of* DePuy Orthopaedics, Inc, Warsaw, IN; with permission.)

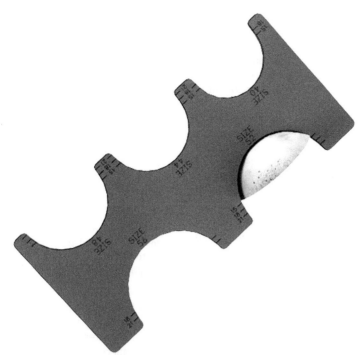

Fig. 4. Once removed, the humeral head fragment is measured to aid in prosthetic head selection. (*Courtesy of* DePuy Orthopaedics, Inc, Warsaw, IN; with permission.)

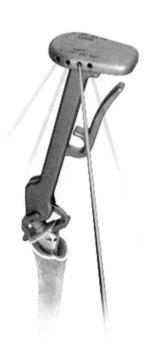

Fig. 5. Version can be established by using the alignment rod in the stem inserter and aligning it with the forearm. In most cases 30° of retroversion is acceptable. (*Courtesy of* DePuy Orthopaedics, Inc, Warsaw, IN; with permission.)

extent of the bicipital groove), and a trial head and matching collar are placed on the trial stem. The head size is determined by measuring the excised head. The neck length includes the width of the collar (ie, approximately 3 mm). For example, when a 48 × 18 head is seated on the stem with its accompanying collar, the collar plus the neck length of the head is 18 mm. Although offset heads and collars are available, the comminution of the tuberosities usually allows for centered components, making up any offset between the stem and the tuberosities with cancellous graft obtained from the excised head.

The humerus is reduced in to the glenoid and the greater tuberosity is reduced to the collar using the previously placed traction suture. Although the lesser tuberosity fragment can also be reduced, the greater tuberosity is the most critical to restore anatomically. Therefore, the traction suture in the greater tuberosity fragment is used to pull the tuberosity anteriorly to the collar in the region of most lateral portion of the stem, which should be approximately 1 cm posterior to the posterior border of the bicipital groove. Fluoroscopy is then used to evaluate stem height, tuberosity to head distance, and reduction of the tuberosity to the shaft. Ideally the tuberosity is either reduced anatomically to the shaft or overlaps it slightly (ie, 2–3 mm), and the head to tuberosity distance is approximately 1 cm. If the stem appears to be too low or too high, the humerus can be redislocated and a trial with either a −5 or +5 epiphysis can be tested.

When the stem height and configuration, head size, and collar size are satisfactory, the trial component is removed and a real component is placed. The component is assembled completely on the back table before insertion. The selected diaphysis and epiphysis are assembled and a heavy, nonabsorbable suture is passed through the hole on the medial portion of the stem for potential later use as a cerclage suture around the tuberosities. After impacting the collar onto the stem taper, sutures for tuberosity fixation are placed. Starting at approximately the midportion of the collar, 3 evenly spaced mattress sutures from anterior to posterior are placed through the holes in the collar with the 2 free ends exiting the superior surface of the collar from adjacent holes. These ends will be used to fix the greater tuberosity to the collar. Two additional mattress sutures are passed in a similar fashion through evenly spaced holes in the anterior half of the collar for lesser tuberosity fixation (**Fig. 6**). All sutures are heavy, nonabsorbable material. The head is then impacted onto the taper and will come to rest just above the collar. Two drill holes are placed on either side of the bicipital groove approximately 1 cm distal to the surgical neck fracture line. A heavy nonabsorbable suture is placed in each pair of holes so that the free ends exit the extramedullary surface of the humerus. These ends will be used later to help stabilize the tuberosities (**Fig. 7**). The stem is then inserted into the humerus, aligning the anterior fin with the previously placed mark on the shaft. It is carefully impacted. Overzealous impaction should be avoided to prevent splitting

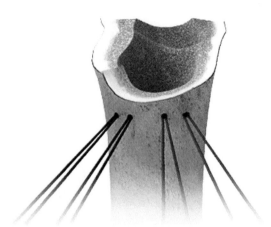

Fig. 7. Additional sutures are placed through drill holes anterior and posterior to the bicipital groove for later use in tuberosity fixation. (*Courtesy of* DePuy Orthopaedics, Inc, Warsaw, IN; with permission.)

of the humeral shaft. The porous coating of the real implant may make complete seating difficult. It is much better to accept stable, slightly incomplete seating rather than to split the humerus, as long as the component remains stable.

Before reducing the humerus, all of the sutures are passed through the greater tuberosity fragment from the deep to the superficial surface of the fragment. These sutures include the posterior limb of the potential cerclage suture from the medial hole in the stem, and all 3 mattress sutures from the posterior half of the collar (**Fig. 8**). Passage of these sutures can be facilitated by using large free needles. The cerclage suture is passed through the most posteromedial portion of the greater tuberosity. The mattress sutures from the collar are most easily passed, starting with the most posteromedial suture and working anterolaterally. The sutures should be passed exactly at the bone-tendon junction or even through the bone 1–2 mm from the bone-tendon junction. The most anterior limb of the most anterior suture should be located at the most anterior extent of the greater tuberosity, adjacent to the previously placed traction suture. The humerus is then reduced.

The greater tuberosity is then reduced using the previously placed traction suture. The most anterior mattress suture from the collar is pulled tight and fluoroscopy is used to check the reduction. Before tying the mattress sutures, bone graft from the resected head is packed between the epiphyseal portion of the stem and the greater tuberosity. The most anterior of the greater tuberosity-collar mattress sutures is tied while the greater tuberosity is held in a reduced position. The position of the tuberosity is again checked to ensure it is acceptable. The other 2 more posterior

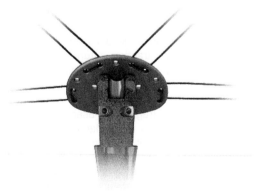

Fig. 6. Before impacting the head, multiple heavy, nonabsorbable sutures are placed through the collar in a mattress configuration for use in securing the tuberosities. (*Courtesy of* DePuy Orthopaedics, Inc, Warsaw, IN; with permission.)

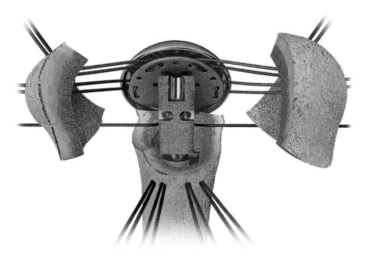

Fig. 8. Before reducing the humerus, the previously placed sutures are passed through the bone-tendon junction. (*Courtesy of* DePuy Orthopaedics, Inc, Warsaw, IN; with permission.)

mattress sutures are then tied. The lesser tuberosity is then reduced using the previously placed traction suture. Adequate reduction is confirmed radiographically, which usually requires either an axillary view or a combination of C-arm and humeral rotation. The anterior limb of the potential cerclage suture through the medial hole in the prosthesis is next passed from deep to superficial at the most medial and inferior extent of the lesser tuberosity fragment. The mattress sutures on the anterior half of the collar are then passed from the deep to the superficial surface of the lesser tuberosity fragment exactly at the bone-tendon junction. Care must be taken when passing all anterior sutures to avoid the axillary and musculocutaneous nerves. Bone graft from the head is packed between the tuberosity and the stem, and the deep limb of the previously placed traction suture is passed through the bone-tendon junction of the greater tuberosity fragment at its most anterior edge. This suture is then tied so that the lesser and greater tuberosity fragments are brought together anatomically at the level of the collar. This reduction can be aided by using a reduction clamp. The anterior mattress sutures are then tied. The traction suture on the greater tuberosity fragment is then used to close the split at the anterior edge of the supraspinatus tendon.

Ideal tuberosity placement is at the periphery of the head, abutted against the collar. In the senior author's experience, the tuberosity cerclage suture from the medial hole in the prosthesis around both tuberosities has a tendency to pull the tuberosities, especially the greater tuberosity, under the head and collar toward the stem. This action results in relative overreduction of the tuberosity.

The cerclage suture is therefore approximated, not overtightened, around the prosthesis and tuberosities, and temporarily clamped with a needle driver. Fluoroscopy is used to check the reduction of the tuberosities, especially the greater tuberosity. If no tendency toward overreduction of the tuberosity is identified, the cerclage suture is tied. If there is a tendency of the greater tuberosity to be pulled under the collar, the cerclage suture is removed and not used. A heavy nonabsorbable suture passed through each tuberosity fragment can be used to approximate the inferior portions of the tuberosity fragments instead of the cerclage suture in this scenario.

The final step is to place and tie the longitudinal sutures from the shaft. The sutures posterior to the bicipital groove are taken superiorly and passed through the bone-tendon junction of the greater tuberosity; the sutures anterior to the bicipital groove are taken superiorly and passed through the bone-tendon junction of the lesser tuberosity. These sutures are then tied. Overtightening again should be avoided so that the tuberosities are not overreduced. The position of the tuberosities should again be confirmed with fluoroscopy (**Fig. 9**).

If the medial calcar is comminuted or adequate stability for cementless fixation is not present at the time of initial trial stem insertion, the trial stem is removed and plans are made to cement a stem one size smaller. A fracture jig is available to assist in selecting appropriate stem height and version as well as tuberosity reduction (**Fig. 10**). This jig is placed around the humeral shaft about 1 to 1.5 cm distal to the major surgical neck fracture line. This maneuver may require release of a portion

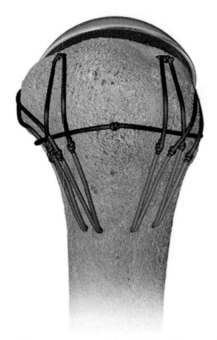

Fig. 9. The sutures are sequentially tied to securely fix the tuberosities in an anatomic position. (*Courtesy of* DePuy Orthopaedics, Inc, Warsaw, IN; with permission.)

of the latissimus tendon as well as the pectoralis major, depending on the location, configuration, and degree of comminution of the fracture. An alignment rod placed in the jig should be aligned with the forearm to obtain 30° of retroversion. The jig is then tightened. The jig should be tightened

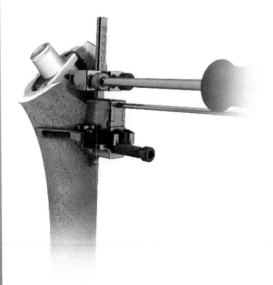

Fig. 10. When cemented fixation is required, a fracture jig is available to assist in selecting the appropriate stem height and allow for tuberosity reduction and trialing. (*Courtesy of* DePuy Orthopaedics, Inc, Warsaw, IN; with permission.)

enough to make it stable but not overtight. The positioning tower is placed onto the jig and the alignment clamp is connected to the hole in the anterior fin of the trial implant. The trial component is then inserted into the humerus and the alignment clamp is slid over the tower. The height of the implant is next determined. An initial rough estimate is obtained using a combination of the size of the greater tuberosity fragment, distance of the medial portion of the trial stem from the medial humerus, and distance from the uppermost portion of the pectoralis major insertion. The alignment clamp is then secured to the tower, the trial collar and head are placed, and the humerus is reduced.

The greater tuberosity is then reduced using a combination of manual manipulation and traction from the previously placed traction suture. Reduction is confirmed with fluoroscopy. The criteria for acceptable stem height and tuberosity reduction are the same as described earlier. The height of the stem can be fine-tuned by sliding it up or down on the fracture jig and tower rather than by using a +5 or −5 epiphysis. When the height, version, head size, and tuberosity reduction are acceptable, the position of the trial stem on the tower is marked. The trial stem is removed with the clamp still attached to it, but the tower and jig are left in place. A real implant is fashioned, complete with the sutures as described earlier for the cementless technique. A cement restrictor is placed distally, the humeral canal is irrigated and dried, and cement is placed in the canal. Antibiotic impregnated cement is routinely used; the cement is not pressurized. The real stem is fitted with the clamp for the jig at the hole in the anterior fin. The stem is inserted into the humeral canal, and the clamp is slid over the tower to the position previously marked with the trial. The clamp is tightened, the excess cement is removed, particularly adjacent to the porous coating, and the cement is allowed to harden. The tuberosities are reduced and secured as already described.

The shoulder is taken through a gentle range of motion to ensure that the tuberosities and prosthesis move as a single unit. Continuity of the axillary nerve is again confirmed by digital palpation. A surgical drain is placed so that it exits the skin of the lateral arm inferiorly near the deltoid insertion, well inferior from the anterior branch of the axillary nerve. The wound is closed in a layered manner, and a sling and sterile dressing are applied (**Fig. 11**).

POSTOPERATIVE CARE

The drain is removed when the output is less than 30 mL per shift, and generally the patient is

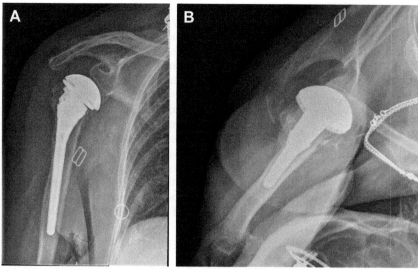

Fig. 11. Postoperative AP (*A*) and axillary (*B*) radiographs of the patient from **Fig. 1**, demonstrating a well-placed hemiarthroplasty with anatomic reduction of the tuberosities.

discharged from hospital on the second postoperative day. The arm is maintained in a sling for 6 weeks after surgery, but passive motion of the shoulder is begun on postoperative day 1. Early passive range of motion is important to minimize postoperative stiffness. However, tuberosity displacement is a devastating complication. In the past, full passive range of motion has been instituted as early as postoperative day 1.[25] However, because of the concern for tuberosity displacement, the senior author has slowed rehabilitation over the first 6 postoperative weeks. The amount of motion is individualized for each patient depending on the bone quality of the tuberosities and the stability of the tuberosity fixation as assessed intraoperatively, but the authors generally start with pendulum exercises, supine passive forward elevation to 90°, and external rotation to neutral. The patient is typically seen in the office at 2 weeks, 4 weeks, 6 weeks, 3 months, 6 months, and 1 year postoperatively, with radiographs on each visit.

Passive range of motion is progressed over the first 6 weeks, starting on the first postoperative visit at 2 weeks. Supine passive forward elevation is advanced to 130° and external rotation to 30° when the patient is seen at the first postoperative office visit at 2 weeks. At 4 weeks postoperatively, full passive range of motion is instituted. An overhead pulley, passive stretching, and active range of motion are initiated at 6 weeks, and strengthening is added at 3 months postoperatively. This progression is obviously dependent on maintenance of tuberosity position and progressive radiographic union, and must be individualized. The intensity and duration of structured rehabilitation

in an office setting should also be individualized according to motion progression and patient compliance. However, in general, patients add formalized rehabilitation at a therapy facility to their home exercises at 4 to 6 weeks postoperatively, and continue for 3 to 4 months. Home exercises continue for approximately 6 to 12 months postoperatively, and recovery generally plateaus at 1 year postoperatively.

RESULTS

Hemiarthroplasty is a reliable procedure for pain relief, but patient function remains a challenge. Functional results are variable, and restoration of full preoperative function in a patient is rarely obtained. In a series of 808 patients at a mean of 3.7 years of follow-up, Kontakis and colleagues[26] reported mean active forward flexion of 105°. Abduction averaged 92° and external rotation averaged 30°. The average Constant score for a subgroup of 560 patients was 56. Antuna and colleagues[27] reported on more long-term results (mean 10.3 years) in 57 patients. The mean active forward elevation in their patients was 100°, with satisfactory results in 27 patients and unsatisfactory results in 30.

Correct height of the implant and healing of the tuberosities in anatomic or near anatomic position is the key to postoperative function.[28] Patients with a properly placed implant and tuberosities that have healed in the correct position can often achieve near normal function. However, nonanatomic placement of the implant or malunion or nonunion of the tuberosities typically leads to function below shoulder level (**Fig. 12**).

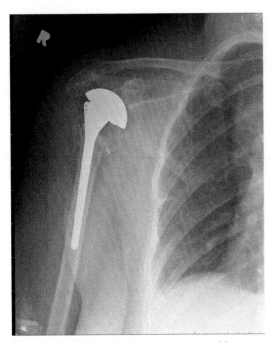

Fig. 12. AP radiograph of a 4-part proximal humerus fracture treated with hemiarthroplasty whereby the hemiarthroplasty stem was placed too superiorly, leading to failure of the rotator cuff and anterior-superior subluxation of the implant. The patient had minimal pain but was limited to waist-level function.

Kontakis and colleagues[26] also reported a 2.2% rate of infection and a 6.8% incidence of proximal migration of the humeral head. The most common complication remains tuberosity malunion, nonunion, and resorption. Bigliani and colleagues[29] reviewed a series of 29 failed hemiarthroplasties, and identified tuberosity-related complications as the most common cause of failure. As detailed herein, malrotation (especially too much retroversion) or inaccurate height (especially too high) of the implant and malposition of the tuberosities (especially the greater tuberosity) can have a substantial detrimental effect on successful healing of the tuberosities and outcome.[28] Reverse shoulder arthroplasty (RSA) can be used as a salvage procedure for patients who develop a tuberosity-related complication following hemiarthroplasty for fracture. However, the results of RSA in this setting are significantly inferior to the results of RSA for treatment of rotator cuff tear arthropathy or as a primary procedure for proximal humerus fractures.[30]

SUMMARY

Displaced proximal humeral fractures requiring treatment with hemiarthroplasty are challenging cases. Pitfalls exist in the management of this injury from the preoperative planning stage, through the operation itself, and the postoperative course. Proper evaluation of both the patient and fracture, and thorough counseling of the patient and family preoperatively are essential. Intraoperatively, obtaining proper humeral height and version, as well as proper tuberosity position and fixation are the most important and challenging aspects. Postoperative vigilance to possible problems and adherence to a structured, progressive rehabilitation plan are also important in obtaining a satisfactory outcome. Identifying and avoiding the potential pitfalls in every step of the management is key to obtaining a satisfactory outcome.

REFERENCES

1. Green A, Norris T. Part II: proximal humeral fractures and fracture dislocations. In: Browner BD, Jupiter JB, Levine AM, et al, editors. Skeletal trauma. 4th edition. Philadelphia: Saunders; 2009. p. 1623–755.
2. Neer CS II. Displaced proximal humeral fractures: II. Treatment of three-part and four-part displacement. J Bone Joint Surg Am 1970;52(6):1090–103.
3. Roux A, Decroocq L, El Batti S, et al. Epidemiology of proximal humerus fractures managed in a trauma center. Orthop Traumatol Surg Res 2012;98(6):715–9.
4. Solberg BD, Moon CN, Franco DP, et al. Locked plating of 3- and 4-part proximal humerus fractures in older patients: the effect of initial fracture pattern on outcome. J Orthop Trauma 2009;23(2):113–9.
5. Sirveaux F, Navex G, Roche O, et al. Reverse prosthesis for proximal humerus fracture, technique and results. Techniques in Shoulder and Elbow Surgery 2008;9(1):15–22.
6. Codeman EA. The shoulder. Boston: Thomas Todd Co; 1934.
7. Hernigou P, Duparc F, Hernigou A. Determining humeral retroversion with computed tomography. J Bone Joint Surg Am 2002;84(10):1753–62.
8. Bioleau P, Walch G. The three dimensional geometry of the proximal humerus, implications for surgical technique and prosthetic design. J Bone Joint Surg Br 1997;79:857–65.
9. Iannotti JP, Gabriel JP, Schneck SL, et al. The normal glenohumeral relationships: an anatomical study of one hundred and forty shoulders. J Bone Joint Surg Am 1992;74:491–501.
10. Murachovsky J, Ikemoto RY, Nascimento LG, et al. Pectoralis major tendon reference (PMT): a new method for accurate restoration of humeral length with hemiarthroplasty for fracture. J Shoulder Elbow Surg 2006;15(6):675–8.
11. Bioleau P, Bicknell RT, Mazzoleni N, et al. CT scan method accurately assesses humeral head retroversion. Clin Orthop Relat Res 2008;466(3):661–9.

12. Neer CS II. Displaced proximal humeral fractures: I. Classification and evaluation. J Bone Joint Surg Am 1970;52(6):1077–89.

13. Muller ME, Nazarian S, Koch P, et al. The comprehensive classification of fractures of long bones. Berlin: Springer Verlag; 1990. p. 120–1.

14. Hertel R, Hempfing A, Stiehler M, et al. Predictors of humeral head ischemia after intracapsular fracture of the proximal humerus. J Shoulder Elbow Surg 2004;13:427–33.

15. Majed A, Macleod I, Bull AM, et al. Proximal humeral fracture classification systems revisited. J Shoulder Elbow Surg 2011;20:1125–32.

16. Hagg O, Lundberg B. Aspects of prognostics factors in comminuted and dislocated proximal humerus fractures. In: Batenab JE, Welsh RP, editors. Surgery of the shoulder. Philadelphia: BC Decker; 1984.

17. Goldman RT, Koval KJ, Cuomo F, et al. Functional outcome after humeral head replacement for acute three- and four- part proximal humeral fractures. J Shoulder Elbow Surg 1995;4(2):81–6.

18. Lim EV, Day LJ. Thrombosis of the axillary artery complicating proximal humeral fractures. J Bone Joint Surg Am 1987;69:778–80.

19. Jobe CM, Phipatanakul WP, Coen MJ. Gross anatomy of the shoulder. In: Rockwood CA Jr, Matsen FA III, Wirth MA, et al, editors. The shoulder. 4th edition. Philadelphia: Saudners; 2009. p. 33–101.

20. Visser CP, Coene LN, Brand R, et al. Nerve lesion in proximal humeral fractures. J Shoulder Elbow Surg 2001;10(5):421–7.

21. Bloom MH, Obata WG. Diagnosis of posterior dislocation of the shoulder with use of Volpeau axillary and angle up roentgenographic views. J Bone Joint Surg Am 1967;49:943–9.

22. Wall B, Nove-Josserand L, O'Connor DP, et al. Reverse total shoulder arthroplasty: a review of results according to etiology. J Bone Joint Surg Am 2007;89:1476–85.

23. Lee TQ, Black AD, Tibone JE, et al. Release of the coracoacromial ligament can lead to glenohumeral laxity: a biomechanical study. J Shoulder Elbow Surg 2001;10:68–72.

24. Flatow EL, Bigliani LU, April EW. An anatomic study of the musculocutaneous nerve and its relationship to the coracoids process. Clin Orthop Relat Res 1989;244:166–71.

25. Bohsali KI, Wirth MA. Fractures of the proximal humerus. In: Rockwood CA Jr, Matsen FA III, Wirth MA, et al, editors. The shoulder. 4th edition. Philadelphia: Saudners; 2009. p. 295–333.

26. Kontakis G, Coutras C, Tosunidis T, et al. Early management of proximal humeral fractures with hemiarthroplasty. J Bone Joint Surg Br 2008;90(11):1407–13.

27. Antuna SA, Sperling JW, Cofield RH. Shoulder hemiarthroplasty for acute fractures of the proximal humerus: a minimum five-year follow-up. J Shoulder Elbow Surg 2008;17(2):202–9.

28. Boileau P, Krishnan SG, Tinsi L, et al. Tuberosity malposition and migration: reasons for poor outcomes after hemiarthroplasty for displaced fractures of the proximal humerus. J Shoulder Elbow Surg 2002;11(5):401–12.

29. Bigliani LU, Flatow EL, McCluskey GM, et al. Failed prosthetic replacement in proximal humeral fractures. Orthop Trans 1991;15:747–8.

30. Levy J, Frankle M, Mighell M, et al. The use of the reverse shoulder prosthesis for the treatment of failed hemiarthroplasty for proximal humeral fracture. J Bone Joint Surg Am 2007;89(2):292–300.

Operative Techniques in the Management of Scapular Fractures

Peter A. Cole, MD[a,b,*], Jonathan R. Dubin, MD[a],
Gil Freeman, MD[a]

KEYWORDS

- Scapula fractures • Judet approach • Open reduction with internal fixation • Scapula
- Scapula reduction techniques

KEY POINTS

- The underlying principle in the treatment of scapula fractures is that deformity and dysfunction are related as with all other fractures; therefore, restoring length, alignment, and rotation to the scapula improves outcomes.
- An accurate diagnostic approach to scapula fractures requires interpretation of good shoulder radiographs and a three-dimensional (3D) computed tomography scan to measure medialization at the lateral border, glenopolar angle, and scapular angulation.
- Extended approaches to the scapula offer excellent visualization posteriorly and should be used for complex fracture patterns or when surgery is delayed for longer than 10 days. Otherwise, more limited muscle-sparing approaches can be used that may expedite rehabilitation.
- There are many techniques for reduction of the lateral border, and these are paramount because it is this maneuver that is pivotal in accomplishing the surgical goals. The lateral pillar must be restored in neck and body fractures and, subsequently, rotational corrections at the medial border can be effected.
- The fixation montage should restore stability to the ring around the border of the scapula, from the lateral border to the spine, vertebral border, and inferior angle, so that the patient can rehabilitate effectively with immediate range of motion.

INTRODUCTION

The management of scapula fractures has evolved over recent years as new techniques and approaches have been promulgated.[1–5] Often the result of a violent, high-energy mechanism, these injuries were often either missed or neglected in favor of managing higher acuity disorders.[6–8] There is a 10% to 15% mortality in patients with scapula fractures, most commonly from a concomitant cranial injury or pulmonary compromise and sepsis.[9–11]

A systematic review by Zlowodzki and colleagues[12] found that, although 80% of intra-articular glenoid fractures are treated operatively, 99% of isolated body fractures received conservative therapy, at least in the first few years of this millennium. However, the field is changing rapidly, given that new reports and clinical studies published in the peer-reviewed literature have called

Funding Sources: Nil.
Conflict of Interest: Dr Cole receives consulting fees/honoraria from AONA and AO International, is a consultant to J&J (Synthes-Depuy), and has shares with BoneFoams Inc, LLC; J.R. Dubin and G. Freeman, none.
[a] Department of Orthopaedic Surgery, Regions Hospital, 640 Jackson Street, St Paul, MN 55101, USA;
[b] Department of Orthopaedic Surgery, University of Minnesota, Minneapolis, MN, USA
* Corresponding author. Regions Hospital, University of Minnesota, 640 Jackson Street, St Paul, MN 55101.
E-mail address: peter.a.cole@healthpartners.com

into question the dogma that all scapula fractures do well without operative management.[10,13–18]

Nordqvist and Petersson[14] published the long-term results of nonoperatively treated scapula fractures and showed that 50% of patients with residual scapula deformity had shoulder symptoms. Cole and colleagues[13] also recently published the outcomes of presurgical and postsurgical correction of extra-articular malunions of the scapula, showing a significant increase in strength and range of the shoulder, as well as an average 29-point improvement in the DASH (disabilities of the arm, shoulder, and hand) score at a mean follow-up of 3 years. As evidence mounts and the techniques improve, surgeons are becoming familiar with safe approaches, and accepting the concept of restoration of proper anatomy to achieve proper function.

ANATOMY AND BIOMECHANICS

An understanding of anatomy and biomechanics of the scapula is paramount for undertaking surgery of scapula fractures. Detailed descriptions can be found in an article by Cole[19] in the January 2002 *Orthopedic Clinics of North America*. In brief, the scapula is a triangular bone that, in its midsection between the scapula borders, is wafer thin. There are 18 muscles that cross, originate, or insert on its borders, causing thickenings of the cortical bone that can provide purchase for screw fixation. In addition, there exists a rich vascular network, including the circumflex scapular artery along the lateral border, and a robust muscular envelope providing a salubrious biology for fracture healing; thus, nonunions are rare. The suprascapular nerve is also important to identify and protect in a posterior approach, because it traverses the spinoglenoid notch from the base of the supraspinatus fossa where it emanates from the suprascapular notch to innervate the infraspinatus (**Fig. 1**).[20] Traction on this nerve can cause rotator cuff weakness and should be avoided during the operation. This requirement makes it difficult to visualize the glenoid without either a tenotomy of the posterior rotator cuff or working between the interval of the teres minor and infraspinatus muscles.

Despite the various ways the scapula can fracture, evidence suggests that most of these injuries can be codified into 3 main types. Using 3D computed tomography (CT) mapping techniques, Armitage and colleagues[21] found in a series of operative scapula fractures that 68% of fractures involved the inferior glenoid, 17% had an intra-articular component, and 22% entered the spinoglenoid notch. In addition, of the fractures

involving the inferior glenoid, most had their exit points on the superomedial border at the base of the scapula spine, and 44% had an exit at the inferomedial one-third of the vertebral border. This knowledge allows surgical planning and understanding the nature of the fracture (**Fig. 2**).

Restoring the anatomy of the scapula facilitates a return of its biomechanical function.[22] At its most basic level, the scapula serves to maintain the arm's position in space. Several investigators have likened the relationship of the glenoid to the humeral head to that of a seal balancing a ball on its nose: the muscles must constantly fire and adjust to accomplish this precise feat. Furthermore, it has recently been postulated that maintaining the rotator cuff muscles at a normal tension relative to the Blick curve optimizes dynamic stability of the glenohumeral joint. Thus, by correcting the anatomy, the surgeon improves a patient's biomechanical function.

INDICATIONS AND PREOPERATIVE PLANNING

The indications used for surgery at our institution have previously been published. These indications include the following:

1. Intra-articular step-off or gap greater than or equal to 4 mm
2. Lateral border offset (medialization) greater than 20 mm on anteroposterior view
3. Angular deformity greater than or equal to 45° seen on the scapular Y view
4. Lateral border offset greater than 15 mm and angular deformity greater than 30°
5. Glenopolar angle less than or equal to 22°
6. Displaced double lesions of the superior shoulder suspensory complex
   a. Both clavicle and scapula displaced greater than or equal to 10 mm
   b. Complete acromioclavicular dislocation and scapula fracture displaced greater than or equal to 10 mm

Fig. 3 shows the measurement technique to determine such indications.[23]

Because of the nature of the mechanism of injury leading to scapula fractures, patients require a thorough preoperative evaluation, often with a multidisciplinary approach because of the polytraumatized nature of most of these patients. It is imperative that the associated life-threatening injuries receive priority,[8,9,24–26] and these commonly include hemopneumothorax, cranial and spinal, as well as ipsilateral extremity injuries. The associated injury rate in displaced operative scapula series is as high as 90%.[27,28] In addition, a comprehensive secondary survey performed and

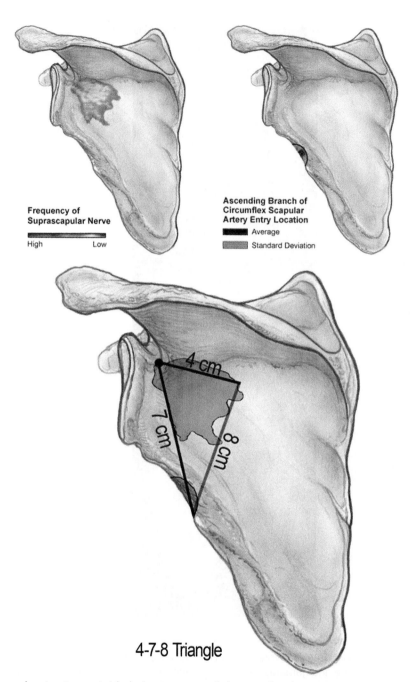

Frequency of
Suprascapular Nerve

High   Low

Ascending Branch of
Circumflex Scapular
Artery Entry Location
■ Average
■ Standard Deviation

4 cm

7 cm

8 cm

4-7-8 Triangle

Fig. 1. Neurovascular structures at risk during exposure of the scapula. The 4-7-8 triangle showing the danger zone between the spinoglenoid notch, the suprascapular bundle, and the circumflex scapular artery. (*From* Wijdicks CA, Armitage BM, Anavian J, et al. Vulnerable neurovasculature with a posterior approach to the scapula. Clin Orthop Relat Res 2009;467(8):2011–7; with permission.)

documented by the orthopedic team is essential to rule out other injuries that may require orthopedic care. Of particular concern is the strong incidence of brachial plexus palsy, approximately 12.5% associated with scapular fractures,[11] and about a 50% ipsilateral extremity injury rate.[8,14,27–32] A

neurologic examination can be challenging in these patients because of intubation in many cases, pain, and ipsilateral fractures, but nevertheless should be completed with vigilance, because the neurologic status can adversely affect outcome.

Inferior Glenoid Neck

Spinoglenoid Notch

Glenoid Articular Surface

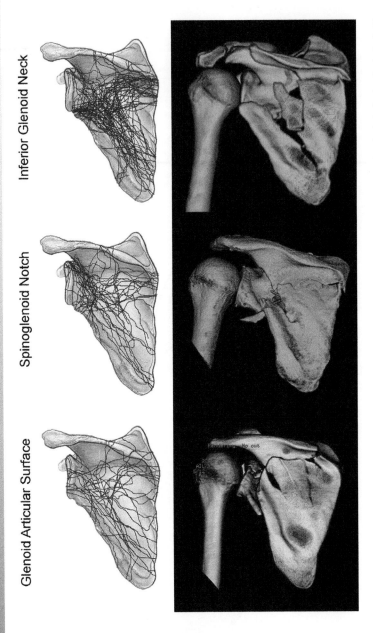

Fig. 2. Scapula fracture map indicating how fractures patterns occur in the scapula body and neck. Note that there is more randomness to the fracture patterns in the intra-articular glenoid variants. (*From* Armitage BM, Wijdicks CA, Tarkin IS, et al. Mapping of scapular fractures with three-dimensional computed tomography. J Bone Joint Surg Am 2009;91(9):2222–8. Fig. 4; with permission.)

The preoperative evaluation also involves a soft tissue assessment of the integument, because many of the fractures occur from a blow to the superior shoulder, which can be associated with abrasions. We prefer to defer surgery until abrasions have completely epithelialized to reduce risks of infection, and, to date, we have not had an infection for this surgery, an astounding statistic that happens to mimic the literature on operative series. Abrasions may take 3 to 4 weeks to resolve, which is enough time for the scapula to form significant callus. Results of surgery in 22 such delayed patients having open reduction with internal fixation were associated with good outcomes as assessed with DASH, as well as range of motion and strength.[33] A daily Hibicleanse scrub is used to reduce the bacterial load over the compromised area. Neither topical nor oral antibiotics are necessary during this phase.

Preoperative planning also must include an assessment of the fracture radiographically and preferably with CT 3D reconstructions both to assess deformity and plan surgical approaches. It is useful to obtain an anteroposterior view of the opposite shoulder to measure the normal glenopolar angle, to compare the restored fractured side with regard to this important alignment variable, which is discussed later.

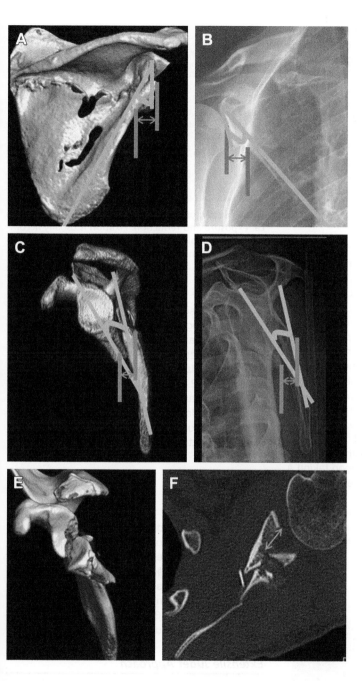

Fig. 3. Measuring displacement in scapula fractures. (*A*, *B*) Glenopolar angle. (*C*, *D*) Angulation (*E*, *F*) Articular step off.

Surgical Approaches

The chosen surgical approach depends on fracture location, complexity, and chronicity. Less invasive approaches are preferred when feasible, but are technically more demanding. There is an unstudied belief that patients rehabilitate faster and have less pain with more limited dissection. The scapula heals quickly because of the rich local blood supply, but surgery is often delayed because of the treatment of other critical injuries

or lost time in transferring the patient to an expert. Therefore, the extensile approach is utilitarian and often used for such situations, because complete exposure of the scapula may be necessary in such circumstances to mobilize callus.

Posterior Approaches

Although the posterior approach has been considered the workhorse for any fracture involving the scapula body or neck,[34] there have recently been several nuances to the posterior approach that have been described. A posterior approach should be used except in the case of anterior glenoid fractures, or superior glenoid fractures involving the coracoid, or isolated process fractures.

Variations on posterior approaches include (1) extensile Judet approach,[35] (2) modified Judet approach,[2] and (3) the minimally invasive direct approach.[1] The senior author (PAC) is now more frequently using an open Judet approach, which spares the deltoid from takedown allowing full access, and has also developed the minimally invasive technique for fractures that are acute and simple.[1] In all cases, the setup and equipment are the same.

The patient is positioned on a bean bag in the lateral decubitus position. A triangular BoneFoam positioner (BoneFoam Inc, Plymouth, Minnesota) is placed on a hand table to allow the ipsilateral extremity to be prepped and draped free and manipulated as necessary during the case (**Fig. 4**), which facilitates manipulation during the operation, as well as allowing the patient to flop slightly forward, which is instrumental in improving the surgeon's visualization and access to the scapula. The forequarter is prepped from midchest to midback, and from the neck to the flank. Should the patient also possess an ipsilateral clavicle fracture, this can be addressed without reprepping and draping by simply maneuvering the arm out of the so-called floppy-forward position, and the surgeon taking a cephalad and anterior position to execute this part of the surgery.

The following implants and instrumentation are useful for surgical exposure and reduction of the fractures and represent the preference of the senior author (**Fig. 5**):

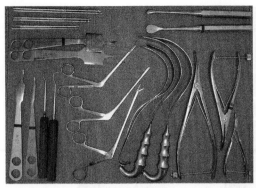

Fig. 5. Retractors and instrumentation used for surgical exposure and reduction. Fixation is usually accomplished with plates from the locking minifragment modular set, and occasionally the small fragment set.

- 2.0-mm, 2.4-mm, and 2.7-mm plates for most cases
  - Although locking implants may be useful, they are not necessary. They help to decrease the need for longer plates and minimize incision sizes.
  - Both 2.7-mm reconstruction plates for the spine and vertebral border and angle of the scapula as well as 2.7-mm dynamic compression (dc) plates for the lateral border.
- Small external-fixator set with 4 mm Schanz pins

Shoulder hook
- Cobb elevator
- Large and medium Hohmann retractors and Deaver retractors
- Lamina spreaders of various sizes; pituitaries of various sizes; #2 braided nonabsorbable sutures, as well as #1, 0, 2-0 absorbable braided sutures, and an absorbable monofilament for the skin, and a 3.2-mm to 6.4-mm (1/8-inch to 1/4-inch) self-suction drain

Extensile Judet Approach

The extensile Judet approach requires elevation of a flap, inclusive of the infraspinatus and teres minor, and is limited by the excursion of the suprascapular nerve (**Fig. 6**). The deltoid is classically mobilized with this flap from the scapula spine. Great care should be taken to minimize such retraction. This approach is required when expecting to encounter abundant callus or a severely comminuted fracture with multiple exit points through the borders that require visualization of the scapular body. Exposure of the articular surface is not possible without over-retracting the

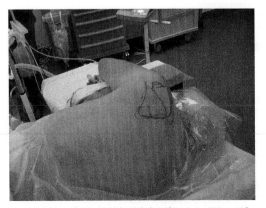

Fig. 4. Floppy-forward lateral decubitus position. Blue line indicates typical incision for the Judet posterior approach.

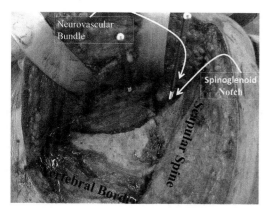

Fig. 6. View with extensile Judet exposure. There is a 4.0-mm Schanz pin in the neck fragment and one in the lateral border distal fragment.

muscle flap containing the neurovascular bundle, and therefore should not be attempted.

An angled incision is made 1 cm caudal to the scapular spine, beginning at its most lateral extent. It is then carried medially to the vertebral border of the scapular body, and then curved inferiorly toward the inferior pole. It is shaped like a boomerang, except with a more acute bend. Dissection is sharply carried to the fascia with the intention of maintaining full-thickness flaps. Next, the posterior deltoid is sharply taken from its origin on the scapular spine, being vigilant to maintain a cuff of fascia for later repair through drill holes. The infraspinatus is then sharply reflected from its origin on the medial border of the scapula. A Cobb elevator is then used to carefully elevate this large muscular flap from the posterior scapula. The suprascapular nerve is encountered medially as it enters the field of view from the spinoglenoid notch.[20] It runs with its respectively named vascular structures and is surrounded in fatty tissue.

A blunt Hohmann or small Deaver retractor can then be placed over the lateral border to facilitate visualization. The circumflex scapular artery is located at the base of the neck on average 4 cm inferior to the articular surface,[20] and, if encountered, should be ligated or coagulated because it will bleed briskly. The large muscular subscapularis on the anterior surface of the scapula provides a rich blood supply to the fracture, which may be responsible for the nearly 100% union rates initially reported in the published literature.

Modified Judet Approach

This approach is best reserved for fractures that are less than 10 days old and do not require visualization of the posterior scapula (ie, minimal comminution). The major advantage of this approach is that it avoids elevation of the posterior musculature by using the intermuscular interval between the teres minor and the infraspinatus (**Fig. 7**).

Positioning, prep, and instrumentation requirements match those of the extensile approach. The incision begins in a similar fashion; however, care is taken to bring the dissection to the level of the investing fascia of the infraspinatus and posterior deltoid. The fascia is then incised in line with the limbs of the incision, and a full-thickness fasciocutaneous flap is elevated from medial to lateral. The interval between the teres minor and the infraspinatus is identified and bluntly opened with a finger. Appropriately placed retractors allow visualization of the lateral border. Reduction and stabilization can then proceed. Closure is performed in a layered fashion with braided, absorbable sutures.

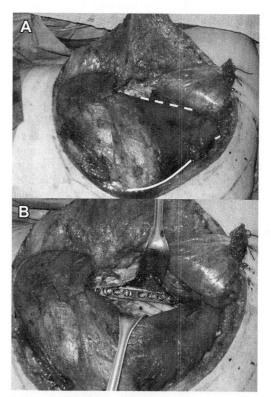

Fig. 7. Modified Judet approach. (*A*) Full-thickness fasciocutaneous flap retracted laterally (top of the image). Posterior deltoid is released from the scapular spine and tagged with a black suture. Dotted line indicates interval between teres minor and infraspinatus. Solid line shows planned release site of teres minor and some latissimus dorsi from medial border. (*B*) Visualization and plating in the internervous plane between infraspinatus and teres minor allowing exposure of the lateral border and neck.

Minimally Invasive Approach

The minimally invasive approach is best reserved for acute fractures that are safe for surgical intervention less than 10 days out from injury, and are simple patterns (2 exit points). Preservation of the integrity of the soft tissue is the main advantage of this approach, but should not compromise the goal of restoring length, alignment, and rotation of the scapula (**Fig. 8**).

The setup and instrumentation are the same as described for the other posterior approaches. The technique requires dual incisions, each centered on the medial and lateral fracture exit points. The lateral incision usually represents a straight, 5-cm to 6-cm incision from the glenoid neck tracking down the lateral edge of the scapular body. The dissection is carried down to the fascia, which is then incised at the inferior border of the deltoid. The subdeltoid space is opened bluntly with a digit, and an appendiceal retractor inserted to reflect the posterior head, allowing direct visualization of the infraspinatus and teres minor. Next, the interval between these two cuff muscles is bluntly developed. With appropriate retractor placement, adequate visualization is achieved.

The medial border is approached with a 5-cm to 6-cm incision centered on the fracture exit point. The fascia is incised, and the dissection is carried sharply down to bone. Taking care to minimize soft tissue stripping, a limited portion of the musculature is sharply elevated off its origin to allow enough visualization for fracture reduction and stabilization. A cuff of fascia is left to allow for robust suture closure through drill holes.

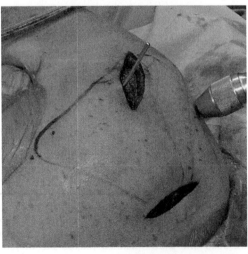

Fig. 8. Two-incision, minimally invasive approach. A Schanz pin is seen in the scapular neck as a reduction aid. In addition, a percutaneously placed Schanz pin is placed superiorly.

Surgical Exit and Wound Closure

A #1 braided suture is used for closing the deep layer. The suture is passed through the full thickness of the deltoid fascia and closed through drill holes in the scapular spine. The same is done for the infraspinatus, which is reattached to the medial border of the scapula. A medium-sized drain is frequently used, taking care to have it exit anteriorly and proximally to keep the drain hole from being in a dependent position with respect to gravity, thus minimizing drainage. A layered closure with 2-0 absorbable braided suture and a running subcuticular stitch is performed.

REDUCTION TECHNIQUES AND METHODS OF STABILIZATION

To achieve an acceptable outcome, restoration of alignment is critical because function and form are directly related. The most important and difficult part of the reduction is usually that of the lateral border because the deforming forces on the individual fragments typically cause worse displacement at this site, and because of the need to work around the muscular flaps.

The senior author has devised 5 tactics that facilitate reduction of the lateral border. These can be used separately or in combination:

1. A Schanz pin is used in the glenoid neck. This pin becomes the joystick for the proximal fragment, and allows for derotation and translation of the neck segment, to help it align with the distal lateral border segment. A 4.0-mm or 5.0-mm Schanz pin is used for this purpose, and a T-handled chuck is nearly essential in delayed cases.
2. A shoulder hook is used in a pilot drill hole on the distal fragment at the lateral border. This maneuver allows the surgeon to joystick the distal fragment to the proximal fragment to align the lateral border.
3. A pointed bone tenaculum is used though drill holes across the primary fracture line at the lateral border.
4. A lamina spreader is inserted between the proximal and distal fragments to mobilize the fragments to achieve adequate reduction. After more than a few days, the soft tissue callus forms, and after a couple weeks the well-developed harder callus takes shape and these must be overcome with osteoclasis and mobilization with a lamina spreader.
5. A small Ex-Fix with 4.0-mm Schanz pins is used to maintain a reduction or maintain length in situations in which application of the pointed bone tenaculum to clamp the fracture is

impossible either because of the orientation of the fracture line or, more commonly, because of comminution.

Before attempting fracture manipulation, adequate visualization must be achieved, and the fracture edges must be clearly delineated by removing soft tissue from the edges. Soft tissue in this case includes the callus, which forms rapidly in these injuries. Again, a lamina spreader is useful to mobilize fragments from callus and soft tissue adhesions or contracture. The senior author's preference is to save any callus and use it for graft before closure; it is a valuable free source of bone morphogenic proteins and biologic enhancers.

Fracture manipulation is commenced next with an understanding of the common deformities. The proximal fragment is often medialized and flexed compared with the remaining body. To align these pieces and restore angulation and glenopolar angle, an attempt is first made with direct techniques. The author prefers to try applying a medially directed force with a shoulder hook against the lateral border (**Fig. 9**). If able to achieve an acceptable reduction, then stabilization can be obtained with a 4-hole 2.4-mm locking reconstruction plate. Care should be taken to place a provisional fixation device medial enough to allow for the stouter, 2.7-mm limited contact dynamic compression plate (LC-DCP) to be placed along the thicker, lateral border for definitive stabilization.

Another technique for reduction uses point-to-point reduction forceps to manipulate the fragments into acceptable reduction. Strategically placed drill holes, often in a serial fashion, can be placed to assist in clamp placement. A lamina spreader can also be used between the fragments

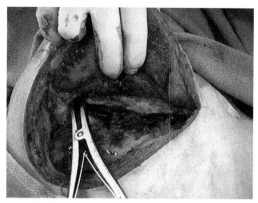

Fig. 10. Lamina spreader inserted into the fracture for mobilization of fragments and osteoclasis of callus.

to free adhesions and mobilize the fracture fragments (**Fig. 10**). A 3.5-mm cortical screw can sometimes be inserted into the glenoid component to be used as a post to push against with the lamina spreader. A combination of these techniques is often used to achieve final reduction of the lateral border. If an acceptable reduction is still not obtained, then a mini–Ex-Fix with 4.0-mm Schanz pins can be applied to restore and hold alignment (**Fig. 11**).

The senior author prefers to perform simultaneous reduction of the medial and lateral borders. The medial border is often reduced similarly, with drill holes, a shoulder hook, and point-to-point clamps. Provisional and definitive stabilization of the medial border involves a novel technique in which a contoured 12-hole 2.4-mm locking reconstruction plate is clamped to the scapula with 2 pediatric Kocher clamps. One tine of the clamp slips

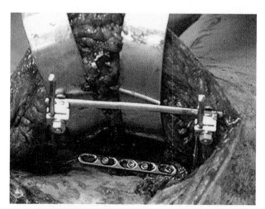

Fig. 11. Mini–Ex-Fix applied to 4.0-mm Schanz pin to maintain length and alignment while definitive fixation is being applied with a minifragment plate(s). Top of the image is lateral and right is the patient's head. One pin is placed into the scapular neck fragment, the other into the lateral body.

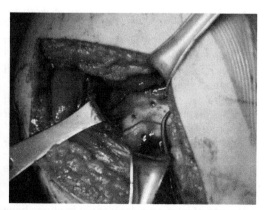

Fig. 9. Reduction technique with shoulder hook and point-to-point clamps. Pilot holes are clearly visualized. In addition, a point-to-point clamp closes the primary fracture line (lower right corner).

deep to the scapula, and the opposite side clamps the plate to the dorsal surface of the scapula. Contouring this plate is challenging, and is best performed with the same two pediatric Kocher clamps. The nose of each clamp is inserted into appropriate holes in the plate to allow for the significant twist and bend that adapts the plate to rest under, and thus provide fixation into, the scapular spine (**Fig. 12**). Screws along the medial border measure 8 to 10 mm and often provide only a unicortical feel when drilling, which should be remembered to prevent iatrogenic injury to the thoracic cavity.

Definitive fixation can depend on the fracture pattern; however, with the most common variants, a planned systematic approach can be expected. Along the lateral border a 2.7-mm LC-DCP plate of the appropriate length can be placed, which allows for a stouter plate that can accept locking screws. Although the bone in this area can be dense, it may not be thick, with screws measuring between 10 and 12 mm. The 2.4-mm reconstruction plate that was used for provisional fixation is left for additional stability (**Fig. 13**).

Fractures through the inferior angle of the scapula, although not as common, do occur, which provides an important key to restoring the relationship of the lateral borders and glenoid to the remainder of the body. It is the senior author's preference to use a small fragment of 3.5-mm locking T-plate, which provides the most screws

in the distal fragment, and this area can often accommodate the larger plate.

WOUND CLOSURE AND POSTOPERATIVE MANAGEMENT

If there is an ipsilateral clavicle fracture, then at this point the patient is brought out of the floppy-forward position by bringing the arm back along the side. The surgeon then can take a position at the top of the bed and commence management of the clavicle in a standard fashion. Otherwise, closure is begun. C-arm imaging can be challenging, but is not required because direct visualization allows acceptable reduction and fixation.

A drain is passed so as to exit in an anterior and proximal position to decrease drainage from the drain hole by being in a less dependent position. Next, the deep fascia of the posterior deltoid is closed with #2 braided suture through drill holes in the scapular spine. Likewise, the fascia between the cuff and rhomboids is reapproximated at the medial border via #2 braided suture and drill holes. Before leaving the operating room, it is important to perform a manipulation of the shoulder before the patient is awake to release the adhesions that have formed from the period of immobilization.

After surgery, active and passive range of motion are not restricted expect in the rare instance that a posterior rotator cuff tenotomy was performed. In this instance, active external rotation and passive internal rotation are restricted. At 6 weeks, full motion should be restored and light strengthening can begin. If motion is suboptimal, then a discussion is had with the patient about aggressive physical therapy and the possibility of manipulation under anesthesia.

Postoperative management:
- A sling or shoulder immobilizer is worn for comfort
- The drain is removed when output is less than 15 mL per 8-hour shift
- Full passive and active range of motion begin immediately after the operation
- Shoulder strengthening with 1.5 to 2.5 kg (3–5 lbs) resistance is started 4 weeks after surgery
- All restrictions are lifted at 12 weeks after surgery

OUTCOMES

Outcomes of intra-articular glenoid fractures have been reported in several large series. In a series of 27 patients, Mayo and colleagues[29] found that 22 patients experienced good or excellent

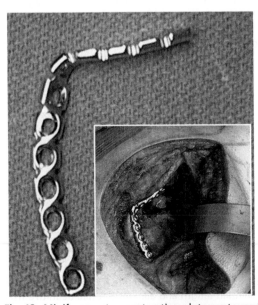

Fig. 12. Minifragment reconstruction plate contoured to the undersurface of the scapular spine and medial border of the scapula. Pediatric Kocher clamps assist in the bending and twisting.

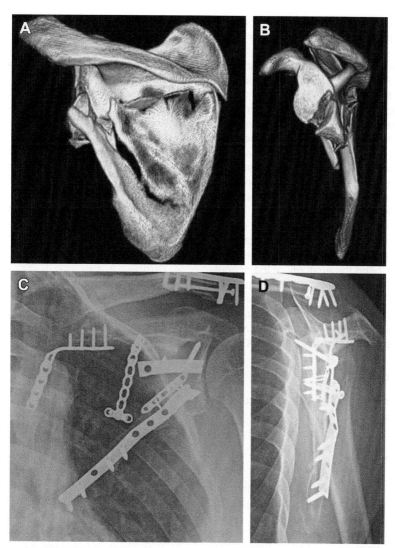

Fig. 13. Case example: this patient sustained a high-energy injury to the scapula. (*A, B*) Preoperative CT scan showing extensive comminution and medialization. (*C, D*) Postoperative radiographs showing restoration of the scapular architecture.

results, and that bad outcomes were related to severe neurologic injury. Likewise, Anavian and colleagues,[27] in the largest published series from our group, reported functional outcomes and DASH scores for 33 patients. After a mean of 25 months after surgical intervention, 91% of patients achieved a DASH of 10. 8 and an average range of shoulder motion comparable with the contralateral limb. However, strength was decreased in the operated extremity, with both flexion and external rotation strength being about 70% of the normal side. However, this was in the presence of a documented neurologic injury in 31% of cases.

More controversial is the treatment of displaced extra-articular fractures of the scapula. Recent

literature shows the deficits of conservative therapy in significantly displaced scapular body and neck fractures, as well as the advantages of surgical open reduction and internal fixation to restore realignment. Ada and Miller[15] found that patients with glenoid medialization greater than 9 mm or angulation greater than 40° had high rates of pain, weakness, and decreased range of motion at 15-month follow-up. Nordqvist and Petersson[14] published similar results after 14-year follow-up in almost 50% of displaced fracture variants. There are subsets of displaced scapula fractures that never return to normal, and the challenge is to understand the proper indications for surgery. Some investigators have identified decreases in as a predictor of poor outcomes.[17,18] Bozkurt and colleagues[17] found a positive correlation between glenopolar angle and constant score ($r = 0.891$, $P<.05$).

The senior author (PAC) recently published the results of a retrospective analysis of 74 patients, which showed 100% union and only 3 malunions.[28] In addition, complications were minimal, with the most common being removal of hardware in 7 patients. Manipulation under anesthesia for adhesions was required in 3 patients. The senior author also recently published the results of the reconstruction of 5 scapular malunions.[13] At 15-month follow-up, all patients had significantly decreased pain after surgery, improved motion and strength, and were satisfied with their results.

In conclusion, the acute management of scapula fractures is evolving. Recent literature is proving that restoring the anatomy of the scapula in a select group of patients with injury patterns meeting strict operative indications can yield significantly better outcomes for patients. Novel approaches and surgical techniques discussed in this article have greatly facilitated this task.

ACKNOWLEDGMENTS

We thank Aaron Jacobson, DC, for his substantial contributions.

REFERENCES

1. Gauger EM, Cole PA. Surgical technique: a minimally invasive approach to scapula neck and body fractures. Clin Orthop Relat Res 2011;469(12): 3390–9.
2. Obremskey WT, Lyman JR. A modified Judet approach to the scapula. J Orthop Trauma 2004; 18(10):696–9.
3. Jones CB, Cornelius JP, Sietsema DL, et al. Modified Judet approach and minifragment fixation of scapular body and glenoid neck fractures. J Orthop Trauma 2009;23(8):558–64.
4. Nork SE, Barei DP, Gardner MJ, et al. Surgical exposure and fixation of displaced type IV, V, and VI glenoid fractures. J Orthop Trauma 2008;22(7):487–93.
5. van Noort A, van Loon CJ, Rijnberg WJ. Limited posterior approach for internal fixation of a glenoid fracture. Arch Orthop Trauma Surg 2004;124(2):140–4.
6. Harris RD, Harris JH Jr. The prevalence and significance of missed scapular fractures in blunt chest trauma. AJR Am J Roentgenol 1988;151(4):747–50.
7. Tadros AM, Lunsjo K, Czechowski J, et al. Causes of delayed diagnosis of scapular fractures. Injury 2008;39(3):314–8.
8. Veysi VT, Mittal R, Agarwal S, et al. Multiple trauma and scapula fractures: so what? J Trauma 2003; 55(6):1145–7.
9. Stephens NG, Morgan AS, Corvo P, et al. Significance of scapular fracture in the blunt-trauma patient. Ann Emerg Med 1995;26(4):439–42.
10. Armstrong CP, Van der Spuy J. The fractured scapula: importance and management based on a series of 62 patients. Injury 1984;15(5):324–9.
11. Thompson DA, Flynn TC, Miller PW, et al. The significance of scapular fractures. J Trauma 1985;25(10): 974–7.
12. Zlowodzki M, Bhandari M, Zelle BA, et al. Treatment of scapula fractures: systematic review of 520 fractures in 22 case series. J Orthop Trauma 2006; 20(3):230–3.
13. Cole PA, Talbot M, Schroder LK, et al. Extra-articular malunions of the scapula: a comparison of functional outcome before and after reconstruction. J Orthop Trauma 2011;25(11):649–56.
14. Nordqvist A, Petersson C. Fracture of the body, neck, or spine of the scapula. A long-term follow-up study. Clin Orthop Relat Res 1992;(283):139–44.
15. Ada JR, Miller ME. Scapular fractures. Analysis of 113 cases. Clin Orthop Relat Res 1991;(269): 174–80.
16. Hardegger FH, Simpson LA, Weber BG. The operative treatment of scapular fractures. J Bone Joint Surg Br 1984;66(5):725–31.
17. Bozkurt M, Can F, Kirdemir V, et al. Conservative treatment of scapular neck fracture: the effect of stability and glenopolar angle on clinical outcome. Injury 2005;36(10):1176–81.
18. Romero J, Schai P, Imhoff AB. Scapular neck fracture–the influence of permanent malalignment of the glenoid neck on clinical outcome. Arch Orthop Trauma Surg 2001;121(6):313–6.
19. Cole PA. Scapula fractures. Orthop Clin North Am 2002;33(1):1–18, vii.
20. Wijdicks CA, Armitage BM, Anavian J, et al. Vulnerable neurovasculature with a posterior approach to the scapula. Clin Orthop Relat Res 2009;467(8): 2011–7.
21. Armitage BM, Wijdicks CA, Tarkin IS, et al. Mapping of scapular fractures with three-dimensional computed tomography. J Bone Joint Surg Am 2009;91(9): 2222–8.
22. Cole PA, Freeman G, Dubin J. Scapula fractures. Curr Rev Musculoskelet Med 2013;6(1):79.
23. Anavian J, Conflitti JM, Khanna G, et al. A reliable radiographic measurement technique for extra-articular scapular fractures. Clin Orthop Relat Res 2011;469(12):3371–8.
24. Baldwin KD, Ohman-Strickland P, Mehta S, et al. Scapula fractures: a marker for concomitant injury? A retrospective review of data in the National Trauma Database. J Trauma 2008;65(2):430–5.
25. Gottschalk HP, Browne RH, Starr AJ. Shoulder girdle: patterns of trauma and associated injuries. J Orthop Trauma 2011;25(5):266–71.

26. Houshian S, Larsen MS, Holm C. Missed injuries in a level I trauma center. J Trauma 2002;52(4):715–9.

27. Anavian J, Gauger EM, Schroder LK, et al. Surgical and functional outcomes after operative management of complex and displaced intra-articular glenoid fractures. J Bone Joint Surg Am 2012;94(7):645–53.

28. Cole PA, Gauger EM, Herrera DA, et al. Radiographic follow-up of 84 operatively treated scapula neck and body fractures. Injury 2012;43(3):327–33.

29. Mayo KA, Benirschke SK, Mast JW. Displaced fractures of the glenoid fossa. Results of open reduction and internal fixation. Clin Orthop Relat Res 1998;(347):122–30.

30. Boerger TO, Limb D. Suprascapular nerve injury at the spinoglenoid notch after glenoid neck fracture. J Shoulder Elbow Surg 2000;9(3):236–7.

31. Solheim LF, Roaas A. Compression of the suprascapular nerve after fracture of the scapular notch. Acta Orthop Scand 1978;49(4):338–40.

32. Egol KA, Connor PM, Karunakar MA, et al. The floating shoulder: clinical and functional results. J Bone Joint Surg Am 2001;83(8):1188–94.

33. Herrera DA, Anavian J, Tarkin IS, et al. Delayed operative management of fractures of the scapula. J Bone Joint Surg Br 2009;91(5):619–26.

34. Lantry JM, Roberts CS, Giannoudis PV. Operative treatment of scapular fractures: a systematic review. Injury 2008;39(3):271–83.

35. Judet R. Surgical treatment of scapular fractures. Acta Orthop Belg 1964;30:673–8.

Treatment of Articular Fractures with Continuous Passive Motion

Laura Lynn Onderko, BS, Saqib Rehman, MD*

KEYWORDS

- Continuous passive motion therapy • Tibial plateau fractures • Articular fractures • Range of motion

KEY POINTS

- In animal studies, continuous passive motion (CPM) has been shown to improve cartilage healing after injury compared with immobilization. Human studies have also shown the improved rate of hemarthrosis clearance with CPM compared with immobilization.
- Clinical studies of CPM have mostly come from the total knee replacement literature. However, its use in joint replacement (which does not rely on cartilage repair) only partially shows the potential benefits of CPM.
- CPM has been used extensively in the postoperative care of articular fractures treated with open reduction and internal fixation, a natural extension of the purported clinical use of early basic science studies. It is believed to help improve cartilage repair, range of motion, and clearance of hemarthrosis. However, little attention has been paid specifically to CPM as a treatment modality.
- Better clinical studies of CPM as a treatment modality for articular fracture management are warranted to determine its potential benefits and to more clearly specify parameters for its use in specific clinical scenarios.

INTRODUCTION

Primarily used to reduce joint stiffness after joint surgery or trauma, continuous passive motion (CPM) therapy works to counteract the pathologic stages of joint stiffness: bleeding, edema, granulation tissue, and fibrosis.[1] This postoperative therapy has been used for a variety of orthopedic surgeries, including the management of total knee arthroplasty, fracture repair, rotator cuff repair, hand rehabilitation, and reconstruction rehabilitation of the anterior cruciate ligament.[2–4] Salter pioneered the use of CPM in the 1980s after observing that the therapy stimulated articular cartilage healing and prevented complications caused by immobilization after injury in rabbit models (**Fig. 1**).[1,5] Further animal studies went on to investigate the role of CPM therapy in reducing joint stiffness after intra-articular injury.[6]

However, whereas studies conducted on animal models show a significant benefit in CPM use after injury, studies performed in a clinical setting show more conflicting results.[6–9] The many variations in clinical CPM protocols could be partially to blame for this lack of agreement, with no standard method of use dictating the number of degrees per day that the machine should advance or the number of hours per day that the treatment should last.[10] Despite this lack of conclusive evidence showing definitive benefits when used clinically, CPM therapy has become standard practice in many centers for postoperative treatment of many joint injuries. However, CPM therapy remains a highly debated treatment, with some recent studies highlighting

Department of Orthopaedic Surgery, Temple University Hospital, 3401 N. Broad Street, Philadelphia, PA 19140, USA
* Corresponding author.
E-mail address: saqib.rehman@tuhs.temple.edu

Orthop Clin N Am 44 (2013) 345–356
http://dx.doi.org/10.1016/j.ocl.2013.04.002
0030-5898/13/$ – see front matter © 2013 Elsevier Inc. All rights reserved.

orthopedic.theclinics.com

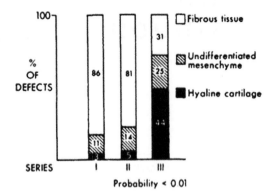

Fig. 1. Improved cartilage repair seen with CPM from animal studies. First index of healing: the nature of the reparative tissue at 3 weeks in the 36 defects in each of the 3 series in adult animals. The bars depict the percentages of the 36 defects in each series that showed predominantly hyaline cartilage, incompletely differentiated mesenchymal tissue, and fibrous tissue. The nature of the reparative tissue in the defects treated with CPM (series III) is superior to that after either immobilization (series I) or intermittent active motion (series II). (*From* Salter RB, Simmonds D, Malcolm B, et al. The biologic effect of continuous passive motion on the healing of full-thickness defects in articular cartilage. J Bone Joint Surg Am 1980;62:1246; with permission.)

the disadvantages of the treatment, such as the need for the patient to stay in bed, the increased costs of maintaining and operating the units, and the extra technical support that patients require from their nurses.[11] With the potential of CPM to facilitate faster recovery, shorten patients' length of stay, and, as a result, reduce costs, many hospitals could benefit from a definitive verdict on the effectiveness of CPM therapy.

Much of the clinical research focuses on the efficacy of this treatment in increasing range of motion and decreasing hospitalization time and postoperative complications after total knee arthroplasty when compared with a regimen focused on physical therapy alone.[12] However, little research exists on the use of CPM for the management of articular fractures. Many articular fractures, such as tibial plateau fractures, can develop stiffness as a sequela.[13] Recovery from this fracture, as an example, is also often further complicated by significant soft tissue injury and can involve collateral ligaments and the anterior and posterior cruciate ligaments.[14] In addition, the significant amount of bleeding associated with the soft tissue injury and fracture of the proximal tibial metaphysis can lead to compartment syndrome, and postoperative complications such as deep vein thrombosis can develop.[14] Given the nature of these possible complications and the proposed benefits of CPM,

which include the potential to decrease hemathrosis and decrease the incidence of deep vein thrombosis in patients with trauma, CPM therapy has may offer many advantages postoperatively.[15] However, our understanding of the efficacy of CPM in the management of articular fractures is not well understood, because few studies have specifically examined CPM in this setting, although its use in patients with total knee arthroplasty has been examined.

In this article, the rationale and basic science evidence for CPM in articular injuries are reviewed and also the clinical evidence in the postoperative treatment of intra-articular fractures.

CPM THERAPY: INVESTIGATING POTENTIAL BENEFITS

The historical progression to the development of CPM started off with early research performed through the 1950s, 1960s, and 1970s, which demonstrated the effects of immobilization compared with joint motion on articular cartilage. These early studies provided evidence of the harmful effects of immobilization, which caused deterioration and articular cartilage loss in animal models. Fibrocartilage replaced the articular cartilage, and adhesions developed after immobilization; after 30 days of immobilization, the cartilage damage could not be reversed like it could be with changes seen in soft tissue. However, this damage could be prevented if immobilization was limited and early exercise was emphasized.[16]

Salter pioneered the use of CPM through his early work starting in the 1970s. He and his colleagues[1] conducted numerous studies on rabbit models and specifically looked at CPM therapy in improving the outcomes in synovial joint injuries. Salter compared CPM therapy with immobilization in his rabbit models, starting CPM immediately after surgery and continuing nonstop for 1 to 4 weeks. He found that the new therapy stimulated healing of the articular cartilage and led to faster and better healing when compared with both immobilization and limited active motion. In looking specifically at intra-articular fractures, CPM therapy stimulated articular cartilage growth and therefore was protective against degenerative arthritis development and resulted in better surgical wound healing. In his 1984 publication Salter summarized his findings and presented an early report on the clinical applications of CPM. In this retrospective study, he observed the effects of CPM for various joint injuries of the hip, knee, ankle, elbow, and finger. Salter's early research summarized in this case study supports the use of CPM therapy in preventing joint stiffness and facilitating healing, specifically for articular cartilage. Early success with rabbit models in the treatment of full-thickness articular cartilage defects, intra-articular fractures, acute septic arthritis, reconstruction of the medial collateral ligament, and lacerations of tendons encouraged the use of CPM therapy in clinical applications. The 9 cases that Salter reviewed used CPM therapy for a variety of injuries (2 intra-articular femur fractures, 1 patellar dislocation, 2 elbow fractures, 1 acetabular fracture, 1 intra-articular finger fracture, 1 hip infection, and 1 case of arthrofibrosis). This is clearly a heterogeneous group of cases. The protocol for CPM therapy followed by and recommended by these case studies indicates immediate postoperative use, starting in recovery and continuing without prolonged interruption for 1 week at 1 cycle per 45 seconds. Success in the clinical setting mimicked the early experimental success with patients treated with the CPM therapy, reporting that they tolerated the treatment well and maintained the increased range of motion achieved through their respective surgical procedures. In addition, the case studies showed no CPM-related complications, periods of prolonged hospitalization, or increase in patient pain or discomfort.[17]

BASIC SCIENCE EVIDENCE
Tendon Strength

Early reports of success with CPM therapy motivated further studies and its benefits on animal models. Loitz and colleagues[18] used rabbit models to investigate the effect of CPM versus immobilization on the mechanical properties of tendons deprived of normal weight-bearing stimulation. This design attempted to mimic the state of tendons after an injury, such as a fracture, which prohibited normal weight bearing. In this experiment, the 26 rabbit models were divided into 2 groups: a control group of 8 rabbits received no treatment and an experimental group of 18 rabbits received CPM to 1 ankle and immobilization for 3 weeks to the other after receiving an articular injury to both ankles without injury to surrounding tendons. The researchers then tested the collagen composition of the tendons and the mechanical properties. The thickness of the dissected tendons was measured with a digital micrometer and the mechanical strength by a servocontrolled electromechanical materials testing system. In addition, samples of the tendons were analyzed for hydroxyproline content. Although the cross-sectional area of control and experimental tendons was similar, averaging 0.9 mm^2 ± 0.2 mm^2, the linear load for the immobilized tendons was found to be 16% less than the control tendons. The value for the CPM-treated tendons was similar to that of the control tendons. In addition, the study found a significant difference in the strength of the control and immobilized tendons, with control tendons 20% stronger than immobilized and 16% stronger than CPM-treated tendons. Looking at tensile strength, these investigators found the control and CPM tendons to be similar, with immobilized tendons showing 25% less strength than both. The composition of the tendons between the groups also differed, although not significantly; the hydroxyproline concentrations of the CPM tendons were 6% greater than both the control and immobilized tendons, showing the increased healing taking place. Overall, the study found the control tendons, as expected, were the strongest of the 3, whereas the tendons coming from the immobilized limbs were the weakest. The tendons taken from injured joints and treated with CPM therapy were in the middle and therefore showed the role of CPM therapy in countering the harmful effects of short-term immobilization.

Joint Motion

Also comparing CPM therapy with immobilization in an animal model, Namba and colleagues[6] focused on treating posttraumatic joint stiffness. This experiment again used rabbit models. After sustaining intra-articular ankle injuries in 2 of their ankles, the 10 rabbits received the 2 different treatments: 1 ankle was treated with immobilization in a cast at 90° flexion and the other with a CPM machine for 3 weeks at 24 hours a day. Evaluating joint stiffness specifically, these investigators found that at 3 weeks the immobilized joint was 2.6 times stiffer than preinjury levels, whereas the CPM-treated joint showed no significant difference when compared with preinjury levels. Although CPM helped maintain joint function after injury, no significant difference was found between the groups in terms of joint swelling.

Wound Healing

The effect of CPM therapy on wound healing is another important consideration in evaluating the treatment. Van Royen and colleagues[19] compared the effects of CPM with cast immobilization in postoperative wound healing. These investigators' histologic and functional tests found that CPM-treated wounds were significantly stronger, and the histologic structure of the collagen fibers showed better organization in the CPM-treated wounds. In this experiment, the investigators used rabbits as their animal models and made skin incisions around the patella and into the knee joint. They then divided the rabbits into 2 groups: the knees of rabbits in the immobilization group were held at 80° flexion for 3 weeks, whereas the CPM group received the therapy for the same duration of time. After 3 weeks of treatment, samples were collected from the healing wound to observe the collagen organization and test the strength. Finding improvements in the strength and healing of the CPM-treated wound, the study concluded that the added tension from the therapy improved the healing of the wounds.

Tissue Repair and Regeneration

Beyond being used to reduce joint stiffness and increasing tendon strength after injury, 2 studies by O'Driscoll and colleagues[20] and Kim and colleagues[21] looked at the potential of CPM therapy to stimulate neochondrogenesis and peripheral nerve repair. Using animal models, O'Driscoll and colleagues found that a periosteum graft put into the knee joints of 30 rabbits showed evidence of articular cartilage growth after 2 weeks in the CPM-treated group when compared with the immobilized group. The CPM group had significantly more cartilage than the immobilization group, 59% of the graft consisting of cartilage compared with 8%, respectively. Using animal models, Kim and colleagues found no statistically significant difference between the CPM group and the immobilization group in average nerve conduction and average fiber density after nerve transection. Therefore, as previous research showing the benefits of CPM therapy suggests, CPM has the potential to stimulate cartilage growth, but does not seem to have any effect on nerve repair.

FREQUENCY AND TREATMENT PARAMETERS: BASIC SCIENCE AND CLINICAL EVIDENCE

As mentioned earlier, CPM is used frequently by clinicians, but there are few guidelines for the timing of treatment, frequency, duration, and other treatment parameters. Studies by Gebhard and colleagues[22] and Shimizu and colleagues[23] further showed the benefits of CPM therapy and also set forth more specific parameters of use. Both studies used animal models to find the ideal number of hours per day needed to obtain the benefits of CPM therapy. Another study by Takai and colleagues[24] looked at the effect of the frequency of the CPM machine cycles on the healing of tendons. This study indicated that the frequency might allow for a shorter duration of use with the same benefits.

Investigating duration of treatment, Gebhard and colleagues[22] looked specifically at joint stiffness, muscle mass, bone density, and regional swelling after intra-articular injury, using rabbit models. Thirty rabbits received an intra-articular injury by a tibial pin drilled into their ankle joints. The rabbits were then divided into 5 groups to receive 4, 8, 12, 16, or 24 hours of CPM each day on 1 injured ankle and immobilization on the other ankle. When not undergoing CPM therapy, the rabbits were immobilized. After 3 weeks, the rabbits were evaluated. In looking at each of the parameters measured, Gebhard and colleagues found that only the rabbits treated with either 16 or 24 hours of CPM therapy had any benefits in reducing joint stiffness. Rabbits that received the shorter duration CPM therapy showed a worsening in mobility, with the CPM-treated limbs as much as 4 times stiffer than immobilized limbs. In terms of swelling, the 24-hour group was the only to show any benefit, although the decrease was not significant. All of the CPM groups increased in muscle mass, being 13% greater than the immobilized limb. However, bone density went against the previous trend, with longer CPM duration having more benefits, and an increase in bone density was observed only in those treated with 12 hours or less of CPM therapy. Bone density data showed a statistically significant inverse relationship between duration and bone density; those treated with 12, 8, and 4 hours of CPM per day had progressively more bone density than those with immobilization or 16 and 24 hours CPM per day. Through their experiments with animal models, Gebhard and colleagues showed the differing effects of CPM therapy on different tissue types and recommended that the therapy be used for at least 16 hours per day to prevent stiffness, reduce swelling, and increase muscle mass, without having detrimental effects on bone density.

Shimizu and colleagues[23] also focused on the dose-response relationship of CPM therapy. The study again used rabbit models, and in both knees of all 34 rabbits, the investigators exposed the knee joint and dislocated the patella as well as creating holes in the articular bone of the femur. Postoperatively, the rabbit subjects were divided into groups based on the number of hours per day that they would receive CPM treatment. All CPM machines were set at the same arc and cycle duration and the same immobilization cast, set at 90° flexion, was used. Ten rabbits received CPM therapy 24 hours a day; 6 rabbits received CPM for 8 hours a day and immobilization for the remaining time on 1 joint and CPM for 2 hours a day with immobilization on the other; 7 rabbits remained immobilized for the full 2 weeks; 9 rabbits were allowed normal cage activity for the full duration; and 5 rabbit knees received immobilization for 1 week followed by 1 week of 24-hour-a-day CPM therapy. After treatment, the rabbits were allowed normal cage activity for an additional 5 weeks before being evaluated. Shimizu and his colleagues examined mobility, histologic features, and the extent of cartilage repair. Although no significant difference was found in passive mobility, visual and histologic analysis of the joints treated with CPM for 24 hours per day and for 8 hours a day showed better repair and healing compared with the immobilized and cage activity groups. In addition, CPM conducted after 1 week of immobilization did not overcome the initial harm caused by immobilization. The findings led the group to recommend that CPM therapy should be started as soon as possible and that the most favorable results are achieved when CPM is performed for 8 to 24 hours a day, although brief periods of immobilization left no ill effects.

Takai and colleagues[24] suggested that the cycles per minute of the CPM machine might allow for shorter durations of use. In their study, they used dogs as the animal model and after flexor tendon injury and repair, the dogs were divided into 2 treatment groups. One group received CPM therapy for 5 minutes per day at 12 cycles per minute, whereas the second group received the same therapy for 60 minutes a day at 1 cycle per minute. These parameters resulted in the same number of cycles per day, but at different frequencies. After harvesting the tendons, the gliding function and strength of the tendons were evaluated at 3 weeks and 6 weeks. Although the function of the tendons was the same for both groups, the tendon strength of the higher-frequency group was significantly greater. Therefore, although duration of CPM therapy is an important variable in the effectiveness of the therapy, the frequency of cycles might have an even greater effect on outcome.

Another important parameter that, like the others discussed earlier, remains unstandardized is the number of days that the patient must use the CPM machine to obtain any benefits. Several clinical studies have looked at this variable. One study[25] determined that 3 days of CPM therapy was sufficient after looking at effects of the therapy on 2 groups of patients. The first group experienced postoperative knee or elbow stiffness that existed for some time before therapy, whereas the second group used CPM therapy immediately after the injury. After only 3 days of therapy, the first group saw significant improvements in range of motion, which was maintained on follow-up, whereas the second group regained their preinjury range of motion with the reduced CPM therapy duration as well. Other studies looked at patients after total knee arthroplasty. In a study by Bennett

and colleagues,[26] an early-flexion CPM group started at a greater degree of flexion in recovery and continued the treatment for 7 days, comparing the outcome with a standard CPM group and a control with no CPM therapy. Overall, the early-flexion group showed significantly greater range of motion early on, but the groups showed similar results after 1 year of follow-up. Similarly, other studies comparing the number of hours per day dedicated to CPM therapy found no significant difference in the range of motion of the patients with total knee arthroplasty.[10,27] Overall, the literature suggests that no consensus has been reached on the optimum number of hours per days and the number of days that the CPM therapy should be administered.

MECHANISMS OF ACTION

Whereas these previous studies showed the potential benefits of CPM therapy, O'Driscoll and colleagues[7] investigated the mechanism behind the beneficial effects of CPM therapy. These investigators hypothesized that clearance of blood from the joint with CPM can facilitate recovery and reduce stiffness. In this experiment using rabbit models, 7 of the 17 received labeled erythrocyte injections into their knees and were scanned that day and subsequently on days 1, 2, 3, 4, and 7. Nine rabbits were injected with unlabeled blood as controls. After the injections, 1 knee was immobilized, and the other underwent CPM therapy continuously for 7 days. After 7 days of treatment, the knee joints of the rabbits were dissected and examined. The results from the scans taken during the treatment showed that after 48 hours of CPM therapy the knee synovial fluid was clear compared with the fluid taken from the immobilized joint, which was bloody. Overall, the rate of clearance was twice as fast in the CPM-treated joint as in the cast immobilized joint, with the clearance of 50% of the blood occurring in 2.2 days compared with 5.5 days, respectively (**Fig. 2**). In looking at the joint after 7 days, 7.1% of the original injected number of erythrocytes were found in the CPM-treated knee comparison with 13.2% found in the immobilized knee. The investigators explained this difference by postulating that during CPM treatment, the intra-articular pressure in the joint is increased and decreased, creating a pumping effect that aids in clearance.

By measuring the intra-articular pressure of a human knee during CPM therapy in a separate study, Pedowitz and colleagues[28] supported the hypothesis put forth by O'Driscoll and colleagues. In a study with 16 patients, the CPM machine was set at 0° to 90° of flexion, with 1 cycle per

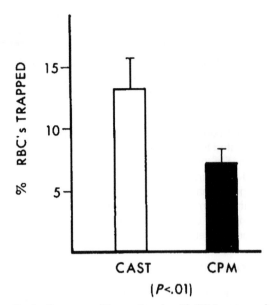

Fig. 2. Clearance of hemarthrosis with CPM compared with cast immobilization of the knee. The bars represent the percentages of injected [111]indium-labeled erythrocytes that remained trapped in the synovium after 7 days. Treatment by CPM decreased this trapping by approximately 50%. Values are expressed as mean ± 1 standard of error of the mean. RBCs, red blood cells. (*From* O'Driscoll SW, Kumar A, Salter RB. The effect of continuous passive motion on the clearance of a hemarthrosis from a synovial joint: an experimental investigation in the rabbit. Clin Orthop 1983;176:309; with permission.)

150 seconds. After taking pressure measurements at full extension and flexion for 3 complete cycles for 90 minutes, the investigators found that the pressure was greatest at the extremes of joint flexion and extension. The minimum pressure occurred at 30° to 60° of flexion (**Fig. 3**). These cyclic pressure gradients both aid in fluid clearance and help stimulate tissue healing, explaining the benefits seen with CPM therapy.

CLINICAL EVIDENCE FOR CPM IN MANAGEMENT OF ARTICULAR FRACTURE

Clinical use of CPM has been investigated, with mixed results, in the total knee arthroplasty literature, but the full benefit of CPM would theoretically be seen with treatment of injury of the articular cartilage, in accordance with the animal data discussed earlier. For many periarticular fractures, early motion is emphasized to prevent fracture disease, as popularized by the Arbeitsgemeinschaft für Osteosynthesefragen (AO) movement. However, specific details about the clinical efficacy of CPM machines for management of particular articular fractures, with regard to the optimal timing, duration, frequency, and motion parameters, is not well studied. In the next section, the clinical literature is reviewed in an attempt to address this situation. However, although CPM is used frequently for these injuries, few studies have specifically investigated CPM.

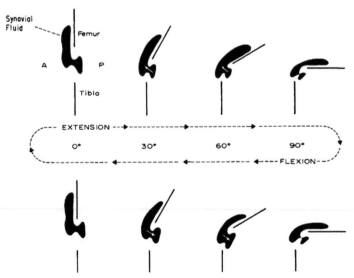

Fig. 3. Intra-articular fluid flow during CPM, consistent with "physiologic compartmentation" of the human knee. A, anterior; P, posterior. (*From* Pedowitz R, Gershuni D, Crenshaw A, et al. Intraarticular pressure during continuous passive motion of the human knee. J Orthop Res 1989;7(4):536; with permission.)

AN EXAMPLE OF THE BENEFITS OF EARLY MOTION: TIBIAL PLATEAU FRACTURES

Tibial plateau fractures represent a periarticular fracture group for which surgery is frequently performed, and early motion is typically recommended. Gausewitz and colleagues[29] reviewed the treatment of 122 acute tibial plateau fractures to determine the effects of early mobilization in rehabilitation. Although the earlier studies showed benefits for early motion, certain risks such as loss of fracture reduction, failure of internal fixation, and compromised healing remained. Dividing patients into groups based on the amount of time that they spent immobilized, Gausewitz and colleagues measured overall outcome by analyzing knee flexion, loss of fracture reduction, hospital length of stay, and ligamentous laxity. The review of patients and results revealed that patients treated without surgical intervention and immobilized for up to 6 weeks regained full range of motion. However, patients treated surgically with open reduction and internal fixation (ORIF) developed stiffness after only 2 weeks of immobilization. Although the range of motion measurements was not statistically significant, after 2 to 6 weeks of immobilization, 4 of the 13 patients had flexion of less than 105° and 3 had flexion contractures compared with the group that received immediate motion, which had only 1 flexion contracture and 1 patient with less than 105° flexion. Despite the improvements in range of motion in the patients with shorter immobilization times, the patients' length of stay was found to be longer. The 23 patients with less than 2 weeks of immobilization stayed an average of 18.1 days compared with those with greater than 2 weeks of immobilization, who stayed an average of 5.7 days. However, these values could be a misrepresentation of drawbacks to the treatment, because the longer stay of the patients with earlier mobilization was often caused by the use of traction and a cast brace compared with patients who were simply discharged in a cast. The primary impact of the study was to highlight the benefits of early mobilization for surgically treated fractures in recovering and maintaining range of motion.

Blokker and colleagues[30] also related patient outcome to immobilization time in patients recovering from tibial plateau fractures. In their review, they considered adequacy of reduction, immobilization time, fracture type, treatment method, and overall result when evaluating patient outcome. However, the results of this review could not support the earlier findings that showed the strong relationship between early motion and better outcome in the patient. Patients were reported to have a satisfactory outcome if they achieved a range of motion of at least 90° flexion, a lack of extension of less than 10°, and had returned to full activity with occasional mild pain or ache. Seventy-five percent of the 60 patients evaluated reported a satisfactory result. No difference was found in outcome in patients who started knee movement in the first 2 weeks compared with those who started after. However, the investigators also recognized that if motion was started by the first or second day of recovery rather than within the first 2 weeks, the results might have been more favorable for early motion. In addition, the assessment of satisfactory versus unsatisfactory result was performed 3 years after the injury, and no intermediate assessments were included. Therefore, the possibility existed that some more significant differences between the group that received early mobilization and the group immobilized for more than 2 weeks could have been observed.

In a similar study involving tibial plateau fractures, Lachiewicz and colleagues[31] focused on cases treated surgically with ORIF. This study reviewed the cases to determine the factors that influenced clinical and radiographic outcomes. The 43 fractures evaluated received several different postoperative treatments, with 17 receiving CPM therapy, 12 having a long leg cast for 6 weeks because of ligament injuries, 6 in a knee immobilizer for 6 weeks, and 16 receiving instruction in range-of-motion exercises. However, with the focus of the study not being on postoperative treatments, the patients were not further divided up or analyzed based on these various treatments specifically. Overall, the investigators found that 35 of the 43 had excellent results, with bicondylar fractures presenting the most difficulties. Patients who experienced this type of fracture were found to have an 18° decrease in range of motion compared with other patients. Ten of the 15 patients were in an immobilizer for more than 3 weeks. In addition, other patients treated postoperatively with an immobilizer for more than 3 weeks also experienced a decreased mean range of motion, measuring 14° lower than those in an immobilizer for a shorter period. This difference was found to be statistically significant. Lachiewicz and colleagues show preliminary support for the use of early CPM in the treatment of tibial plateau fractures.

In a prospective study, Gaston and colleagues[32] evaluated knee function during recovery of a fracture of the tibial plateau. Fifty-one of the 63 patients were treated surgically with internal fixation, whereas another 5 were treated with a combination of internal and external fixation and 7 were treated nonoperatively. Gaston and colleagues tested joint movement and muscle function at 3, 6, and 12 months. At 12 months, only 14% had regained normal quadriceps muscle strength, whereas 30% had normal hamstring muscle strength. In addition, 21% suffered from residual flexion contractures. All the patients underwent standard physical therapy treatment for 12 weeks after surgery. The study outlined the slow recovery process after fractures of the tibial plateau. Whereas 82% of the patients had achieved 100° of knee flexion, 21% still had extension deficits greater than 5°, and this deficit was especially pronounced in patients older than 40 years. These deficits have an impact on daily life for patients, with a minimum of 65° of flexion needed for the swing phase of normal gait, a 90° minimum needed to descend stairs, and 105° necessary for getting up from a chair.

In a separate retrospective study,[33] outcomes were measured differently by using Hospital for Special Surgery and Lysholm scores after tibial plateau fracture treatment along with CPM. In this study, the knee was immediately placed in CPM, although the specifics of the CPM protocol were not included in the study. The study showed a significant decrease in activity as a result of knee complaints in the first 2 to 3 years after the injury; however, at 3 to 6 years after injury, these scores had increased to show good function and a return to preinjury activity levels. This trend reversed itself after 6 years of follow-up, although with patients again deteriorating as a result of an increase in arthritis. In contrast to the previous study, which found that age predicted a worse outcome, this study, which relied more on patient self-evaluation, found that the younger patients felt more impaired by the injury.

The results from these 2 studies highlight the long recovery process that patients with tibial plateau fractures face, and the lack of consensus on postoperative treatment between the 2 further supports the need for more directed research.

CLINICAL DATA FOR ARTICULAR FRACTURES AND CPM

Several studies have recommended, without clear evidence, that CPM and early passive motion are important for recovery.[34,35] In this section, clinical studies in which CPM was used for articular fractures as part of the treatment are reviewed.

Proximal Tibia Fractures

Tibial eminence fractures are frequently treated with arthroscopic methods and fixation, with CPM used frequently postoperatively. Osti and

colleagues[36] reported 10 patients in which this was performed, and CPM was used postoperatively. No specific data regarding timing, frequency, or other parameters for the CPM were provided. Patients achieved full extension and flexion between 125° and 135°. In a separate study,[37] CPM was also used in 32 patients with tibial eminence fractures treated with arthroscopic fixation starting on postoperative day 1. Near full range of motion was achieved in all patients.

CPM therapy was used in some patients postoperatively treated with arthroscopic-assisted tibial plateau fracture fixation, as reported by Caspari and colleagues.[38] Twenty-nine patients were treated in this case series, but there was no indication of how many patients were treated with CPM, or why it was chosen for those patients. In a similar study,[39] arthroscopic-assisted tibial plateau fracture fixation was performed in 9 cases with CPM used postoperatively. Although no particular parameters were described, CPM was used for 5 days postoperatively and "clinical function was quite satisfactory," without more detail provided. Ohdera and colleagues[40] compared arthroscopic with open reduction methods for treatment of tibial plateau fractures with CPM used for all patients postoperatively. Parameters for the CPM were not described, nor was the timing ("several days after surgery"). In a similar study,[41] 25 patients with tibial plateau fractures from skiing injuries treated with arthroscopic reduction techniques were managed with CPM postoperatively. Again, no specific information was provided regarding the timing, frequency, or CPM parameters used other, than that it was used in the hospital postoperatively.

CPM therapy was also used postoperatively from 0° to 30° in 4 patients with severe bicondylar tibial plateau fractures treated with combined anterior and posterior ORIF methods.[42] In another study,[43] CPM was used immediately postoperatively and continued for 2 weeks at home, if indicated, for bicondylar tibial plateau fractures treated with ORIF. Carlson[44] described his experience with dual-incision posterior ORIF of bicondylar tibial plateau fractures in 8 patients who also had CPM postoperatively. These patients were treated with CPM postoperatively in the hospital and continued until knee flexion was near 90°. No other specific information regarding the CPM was provided in Carlson's report. There do not seem to be any particular problems with CPM use in elderly individuals, as reported by Biyani and colleagues[45] after ORIF of tibial plateau fractures. In this particular study, CPM with cast bracing was compared with cast bracing alone postoperatively, with no significant difference in clinical outcomes. However, there was no indication as to when CPM was chosen, and there were multiple fracture patterns, with different surgeons and surgical approaches, making it difficult to draw conclusions regarding the efficacy of CPM for these patients.

Distal Femur Fractures

Similar to treatment of tibial plateau fractures, surgeons have used CPM postoperatively after treatment of distal femur fractures. Shewring and Meggitt[46] reported on 21 cases of distal femur fractures treated with the AO dynamic condylar screw and CPM started on the second postoperative day. CPM was used twice a day for 2 weeks. Unicondylar femur fractures treated by ORIF in 16 cases in a separate study were also treated with CPM on the first postoperative day.[47] No other data regarding the specifics of the CPM treatment were provided. Other intra-articular femur fractures such as the Hoffa fracture have been treated with ORIF followed by CPM.[48]

Elbow Fractures

The elbow is particularly prone to developing stiffness after trauma and surgery. CPM has therefore been looked to as a possible treatment after both fracture fixation and surgery for release of arthrofibrosis. Frankle and colleagues[49] reported 21 patients with elbow dislocations and radial head fractures treated by ORIF and benign neglect, depending on the severity of the injury. Early motion was performed in all patients, with CPM in only 2 patients. No additional data regarding the CPM were given in this study. Athwal and colleagues[50] reported on 37 patients who underwent ORIF for AO/OTA (Orthopaedic Trauma Association) type C distal humerus fractures, with some patients also having postoperative CPM treatment. No specific data regarding timing, frequency, or CPM parameters were provided.

Other Articular Fractures

CPM has also been used extensively for postoperative management of articular fractures of the ankle, hip, shoulder, and fingers, in addition to the knee and elbow, which have already been discussed. Acetabulum fractures frequently lead to hip stiffness after traumatic arthritis, for instance, and can be potentially helped with postoperative CPM.[51,52] For instance, Brumback and colleagues[51] reported on 58 patients with posterior acetabulum fracture dislocations treated with ORIF and CPM, and many cases also had postoperative skeletal traction, although specific data regarding the CPM were not provided. CPM was

the focus of 1 particular study of ankle fractures treated with ORIF; Farsetti and colleagues[3] described a retrospective series of 22 patients, each of whom underwent ORIF of a malleolar ankle fracture and had 10 years of follow-up. In the first group, CPM was applied immediately postoperatively and for 3 weeks. In the second group, a plaster splint or cast was applied for 3 weeks. Patients with CPM had higher American Orthopaedic Foot and Ankle Society scores and fewer cases of osteoarthritis at 10 year follow-up than patients treated in a cast. Although this was not a controlled study and had few patients, it does show the potential functional benefits of CPM compared with immobilization.

Sequelae of Articular Fractures: Arthrofibrosis and Heterotopic Ossification

Although it is not the focus of this article, CPM is also used frequently postoperatively after open or arthroscopic treatment of arthrofibrosis of the elbow. Duration of treatment is reported from 1 to 6 weeks postoperatively, although we are not aware of any studies that have investigated CPM specifically.[53–57] Bae and colleagues[54] were particularly aggressive and liberal with CPM treatment, applying this in the recovery room after a medial elbow release and using it for 23 hours a day for 3 weeks, followed by nighttime use for an additional 3 weeks in addition to physical therapy throughout this time. Alternatively, Kraushaar and colleagues[58] did not believe that CPM was needed in a series of 12 patients with posttraumatic elbow flexion contracture treated with an open lateral release technique.

Contractures of the knee are occasionally treated with Judet quadricepsplasty, and CPM is frequently used postoperatively, as described by Ali and colleagues[59] in 10 patients in whom CPM was used. In this study, immediate CPM at a slow rate was applied from 0° to 60° under epidural control and ice packs. The range of motion and rate (speed) of the CPM were gradually increased up to maximal possible flexion.

SUMMARY

CPM therapy clearly has some basic science and animal data to support its use in the management of articular cartilage lesions, which can be extrapolated clinically to the treatment of articular fractures. Most clinical studies looking specifically at CPM treatment come from the total joint replacement literature, in which patients without articular cartilage lesions are treated. The goals in these cases are not to improve articular cartilage repair but to improve range of motion, and results have been mixed. Although CPM is used in other cases, such as articular fractures, ligament reconstruction, surgery for articular cartilage repair, and surgery for arthrofibrosis release, it has not been well studied as a treatment of these indications. Few studies have looked at CPM as a treatment modality with articular fractures, so there is little guidance regarding the recommended time of onset, rate, duration, and other parameters that should be used. The heterogeneity of articular fractures, along with the multitude of surgical treatment factors that can affect range of motion, cartilage repair, and functional outcomes, make it difficult to study CPM from the available data in the literature. Meaningful information could be obtained from a narrow injury subtype, in a randomized controlled study, to determine if CPM is beneficial at all, and if so, how it should be used. It seems that there is enough basic science evidence and reported use of CPM for articular fractures to warrant such a study, because there is still room for improvement in management of articular fractures.

REFERENCES

1. Salter RB. The biologic concept of continuous passive motion of synovial joints. The first 18 years of basic research and its clinical application. Clin Orthop 1989;(242):12.
2. Du Plessis M, Eksteen E, Jenneker A, et al. The effectiveness of continuous passive motion on range of motion, pain and muscle strength following rotator cuff repair: a systematic review. Clin Rehabil 2011;25(4):291–302.
3. Farsetti P, Caterini R, Potenza V, et al. Immediate continuous passive motion after internal fixation of an ankle fracture. J Orthop Trauma 2009;10(2): 63–9.
4. Rosen MA, Jackson DW, Atwell EA. The efficacy of continuous passive motion in the rehabilitation of anterior cruciate ligament reconstructions. Am J Sports Med 1992;20(2):122–7.
5. Salter RB, Simmonds D, Malcolm B, et al. The biological effect of continuous passive motion on the healing of full-thickness defects in articular cartilage. J Bone Joint Surg Am 1980;62:1232–51.
6. Namba RS, Kabo JM, Dorey FJ, et al. Continuous passive motion versus immobilization. The effect on posttraumatic joint stiffness. Clin Orthop 1991;(267):218.
7. O'Driscoll SW, Kumar A, Salter RB. The effect of continuous passive motion on the clearance of a hemarthrosis from a synovial joint: an experimental investigation in the rabbit. Clin Orthop 1983;176:305.
8. O'Driscoll S, Kumar A, Salter R. The effect of the volume of effusion, joint position and continuous passive motion on intraarticular pressure in the rabbit knee. J Rheumatol 1983;10(3):360.
9. McCarthy MR, O'Donoghue PC, Yates CK, et al. The clinical use of continuous passive motion in physical therapy. J Orthop Sports Phys Ther 1992;15(3):132–40.
10. Chiarello CM, Gundersen L, O'Halloran T. The effect of continuous passive motion duration and increment on range of motion in total knee arthroplasty patients. J Orthop Sports Phys Ther 1997; 25(2):119–27.
11. Beaupré LA, Davies DM, Jones CA, et al. Exercise combined with continuous passive motion or slider board therapy compared with exercise only: a randomized controlled trial of patients following total knee arthroplasty. Phys Ther 2001;81(4):1029–37.
12. Brosseau L, Milne S, Wells G, et al. Efficacy of continuous passive motion following total knee arthroplasty: a metaanalysis. J Rheumatol 2004; 31(11):2251–64.
13. Papagelopoulos PJ, Partsinevelos AA, Themistocleous GS, et al. Complications after tibia plateau fracture surgery. Injury 2006;37(6):475–84.
14. Krieg JC. Proximal tibial fractures: current treatment, results, and problems. Injury 2003;34(Suppl 1):A2–10.
15. Fuchs S, Heyse T, Rudofsky G, et al. Continuous passive motion in the prevention of deep-vein thrombosis: a randomised comparison in trauma patients. J Bone Joint Surg Br 2005; 87(8):1117–22.
16. McDonough AL. Effects of immobilization and exercise on articular cartilage–a review of literature. J Orthop Sports Phys Ther 1981;3(1):2–5.
17. Salter RB, Hamilton HW, Wedge JH, et al. Clinical application of basic research on continuous passive motion for disorders and injuries of synovial joints: a preliminary report of a feasibility study. J Orthop Res 1983;1(3):325–42.
18. Loitz BJ, Zernicke RF, Vailas AC, et al. Effects of short-term immobilization versus continuous passive motion on the biomechanical and biochemical properties of the rabbit tendon. Clin Orthop Relat Res 1989;244:265–71.
19. van Royen BJ, O'Driscoll SW, Dhert W, et al. A comparison of the effects of immobilization and continuous passive motion on surgical wound healing in mature rabbits. Plast Reconstr Surg 1986; 78(3):360.
20. O'Driscoll S, Salter R. The induction of neochondrogenesis in free intra-articular periosteal autografts under the influence of continuous passive motion. An experimental investigation in the rabbit. J Bone Joint Surg Am 1984;66(8):1248.
21. Kim H, Kerr R, Turley C, et al. The effects of postoperative continuous passive motion on peripheral nerve repair and regeneration. An experimental

investigation in rabbits. J Hand Surg Br 1998;23(5): 594–7.

22. Gebhard J, Kabo J, Meals R. Passive motion: the dose effects on joint stiffness, muscle mass, bone density, and regional swelling. A study in an experimental model following intra-articular injury. J Bone Joint Surg Am 1993;75:1636–47.

23. Shimizu T, Videman T, Shimazaki K, et al. Experimental study on the repair of full thickness articular cartilage defects: effects of varying periods of continuous passive motion, cage activity, and immobilization. J Orthop Res 1987;5(2):187–97.

24. Takai S, Woo SL, Horibe S, et al. The effects of frequency and duration of controlled passive mobilization on tendon healing. J Orthop Res 2005;9(5): 705–13.

25. Laupattarakasem W. Short term continuous passive motion. A feasibility study. J Bone Joint Surg Br 1988;70(5):802.

26. Bennett LA, Brearley SC, Hart JAL, et al. A comparison of 2 continuous passive motion protocols after total knee arthroplasty: a controlled and randomized study. J Arthroplasty 2005;20(2): 225–33.

27. Denis M, Moffet H, Caron F, et al. Effectiveness of continuous passive motion and conventional physical therapy after total knee arthroplasty: a randomized clinical trial. Phys Ther 2006;86(2):174–85.

28. Pedowitz R, Gershuni D, Crenshaw A, et al. Intra-articular pressure during continuous passive motion of the human knee. J Orthop Res 1989;7(4): 530–7.

29. Gausewitz S, Hohl M. The significance of early motion in the treatment of tibial plateau fractures. Clin Orthop Relat Res 1986;(202):135–8.

30. Blokker CP, Rorabeck CH, Bourne RB. Tibial plateau fractures. An analysis of the results of treatment in 60 patients. Clin Orthop Relat Res 1984;(182):193–9.

31. Lachiewicz PF, Funcik T. Factors influencing the results of open reduction and internal fixation of tibial plateau fractures. Clin Orthop Relat Res 1990;(259):210–5.

32. Gaston P, Will EM, Keating JF. Recovery of knee function following fracture of the tibial plateau. J Bone Joint Surg Br 2005;87(9):1233–6.

33. Vandenberghe D, Cuypers L, Rombouts L, et al. Internal fixation of tibial plateau fractures using the AO instrumentation. Acta Orthop Belg 1990;56(2): 431–42.

34. Fenton P, Porter K. Tibial plateau fractures: a review. Trauma 2011;13(2):181.

35. Tscherne H, Lobenhoffer P. Tibial plateau fractures. Management and expected results. Clin Orthop Relat Res 1993;(292):87–100.

36. Osti L, Merlo F, Liu SH, et al. A simple modified arthroscopic procedure for fixation of displaced

tibial eminence fractures. Arthroscopy 2000;16(4): 379–82.

37. Senekovič V, Veselko M. Anterograde arthroscopic fixation of avulsion fractures of the tibial eminence with a cannulated screw. Arthroscopy 2003;19(1): 54–61.

38. Caspari RB, Hutton PM, Whipple TL, et al. The role of arthroscopy in the management of tibial plateau fractures. Arthroscopy 1985;1(2):76–82.

39. Bernfeld B, Kligman M, Roffman M. Arthroscopic assistance for unselected tibial plateau fractures. Arthroscopy 1996;12(5):598–602.

40. Ohdera T, Tokunaga M, Hiroshima S, et al. Arthroscopic management of tibial plateau fractures–comparison with open reduction method. Arch Orthop Trauma Surg 2003;123(9):489–93.

41. Gill TJ, Moezzi DM, Oates KM, et al. Arthroscopic reduction and internal fixation of tibial plateau fractures in skiing. Clin Orthop 2001;383:243.

42. Georgiadis GM. Combined anterior and posterior approaches for complex tibial plateau fractures. J Bone Joint Surg Br 1994;76(2):285–9.

43. Buchko GM, Johnson DH. Arthroscopy assisted operative management of tibial plateau fractures. Clin Orthop 1996;332:29–36.

44. Carlson DW. Posterior bicondylar tibial plateau fractures. J Orthop Trauma 2005;19(2):73–8.

45. Biyani A, Reddy N, Chaudhury J, et al. The results of surgical management of displaced tibial plateau fractures in the elderly. Injury 1995;26(5): 291–7.

46. Shewring D, Meggitt B. Fractures of the distal femur treated with the AO dynamic condylar screw. J Bone Joint Surg Br 1992;74(1):122–5.

47. Ostermann PA, Neumann K, Ekkernkamp A, et al. Long term results of unicondylar fractures of the femur. J Orthop Trauma 1994;8(2):142–6.

48. Papadopoulos AX, Panagopoulos A, Karageorgos A, et al. Operative treatment of unilateral bicondylar Hoffa fractures. J Orthop Trauma 2004;18(2):119–22.

49. Frankle MA, Koval KJ, Sanders RW, et al. Radial head fractures associated with elbow dislocations treated by immediate stabilization and early motion. J Shoulder Elbow Surg 1999;8(4): 355–60.

50. Athwal GS, Hoxie SC, Rispoli DM, et al. Precontoured parallel plate fixation of AO/OTA type C distal humerus fractures. J Orthop Trauma 2009; 23(8):575.

51. Brumback RJ, Holt ES, McBride MS, et al. Acetabular depression fracture accompanying posterior fracture dislocation of the hip. J Orthop Trauma 1990;4(1):42–8.

52. Tannast M, Siebenrock KA. Operative treatment of T-type fractures of the acetabulum via surgical hip dislocation or Stoppa approach. Oper Orthop Traumatol 2009;21(3):251.

53. Kim SJ, Shin SJ. Arthroscopic treatment for limitation of motion of the elbow. Clin Orthop 2000;375: 140–8.

54. Bae DS, Waters PM. Surgical treatment of posttraumatic elbow contracture in adolescents. J Pediatr Orthop 2001;21(5):580–4.

55. Gates H, Sullivan F, Urbaniak J. Anterior capsulotomy and continuous passive motion in the treatment of post-traumatic flexion contracture of the elbow. A prospective study. J Bone Joint Surg Am 1992;74:1229–34.

56. Rymaszewski L, Glass K, Parikh R. Post-traumatic elbow contracture treated by arthrolysis and continuous passive motion under brachial plexus anesthesia. J Bone Joint Surg Br 1994;76:572–6.

57. Breen T, Gelberman R, Ackerman G. Elbow flexion contractures: treatment by anterior release and continuous passive motion. J Hand Surg Br 1988; 13(3):286–7.

58. Kraushaar BS, Nirschl RP, Cox W. A modified lateral approach for release of posttraumatic elbow flexion contracture. J Shoulder Elbow Surg 1999; 8(5):476–80.

59. Ali AM, Villafuerte J, Hashmi M, et al. Judet's quadricepsplasty, surgical technique, and results in limb reconstruction. Clin Orthop 2003;415:214.

PEDIATRICS

Preface
Pediatrics

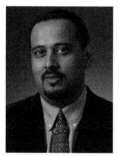

Shital N. Parikh, MD, FACS
Editor

For a long time, *Orthopedic Clinics of North America* has provided timely and focused clinical review articles. The new format would continue the tradition of such articles with each volume containing topics that represent multiple orthopedic specialties. I am proud and excited to be a part of this change and to be part of such a distinguished editorial board. As the section editor for pediatric orthopedics, my goal is to provide the readers with up-to-date and comprehensive review articles related to the clinical practice of orthopedics in children and adolescents.

Pediatric orthopedics has evolved to include various subspecialties like pediatric trauma, pediatric spine, pediatric hand, pediatric sports, neuromuscular disorders, pediatric hip, tumors, and feet. Future articles in *Orthopedic Clinics of North America* would represent all such subspecialties, the topics determined based on emerging knowledge, perceived need, and the scope of clinical practice.

I believe that the analyses and knowledge of complications related to any given topic is the only way to anticipate and avoid them in future. As the number of scoliosis and kyphosis-corrective surgery continues to increase in the United States and around the world, the topic of Complications of Surgical Treatment of Pediatric Spinal Deformities is both important and timely. I hope this article and similar clinical review articles in the future will help readers in their daily practice.

Shital N. Parikh, MD, FACS
Associate Professor of Orthopaedic Surgery
Cincinnati Children's Hospital Medical Center
University of Cincinnati School of Medicine
Cincinnati, OH, USA

E-mail address:
Shital.Parikh@cchmc.org

Orthop Clin N Am 44 (2013) xvii
http://dx.doi.org/10.1016/j.ocl.2013.05.005
0030-5898/13/$ – see front matter © 2013 Published by Elsevier Inc.

orthopedic.theclinics.com

Complications of Surgical Treatment of Pediatric Spinal Deformities

Marios G. Lykissas, MD, PhD[a], Alvin H. Crawford, MD[b],*,
Viral V. Jain, MD[b]

KEYWORDS

- Growing spine • Scoliosis • Kyphosis • Spinal fusion • Complications

KEY POINTS

- Although current orthopedic practice ensures good long-term surgical results, complications occur, with reported prevalences of 15.4% and 0.69% for non-neurologic and neurologic complications, respectively.
- Factors associated with increased risk for neurologic injury in adolescent idiopathic scoliosis are categorized as surgeon dependent and surgeon independent.
- Factors that are responsible for, or contribute to, non-neurologic complications in adolescent idiopathic scoliosis surgical management are prolonged anesthesia time, excessive bleeding, and history of renal disease.
- Pediatric patients requiring surgery for nonidiopathic deformities of the spine are at higher risk for perioperative and long-term complications, mainly because of underlying comorbidities.
- In all patients with nonidiopathic deformities of the spine, a multidisciplinary treatment strategy is helpful to assure optimization of medical conditions before surgery.

INTRODUCTION

When spine surgery is recommended for the correction of a young patient's spinal deformity, many questions arise from the patient and family. In most cases, they wish to know possible complications and the need for additional surgeries. These questions are not easily answered because they are affected by many variables, and the existing information in the literature remains limited, especially for uncommon pathologic conditions and syndromes. Recording complications of the surgical treatment of pediatric deformity of the spine is considered essential for future surgical decision making.

Spine surgery in children and adolescents is uncommon, with an estimated prevalence of 1/100,000 to 10/100,000 among all children.[1] Common surgical indications include intradural or extradural tumors and spinal deformities. Idiopathic scoliosis represents the most extensively investigated deformity of the pediatric and adolescent spine, with several studies reporting on surgical complications and reoperation rates. Although current orthopedic practice ensures good long-term surgical results, complications occur, with reported prevalences of 15.4% and 0.69% for non-neurologic and neurologic complications, respectively, with the latter the most devastating

Funding Sources: There is no funding source.
Conflict of Interest: There is no conflict of interest.
[a] Spine and Scoliosis Service, Hospital for Special Surgery, 535 East 71st Street, New York, NY 10021, USA;
[b] Division of Orthopaedic Surgery, Cincinnati Children's Hospital Medical Center, 3333 Burnet Avenue, MLC 2017, Cincinnati, OH 45229, USA
* Corresponding author.
E-mail address: Alvin.Crawford@cchmc.org

complications and the greatest concern for children undergoing spinal fusion for adolescent idiopathic scoliosis and their parents.[2,3]

Compared with idiopathic scoliosis, pediatric patients requiring surgery for nonidiopathic deformities of the spine are at higher risk for perioperative and long-term complications, mainly because of underlying comorbidities. *Nonidiopathic spinal deformities* is an umbrella term for a variety of syndromic, congenital, pathologic, postsurgical, and neurogenic deformities in both the coronal and sagittal planes. These include but are not limited to connective tissue disorders, such as Marfan syndrome and Ehlers-Danlos syndrome; neuromuscular conditions, such as cerebral palsy, myelomeningocele, muscular dystrophies, and neurofibromatosis (NF); congenital abnormalities of the spine; skeletal dysplasias, such as achondroplasia; mucopolysaccharidoses; and Scheuermann kyphosis. For most of these diagnoses, there are no large studies with sufficient follow-up evaluating complications after surgical intervention for correction of spinal deformity.

This article summarizes the complications of surgical treatment of the growing spine. For each condition associated with spinal deformity, preoperative considerations and intraoperative surgical recommendations are reviewed. Illustrative cases for pediatric spine surgical complications are discussed.

ADOLESCENT IDIOPATHIC SCOLIOSIS
Neurologic Complications

- In 1975, the Scoliosis Research Society (SRS) Morbidity and Mortality Committee published the first significant analysis of 1885 scoliosis cases, with nearly all patients having undergone posterior spinal fusion with Harrington rod instrumentation.[4] Neurologic complications were recorded in 87 patients (0.72%), with 74 patients having spinal cord injury. Although this study was limited by the heterogeneity of diagnoses, it helped to better understand the effects of spinal instrumentation on neurologic function and stimulate the development of intraoperative neurophysiologic monitoring and the wake-up test. The investigators noted that congenital scoliosis, kyphosis, preexisting neurologic deficits, and high magnitude curves were associated with higher complication rates. Among patients with spinal cord injury, approximately one-third (36%) recovered completely, one-third (32%) had partial recovery, and one-third (32%) had no return of function. Prognosis for recovery was better for incomplete spinal cord deficits than complete and improved spinal cord deficits when instrumentation was removed within 3 hours of neurologic deficit diagnosis.

- Coe and colleagues[5] published the most recent analysis of SRS morbidity and mortality data in 2006 that analyzed 58,197 adolescent idiopathic scoliosis procedures performed by SRS members between 2001 and 2003. These investigators noticed that combined anterior and posterior instrumentation and fusion had significantly higher rates of neurologic complications (1.75%) compared with anterior (0.26%) or posterior (0.32%) instrumented spinal fusion alone. Spinal cord injury was recorded in 9 patients treated with combined fusion and 9 patients managed with posterior fusion alone. All spinal cord injuries were incomplete. Complete recovery was noted in 11 patients (7 from the posteriorly fused patients) and incomplete recovery in 6 (2 from the posteriorly fused patients), whereas no neurologic recovery was recorded in 1 patient who underwent combined fusion. Combined fusion was complicated by a dural tear in 0.12% of cases, whereas anterior or posterior fusion alone was associated with dural tear in 0.26% and 0.18% of cases, respectively. Limitations of this study include its retrospective, nonconsecutive character and the fact that it was not limited a priori to diagnosis of adolescent idiopathic scoliosis.

- To overcome these limitations, Diab and colleagues[3] reviewed 1301 consecutive surgically treated adolescent idiopathic scoliosis cases using a prospective database. Neurologic complications included 4 spinal cord injuries, 3 thecal penetrations, and 2 nerve root injuries (1 positional femoral neurapraxia). The overall rate of neurologic complications was 0.69%. The complication rate was reduced to 0.38% when dural tears and positional neurapraxia were eliminated. All neurologic injuries resolved completely within 6 months of the index operation. Three neurologic injury cases were associated with apical sublaminar wires placement. The investigators concluded that neural stretch secondary to large reduction and apical sublaminar wires are major risk factors for neurologic injury. In a meta-analysis addressing surgical outcomes after instrumented posterior spinal fusion that analyzed studies with a minimum follow-up of 5 years, neurologic complications were recorded in 2 of 1136 patients (0.17%).[6] Both patients had been treated with Cotrel-Dubousset construct and suffered from unilateral lower extremity paresis immediately after surgery. Complete neurologic recovery was noted in both patients a few months after the operation. In one, hyperreflexia of the affected lower extremity was found during the last follow-up.

- Factors associated with increased risk for neurologic injury in adolescent idiopathic scoliosis are categorized as surgeon dependent and surgeon independent (**Fig. 1**). Surgeon-dependent factors include type of procedure (with distraction, overcorrection, kyphosis correction, and osteotomy having the highest rates of neurologic injury), approach (with combined approach having the highest rates of neurologic injury), type of instrumentation (with sublaminar wires having the highest rates of neurologic injury), and excessive hemorrhage/prolonged hypotension resulting in decreased spinal cord perfusion.[3,7–9] Surgeon-independent factors include curve magnitude and preexisting neurologic deficit.[10] Most of the neurologic complications are detected intraoperatively as neuromonitoring signal changes and are reversible in a majority of the cases without any long-term sequelae. In cases of intraoperative neurologic change, the authors recommend immediate increase of the mean arterial pressure to 80 mm Hg followed by release of correction, intraoperative imaging to evaluate implant position, steroids administration, and wake-up test if no neurologic improvement is recorded within 30 minutes.

Non-Neurologic Complications

- The overall prevalence of non-neurologic complications associated with surgical management of adolescent idiopathic scoliosis ranges from 0% to 15.4%, whereas the overall reoperation rates range from 3.9% to 26%.[11–15] Non-neurologic complications are categorized as perioperative (intraoperative and postoperative complications occurring during the first postoperative week), early postoperative (occurring between the second and fourth postoperative weeks), and late postoperative complications (occurring after the fourth postoperative week). Perioperative non-neurologic complications include pulmonary, visceral, and urinary complications, excessive hemorrhage, superior mesenteric artery syndrome, and perioperative blindness. Early postoperative complications include ileus, superior mesenteric artery syndrome, wound hematoma, cholololithiasis,

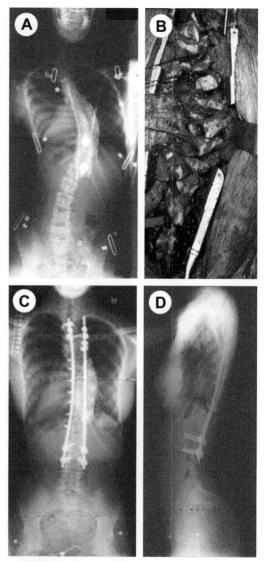

Fig. 1. (A) A 14-year-old girl with progressive adolescent idiopathic scoliosis treated with Harrington instrumentation. During implant insertion removal in another institution, she became completely paralyzed. She had partial recovery of motor function but persistent loss of urinary control. Posteroanterior radiograph shows curve progression after 1 year of bracing. She underwent anterior release and fusion with video-assisted thoracoscopic surgery followed by posterior osteotomies and fusion. (B) Intraoperative image of curve correction with Ponte osteotomies at the apex and fixation with a hybrid construct. (C) Posteroanterior radiograph 3 years after the last surgery shows good curve correction and coronal alignment. (D) Lateral radiograph 3 years after the last surgery reveals good sagittal alignment.

pancreatitis, syndrome of inappropriate antidiuretic hormone secretion, and wound seroma. Pseudarthrosis, implant failure (**Fig. 2**), junctional kyphosis, postoperative

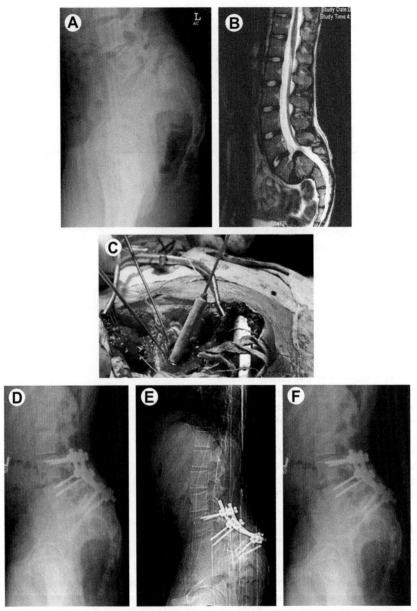

Fig. 2. (*A*) A 12-year-old boy with high-grade spondylolisthesis of L5 on S1. (*B*) Sagittal MRI view of the same patient. (*C*) Intraoperative image shows L5-S1 transacral interbody fusion with the Bohlman and Cook technique using a fibula strut graft. (*D*) Immediate postoperative lateral radiograph demonstrates partial reduction of L5 to S1. (*E*) One year after the index procedure, the lateral radiographic view shows failure of the right S1 screw. At that time, the patient remained asymptomatic but was brought to operating room to prevent any further displacement. (*F*) Lateral radiographic view 6 years after the revision surgery reveals no progression of spondylolisthesis and intact implants.

curve progression, crankshaft phenomenon, implant prominence (**Fig. 3**), late operative site pain, residual rib prominence, and decompensation are considered late complications.

- According to the only level 1 study evaluating non-neurologic complications after surgery for adolescent idiopathic scoliosis, factors that are responsible for or contribute to

non-neurologic complications are prolonged anesthesia time, excessive bleeding, and history of renal disease.[2] No association was found between the prevalence of non-neurologic complications and the number of the levels fused, the type of bone graft, diaphragm detachment, or the approach used (combined anterior and posterior, anterior

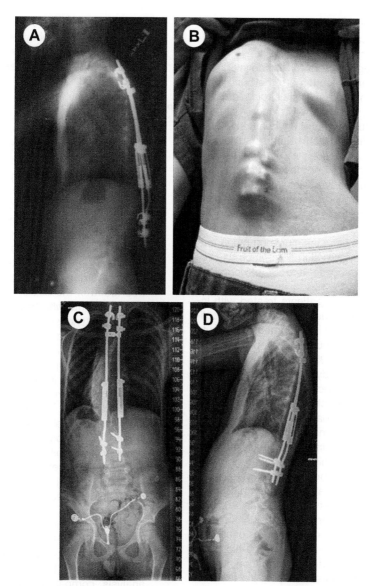

Fig. 3. (*A*) A 10-year-old boy with infantile scoliosis treated with casting and bracing until age 6 years when he was treated with growing rods. Lateral radiograph of the spine shows distal dislodgment of the inferior hooks. (*B*) Clinical image of the same patient demonstrates significant implant prominence. (*C*) Posteroanterior radiograph of the spine immediately after replacement of the distal anchors with pedicle screws. (*D*) Lateral radiograph after pedicle screw fixation.

alone, or posterior alone). Alternatively, the most recent SRS Morbidity and Mortality Committee data revealed that patients who undergo combined anterior and posterior spinal surgery have twice as many complications (10.2%) as patients who have anterior (5.2%) or posterior (5.1%) surgery alone.[5] In regards to the instrumentation type, a recent meta-analysis of midterm to long-term outcomes of surgical management of adolescent idiopathic scoliosis demonstrated that

all-pedicle screw fixation is associated with the lower risk of pseudarthrosis, infection, neurologic deficit, and reoperation compared with Harrington rod and Cotrel-Dubousset instrumentation.[6]

Infection

- Deep infection is one of the most devastating complications, affecting 0% to 9.7% of patients in various series.[11–13,16,17] It is the most common reason for unanticipated repeat surgical intervention after primary spinal fusion for idiopathic scoliosis.[11,15,17] Proposed etiologic factors for the development of deep wound infection are the bulk of the spinal implant system, metallurgic reactions, contamination with low-virulence bacteria, skill of the surgeon, and environmental variables.[18,19] Richards and Emara[16] classified spinal wound infections as early or delayed depending on whether they occur within the first 12 postoperative weeks or 20 weeks after the index procedure, respectively. In early infections, the most common offending organism is *Staphylococcus aureus*, whereas in delayed infections the most commonly isolated organisms are skin flora, such as *Propionibacterium acnes* and *Staphylococcus epidermidis*.[17]

- In a series of 1046 patients treated with instrumented spinal fusion for idiopathic scoliosis, 12.9% had revision surgery with acute or chronic deep wound infections the most common reason (26% of 172 reoperations).[17] A finding of this study was the strong association between the occurrence of deep infection and the approach selected. All infections were recorded in patients who had undergone posterior spinal instrumentation and fusion whereas no infections occurred after anterior surgery. This finding was not substantiated by a more recent study that showed no statistically significant difference in infection rate between patients undergo anterior or posterior spinal fusion for idiopathic scoliosis.[15] A meta-analysis of studies evaluating surgically treated idiopathic scoliosis patients recorded an infection rate of 3.6% in 721 patients.[6] Patients treated with Harrington rods had a higher infection rate of 5.5%, followed by Cotrel-Dubousset construct with an infection rate of 4.3%, and all-pedicle screw fixation with an infection rate of 1.18%.

- Although early infections diagnosed in the setting of an unfused spine or immature fusion are treated with systemic antibiotics and repeated irrigation and débridement, chronic infections require implant removal, spine débridement, and bracing. Loss of correction in both planes should be expected after implant removal and 25% of patients require reinstrumentation in a second stage.[20] An attractive concept in cases of chronic deep infection is the 1-stage rod removal and reinstrumentation/refusion with titanium implants.[21] To prevent deep wound

infection, the authors recommend keeping soft tissues moist with intermittent antibiotic irrigation (every 30 minutes) and performing 3-minute Betadine soaks before final decortication.

Pseudarthrosis

- Pseudarthrosis after instrumented posterior spinal fusion for idiopathic scoliosis has been reported from 1% to 8.9% in some series.[22–25] Development of pseudarthrosis has been associated with the rigidity of implant systems.[14] When 1046 idiopathic scoliosis patients treated in the majority of cases of Texas Scottish Rite Hospital constructs were retrospectively evaluated, 27 pseudarthroses (2.6%) requiring reoperation were recorded.[16] No significant difference was found in the risk of pseudarthrosis between patients who had undergone anterior versus posterior spinal fusion. No pseudarthrosis was recorded in patients treated with combined anterior and posterior approach. In another retrospective case series of 1057 spinal fusions for idiopathic scoliosis, reoperation for pseudarthrosis was performed in 12 patients (11.4%).[13] A significant difference in the pseudarthrosis rate was noted between anteriorly and posteriorly fused patients. No direct conclusions could be made, however, because of the heterogeneity of the implants used, reflecting the evolution of spinal instrumentation from early 1980s to late 1990s.

- According to a systematic review of the literature, the incidence of pseudarthrosis is 3.6% after Harrington rods, 2.8% for segmental hooks, and 7.1% after pedicle screw fixation (**Fig. 4**).[22] A recent meta-analysis compared midterm to long-term correction outcomes and complications of the most commonly used instrumentation systems in idiopathic scoliosis.[6] In 1565 patients who underwent instrumented posterior spinal fusion, 30 patients (1.9%) were found to have pseudarthrosis. Pseudarthrosis was more frequent after Harrington rods (3.1%) compared with Cotrel-Dubousset constructs (1.7%). No case of pseudarthrosis was noted in 254 patients treated with all-pedicle screw fixation.

Curve progression

- Postoperative curve progression is a late complication that may occur proximal or distal to the fusion segment involving the coronal and/or the sagittal plane. It is the third

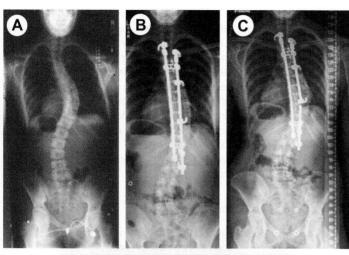

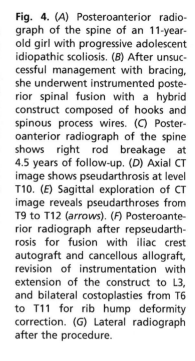

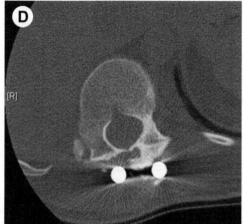

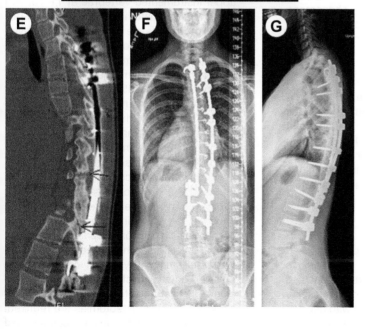

Fig. 4. (*A*) Posteroanterior radiograph of the spine of an 11-year-old girl with progressive adolescent idiopathic scoliosis. (*B*) After unsuccessful management with bracing, she underwent instrumented posterior spinal fusion with a hybrid construct composed of hooks and spinous process wires. (*C*) Posteroanterior radiograph of the spine shows right rod breakage at 4.5 years of follow-up. (*D*) Axial CT image shows pseudarthrosis at level T10. (*E*) Sagittal exploration of CT image reveals pseudarthroses from T9 to T12 (*arrows*). (*F*) Posteroanterior radiograph after repseudarthrosis for fusion with iliac crest autograft and cancellous allograft, revision of instrumentation with extension of the construct to L3, and bilateral costoplasties from T6 to T11 for rib hump deformity correction. (*G*) Lateral radiograph after the procedure.

most common cause of reoperation after infection and pseudarthrosis and may result in loss of shoulder, coronal, or sagittal balance and cosmetic concerns.[14] Adding on of segments cephalad or caudal to the fused spine indicates insufficient length of the index procedure. Curve progression continues until the completion of skeletal growth. When coronal or sagittal imbalance is diagnosed, curve progression is considered significant and extension of the fusion is required. Richards and Emara[16] reported a reoperation rate for curve progression of 1.1%. They found no significant difference in the occurrence of curve progression between patients who had undergone anterior or posterior spinal fusion.

Crankshaft phenomenon

- Crankshaft phenomenon is characterized by progressive 3-D loss of deformity correction within the length of the posterior spinal fusion. It is usually seen in growing children who are fused at an early stage by an isolated posterior approach and it is attributed to continued growth of the vertebral bodies.[26] Risk factors include open triradiate cartilages, Risser stage 0 or 1, girls younger than 11 years, and boys younger than 13 years. Skeletally immature children with congenital scoliosis may have decreased risk for crankshaft phenomenon due to abnormal anterior growth plates. Moreover, crankshaft phenomena have not been recorded in recent series of cerebral palsy children with scoliosis treated with unit rod instrumentation, even in the presence of open triradiate cartilages.[27] Diagnosis is made when 10° or more of progression of the Cobb angle or the rib-vertebral angle within the length of the index fusion is noted on plain films. Management of crankshaft phenomenon includes revision posterior fusion and posterior osteotomies for spinal correction and stabilization along with anterior fusion to arrest deformity progression.

Decompensation

- Loss of the postsurgical ability of the unfused spine to compensate reflects an iatrogenic failure to understand normal alignment and compensatory mechanisms of the spine treated. Risk factors associated with decompensation include failure to identify the curve pattern, failure to select proper fusion levels, derotation, lumbar curve progression after selective thoracic fusion, overcorrection of the thoracic curve, rigid lumbosacral hemicurve, crankshaft phenomenon, and adding on proximal or distal to the fused spine.[28] Depending on the skeletal growth remaining, decompensation is managed either with extension of the instrumented fusion to the lumbar curve down to the stable vertebrae (no sufficient growth remaining) or by using an external orthosis, which may control or even correct the lumbar curve (sufficient growth remaining).

Junctional kyphosis

- Junctional kyphosis is a form of adjacent segment pathology involving kyphosis greater than 10° between the upper or lower instrumented vertebrae and the vertebral body 2 levels above or below, respectively. It has been identified in patients undergoing instrumented fusion for adolescent idiopathic scoliosis and Scheuermann kyphosis. Potential risk factors include type of instrumentation, correction of sagittal imbalance, older age at surgery, surgical correction of thoracic kyphosis more than 50°, fusion to the sacrum, upper or lower instrumented vertebrae, integrity of the posterior ligamentous complex, and combined anterior and posterior surgery.[29] Patients undergo combined anterior and posterior surgery and thoracoplasty; they have an upper instrumented vertebrae at T1–T3; and those without anatomic restoration of normal thoracic kyphosis are at higher risk for developing proximal junctional kyphosis.[29]

- According to a systematic review of the literature, although proximal junctional kyphosis occurs in 17% to 39% of cases after spinal deformity surgery, it has no affect on quality of life.[29] In addition, there is a paucity of literature regarding the natural course of the pathology in long-term follow-up and the methods for addressing proximal junctional kyphosis when it occurs. Postoperative normalization of the global sagittal alignment, avoidance of facetectomies, and maintenance of the interspinous and supraspinous ligaments at the most cephalad and most caudal levels fused have been proposed to minimize junctional kyphosis. In the presence of symptomatic junctional kyphosis, extension of the instrumentation and fusion with or without corrective osteotomies are required. Decompression and fusion are recommended for associated central or neuroforaminal stenosis.

Residual rib prominence

- Idiopathic scoliosis patients' most common presenting complaint is due to the external manifestations of the condition, which include rib hump, asymmetry of shoulder level, prominent scapula, breast and pelvic asymmetry, and back discomfort. Treatment should be able to address all the facets of the deformity. In a study of 502 patients who had undergone instrumentation and fusion for adolescent idiopathic scoliosis, the primary indication for revision surgery was residual rib prominence.[30] It has been demonstrated that costoplasty, combined with pedicle screws and vertebral derotation, may significantly improve rib hump deformity as opposed to pedicle screws and vertebral derotation alone.[31] The theoretic disadvantage of performing a costoplasty is its effect on pulmonary function and the added morbidity from the procedure. Studies showed no significant pulmonary compromise, however, at minimum follow-up of 2 years after costoplasty.[32,33]

Perioperative blindness

- Postoperative visual loss associated with spine surgery is a rare but devastating complication. It may result from ischemic optic neuropathy, central retinal artery occlusion, central retinal vein occlusion, pituitary apoplexy, or cortical ischemia. The incidence of postoperative visual loss after spine surgery ranges from 0.094% to 2.0%.[34,35] In a survey of 400 spine surgeons through the SRS, Myers and colleagues[36] identified 27 unreported complications and reported 1 eye complication for every 100 spinal operations.

COMPLICATIONS RELATED TO SURGICAL MANAGEMENT OF NONIDIOPATHIC SPINAL DEFORMITIES
Cerebral Palsy

- Patients with cerebral palsy are at a high risk for perioperative complications because of underlying comorbidities, such as malnutrition, seizure disorders, respiratory failure, and gastrointestinal disorders. More specifically, it has been found that serum albumin less than 3.5 g/dL and total lymphocyte count less than 1.500 cells/mm³ are associated with higher rates of infection, prolonged intubation, and longer period of hospitalization.[37] Perioperative complications in cerebral palsy

patients include excessive blood loss, atelectasis, bronchopneumonia and aspiration pneumonia, ileus, and urinary tract infections. Wound infections are more frequent than those recorded in idiopathic scoliosis.[38] A multidisciplinary team approach is imperative to improve perisurgical care and decrease complication rates in cerebral palsy patients with spinal deformity, necessitating operative stabilization. Spinal cord monitoring is of value even in nonambulatory children with spastic quadriplegia, because they may benefit from preservation of protective sensation.

Myelomeningocele

- Similarly to cerebral palsy, spinal deformity associated with myelomeningocele continues to present challenges to orthopedic spine surgeons due to the complexity of this patient population. Perioperative complication rates range from 7.5% to 61%.[39,40] Apart from the complications described in cerebral palsy that may affect any child with neuromuscular scoliosis, spine deformity surgery in myelomeningocele patients has significantly higher risk of osteopenic fractures, decubitus ulcers due to insensate skin, and infection, including urinary tract infections, wound infections, and sepsis. Wound closure is often problematic due to scarred and poorly vascularized skin over the defect. Because latex sensitivity is reported in up to 40% of myelomeningocele patients, all these patients should be managed as having latex allergy.[41] Loss of posterior elements may affect the adequacy of fixation, which, in turn, may affect the incidence of pseudarthrosis, implant failure, and loss of correction (**Fig. 5**).[42] The senior author thinks that happiness in the management of myelomeningocele spinal deformity is often a transient experience.

Connective Tissue Disorders

Marfan syndrome

- Approximately 12% of patients with Marfan syndrome develop spinal deformity that requires surgical intervention.[43] Preoperative work-up should address higher operative risks due to aortic dilatation, risk of dissection, anticoagulation for prosthetic cardiac valves, and risk of pulmonary complications.[44] Unique features of Marfan syndrome that may adversely affect the surgical

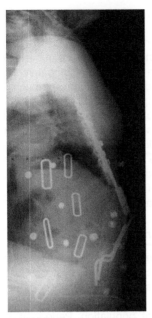

Fig. 5. A 6-year-old female patient with myelomeningocele and lumbar kyphoscoliosis managed with growing rods inserted via the Fackler and Warner technique. Lateral radiograph of the spine shows implant failure.

outcome include dural ectasia, decreased bone mineral density, and thinned posterior elements. According to Jones and colleagues,[45] patients with Marfan syndrome who undergo spinal surgery have increased blood loss, infection rate, pseudarthrosis, failure of instrumentation, and decompensation in both planes. Imaging evaluation with MRI of the entire spine to evaluate for dural ectasia and lumbar CT scan to assess the adequacy of pedicles are indicated before surgery (**Fig. 6**). To avoid decompensation, extension of fusion to stable and neutral vertebrae in both planes, minimization of soft tissue dissection, increased fixation points, and avoidance of extreme correction and selective fusion are recommended.[45]

Ehlers-Danlos syndrome

- Spinal deformity usually involves the classic (type I) and the ocular-scoliotic type (type VI) of Ehlers-Danlos syndrome. Surgical correction is difficult due to stiff deformity and is associated with serious intraoperative complications. Vascular fragility is inherent in Ehlers-Danlos syndrome and, therefore, iatrogenic vascular injury may be inevitable during posterior spinal surgery.[46] Anterior spinal fusion should be performed when deemed essential due to the fragility of the retroperitoneal vessels and the possibility of life threatening hemorrhage. High rate of neurologic complications secondary to combination of vascular fragility and ligamentous laxity has also been reported in one study, but the exact incidence remains unknown.[47]

Scheuermann Kyphosis

- Common complications associated with surgical management of Scheuermann kyphosis include deep wound infection, neurologic dysfunction, pseudarthrosis, implant failure, deformity progression, postoperative pain, and junctional kyphosis. A combined anterior and posterior approach has been recommended to achieve the best deformity correction as well as to minimize the risk of postoperative loss of correction and pseudarthrosis. Combined video-assisted thoracoscopic surgery anterior spinal release and posterior spinal fusion has been shown an effective alternative for the management of more severe and rigid curves with lower morbidity compared with thoracotomy.[48]

- Based on the SRS Morbidity and Mortality database, Coe and colleagues[49] published a significant analysis of 683 spinal fusions for Scheuermann kyphosis with 499 procedures (75%) performed in children. They noted significantly lower complication rates after surgical correction of Scheuermann kyphosis in children (12%) compared with adults (22%). The overall incidence of complications did not differ between the posterior (14.8%) and the same-day anterior-posterior procedures (16.9%). Anterior surgery was associated with the lower complication rates (4.1%). The most common complication was infection (3.8% in pediatric patients). The overall rate of acute neurologic complications was 1.9% and included 2 spinal cord injuries in pediatric patients (0.4%). One pediatric patient (0.2%) died from an unknown cause.

Neurofibromatosis

- The reported incidence of pseudarthrosis after an attempt at spinal fusion in NF type 1 (NF-1) patients ranges between 15% and 38%.[50] The incidence is even higher in the presence of kyphosis of more than 50°. It is suggested that the primary reason for fusion failure is an inadequate anterior procedure. Erosion from enlarging neurofibromas, dural ectasia, and meningoceles may, however, play a role. The best results are obtained

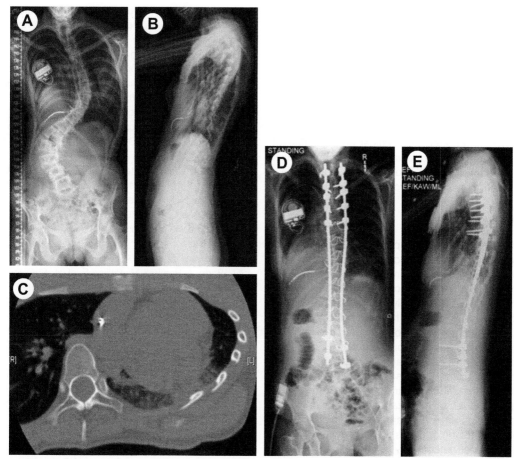

Fig. 6. (*A*) Posteroanterior radiograph of the spine of an 11-year-old girl with Marfan syndrome and significant lordoscoliosis. (*B*) Lateral radiograph of the same patient illustrating significant thoracic lordosis. (*C*) Axial CT image at T6 level shows bilateral absence of fixation point for pedicle screws (thin pedicles). (*D*) Posteroanterior radiograph immediately after scoliosis surgery with hybrid instrumentation. Pedicle screw placement was based on preoperative CT. Extrapedicular screws were used at upper thoracic levels. (*E*) Lateral radiograph immediately after surgery demonstrating improvement in thoracic lordosis.

when a preplanned combined intervertebral fusion and posterior arthrodesis is performed. Despite the circumferential arthrodesis, solid fusion is not obtained in every patient, and some patients require repeat operative procedures.

- A neurologic deficit in patients with NF-1 may be due to spinal cord compression secondary to spinal deformity, rib penetration into the spinal canal, or intraspinal tumors. Paraplegia in young patients is usually caused by spinal deformity and in older patients by tumors. Neurologic impairment is more common in NF-1 patients with kyphosis.
- Rib head dislocation into the spinal canal should be ruled out before any attempt for surgical correction of the spinal deformity because correction may result in spinal cord impingement by the unrecognized dislocated

rib head. Resection of a segment of rib distal to the tip of the transverse process theoretically mobilizes the rib head and decreases the possibility of spinal cord impingement.

- Bleeding during spine deformity surgery as well as postoperative hemorrhage and hematoma formation are not uncommon in NF-1 patients, especially during an anterior approach. Postoperative extradural hematoma causing paraplegia has been described.[51] Meticulous hemostasis using bipolar coagulation and hemostatic agents (ie, thrombin or hemostatic matrix [Floseal, Baxter Healthcare Corp., Fremont, CA]) must be performed during surgery. The authors recommend that a putty of Gelfoam (Baxter), microfibrillar collagen hemostat (Avitene, Davol Inc., Warwick, RI), and thrombin (human powder) is available.

- Progression of the deformity may be noticed after solid spinal arthrodesis. Thus, close follow-up is needed even after successful spinal fusion. In patients who are skeletally immature, anterior spinal fusion in conjunction to the posterior surgery is required to prevent the occurrence of crankshaft phenomenon, which is produced by continuing unbalanced anterior vertebral growth. A rarely reported nonsurgical complication of rupture of a subclavian artery aneurysm was responsible for the only mortality in a spinal deformity surgical group from Cincinnati.[52–54]

SUUMMARY

Surgery in children with spinal deformity is a challenging undertaking. Although current orthopedic practice ensures good long-term surgical results, complications occur. Idiopathic scoliosis represents the most extensively investigated deformity of the pediatric spine, with several studies reporting on neurologic and non-neurologic complications. Nonidiopathic deformities of the spine are at higher risk for perioperative and long-term complications, mainly because of underlying comorbidities. A multidisciplinary treatment strategy is helpful to assure optimization of medical conditions before surgery. Awareness of complications that occur during or after spine surgery is essential to avoid poor outcomes.

REFERENCES

1. Boachie-Adjei O, Cunningham ME. Revision spine surgery in the growing child. In: Akbarnia BA, Yazici M, Thompson GH, editors. The growing spine. Berlin: Springer-Verlag; 2011. p. 487–98.
2. Carreon LY, Puno RM, Lenke LG, et al. Non-neurologic complications following surgery for adolescent idiopathic scoliosis. J Bone Joint Surg Am 2007;89:2427–32.
3. Diab M, Smith AR, Kuklo TR, Spinal Deformity Study Group. Neural complications in the surgical treatment of adolescent idiopathic scoliosis. Spine (Phila Pa 1976) 2007;32:2759–63.
4. MacEwen GD, Bunnell WP, Sriram K. Acute neurological complications in the treatment of scoliosis. A report of the Scoliosis Research Society. J Bone Joint Surg Am 1975;57:404–8.
5. Coe JD, Arlet V, Donaldson W, et al. Complications in spinal fusion for adolescent idiopathic scoliosis in the new millennium. A report of the Scoliosis Research Society Morbidity and Mortality Committee. Spine (Phila Pa 1976) 2006;31:345–9.
6. Lykissas MG, Jain VV, Senthil N, et al. Mid- to long-term outcomes in adolescent idiopathic scoliosis

7. following instrumented posterior spinal fusion: a Meta-analysis. Spine (Phila Pa 1976) 2013;38(2): E113–9.
7. Yeoman PM, Gibson MJ, Hutchinson A, et al. Influence of induced hypotension and spinal distraction on feline spinal somatosensory evoked potentials. Br J Anaesth 1989;63:315–20.
8. Wilburg G, Thompson GH, Shaffer JW, et al. Postoperative neurological deficits in segmental spinal instrumentation. J Bone Joint Surg Am 1984;66: 1178–87.
9. Morbidity and mortality committee report 1974–1979, Scoliosis Research Society. Read at 14th Annual Meeting, Seattle (WA); 1979.
10. Asher M, Lai SM, Burton D, et al. Safety and efficacy of Isola instrumentation and arthrodesis for adolescent idiopathic scoliosis: two- to 12-year follow up. Spine 2004;29:2013–23.
11. Bago J, Ramirez M, Pellise F, et al. Survivorship analysis of Cotrel-Dubousset instrumentation in idiopathic scoliosis. Eur Spine J 2003;12:435–9.
12. Richards BS, Herring JA, Johnston CE, et al. Treatment of idiopathic scoliosis using Texas Scottish Rite Hospital (TSRH) instrumentation. Spine 1994; 19:1598–605.
13. Danielsson AJ, Nachemson AL. Radiologic findings and curve progression 22 years after treatment for adolescent idiopathic scoliosis. Spine 2001;26:516–25.
14. Dickson JH, Erwin WD, Rossi D. Harrington instrumentation and arthrodesis for idiopathic scoliosis: a twenty-one year follow-up. J Bone Joint Surg Am 1990;72:678–83.
15. Luhmann SJ, Lenke LG, Bridwell KH, et al. Revision surgery after primary spine fusion for idiopathic scoliosis. Spine 2009;34:2191–7.
16. Richards BS, Emara KM. Delayed infections after posterior TSRH spinal instrumentation for idiopathic scoliosis. Spine 2001;26:1990–6.
17. Richards BS, Hasley BP, Casey VF. Repeat surgical interventions following "definitive" instrumentation and fusion for idiopathic scoliosis. Spine 2006;31: 3018–26.
18. Ho C, Sucato DJ, Richards BS. Risk factors for the development of delayed infections following posterior spinal fusion and instrumentation in adolescent idiopathic scoliosis patients. Spine 2007;32:2272–7.
19. Theiss SM, Lonstein JE, Winter RB. Wound infections in reconstructive spine surgery. Orthop Clin North Am 1996;27:105–10.
20. Sink EL, Newton PO, Mubarak SJ, et al. Maintenance of sagittal plane alignment after surgical correction of spinal deformity in patients with cerebral palsy. Spine 2003;28:1396–403.
21. Muschik M, Luck W, Schlenzka D. Implant removal for late-developing infection after instrumented

posterior spinal fusion for scoliosis: reinstrumentation reduces loss of correction. A retrospective analysis of 45 cases. Eur Spine J 2004;13:645–51.

22. Westrick ER, Ward WT. Adolescent idiopathic scoliosis: 5-year to 20-year evidence-based surgical results. J Pediatr Orthop 2011;31:S61–8.

23. Willers U, Hedlund R, Aaro S, et al. Long-term results of Harrington instrumentation in idiopathic scoliosis. Spine 1993;18:713–7.

24. Suk SI, Lee CK, Kim WJ, et al. Segmental pedicle screw fixation in the treatment of thoracic idiopathic scoliosis. Spine 1995;20:1399–405.

25. Asher M, Lai SM, Burton D, et al. Safety and efficacy of Isola instrumentation and arthrodesis for adolescent idiopathic scoliosis: two- to 12-year followup. Spine 2004;29:2013–23.

26. Roberto RF, Lonstein JE, Winter RB, et al. Curve progression in Risser stage 0 or 1 patients after posterior spinal fusion for idiopathic scoliosis. J Pediatr Orthop 1997;17:718–25.

27. Smucker JD, Miller F. Crankshaft effect after posterior spinal fusion and unit rod instrumentation in children with cerebral palsy. J Pediatr Orthop 2001;21:108–12.

28. Wodd KB. Postsurgical sagittal and coronal plane decompensation in deformity surgery. In: Vaccaro AR, Regan JJ, Crawford AH, et al, editors. Complications of pediatric and adult spinal surgery. New York: Markel Dekker; 2004. p. 687–708.

29. Kim HJ, Lenke LG, Shaffrey CI, et al. Proximal Junctional Kyphosis (PJK) as a distinct form of Adjacent Segment Pathology (ASP) following Spinal Deformity Surgery: a systematic review. Spine (Phila Pa 1976) 2012;37(Suppl 22):S144–64.

30. Campos M, Dolan L, Weinstein S. Unanticipated revision surgery in adolescent idiopathic scoliosis. Spine 2012;37:1048–53.

31. Lykissas MG, Sharma V, Jain VV, et al. Assessment of rib hump deformity correction in adolescent idiopathic scoliosis with or without costoplasty using the double rib contour sign. J Spinal Disord Tech 2012. [Epub ahead of print].

32. Suk SI, Kim JH, Kim SS, et al. Thoracoplasty in thoracic adolescent idiopathic scoliosis. Spine 2008;33:1061–7.

33. Min K, Waelchli B, Hahn F. Primary thoracoplasty and pedicle screw instrumentation in thoracic idiopathic scoliosis. Eur Spine J 2005;14:777–82.

34. Zimmerer S, Koehler M, Turtschi S, et al. Amaurosis after spine surgery: survey of the literature and discussion of one case. Eur Spine J 2011;20:171–6.

35. Stevens WR, Glazer PA, Kelley SD, et al. Ophthalmic complications after spinal surgery. Spine 1997;22:1319–24.

36. Myers MA, Hamilton SR, Bogosian AJ, et al. Visual loss as a complication of spine surgery. A review of 37 cases. Spine 1997;22:1325–9.

37. Jevsevar DS, Karlin LI. The relationship between preoperative nutritional status and complications after an operation for scoliosis in patients who have cerebral palsy. J Bone Joint Surg Am 1993; 75:880–4.

38. Lonstein JE, Akbarnia BA. Operative treatment of spinal deformities in patients with cerebral palsy or mental retardation. J Bone Joint Surg Am 1983;65:43–55.

39. Ward WT, Wenger DR, Roach JW. Surgical correction of myelomeningocele scoliosis: a critical appraisal of various instrumentation systems. J Pediatr Orthop 1989;9:262–8.

40. Geiger F, Parsch D, Carstens C. Complications of scoliosis surgery in children with myelomeningocele. Eur Spine J 1999;8:22–6.

41. Banta JV, Bonanni C, Prebluda J. Latex anaphylaxis during spinal surgery in children with myelomeningocele. Dev Med Child Neurol 1993;53: 543–8.

42. Ibrahim DT, Sarwark JF. Complications related to the surgical management of patients with myelomeningocele. In: Vaccaro AR, Regan JJ, Crawford AH, et al, editors. Complications of pediatric and adult spinal surgery. New York: Markel Dekker; 2004. p. 677–86.

43. Sponseller PD, Hobbs W, Riley LH III, et al. The thoracolumbar spine in Marfan syndrome. J Bone Joint Surg Am 1995;77:867–75.

44. Sponseller PD. Complications related to the surgical management of patients with skeletal dysplasias and connective tissue diseases. In: Vaccaro AR, Regan JJ, Crawford AH, et al, editors. Complications of pediatric and adult spinal surgery. New York: Markel Dekker; 2004. p. 639–54.

45. Jones KB, Erkula G, Sponseller PD, et al. Spine deformity correction in Marfan syndrome. Spine 2002;27:2003–12.

46. McMaster MJ. Spinal deformity in Ehlers-Danlos syndrome. Five patients treated by spinal fusion. J Bone Joint Surg Br 1994;76:773–7.

47. Vogel LC, Lubicky JP. Neurologic and vascular complications of scoliosis surgery in patients with Ehlers-Danlos syndrome. A case report. Spine 1996;21:2508–14.

48. Herrera-Soto JA, Parikh SN, Al-Sayyad MJ, et al. Experience with combined video-assisted thoracoscopic surgery (VATS) anterior spinal release and posterior spinal fusion in Scheuermann's kyphosis. Spine 2005;30:2176–81.

49. Coe JD, Smith JS, Berven S, et al. Complications of spinal fusion for Scheuermann kyphosis: a report of the scoliosis research society morbidity and mortality committee. Spine 2010;35: 99–103.

50. Crawford AH, Lykissas MG, Schorry EK, et al. Neurofibromatosis: etiology, commonly encountered

spinal deformities, common complications and pitfalls of surgical treatment. Spine Deformity 2012; Preview Issue:85–94.

51. Lonstein JE, Winter RB, Moe JH, et al. Neurologic deficits secondary to spinal deformity. A review of the literature and report of 43 cases. Spine 1980; 5:331–55.

52. Slisatkorn W, Subtaweesin T, Laksanabunsong P, et al. Spontaneous rupture of the left subclavian artery in neurofibromatosis. Asian Cardiovasc Thorac Ann 2003;11:266–8.

53. Takahashi K, Maruyama A, Ainai S, et al. A case of ruptured left subclavian artery associated with von recklinghausen's disease. Kyobu Geka 1989;42: 1036–8 [in Japanese].

54. Souftas V, Tsivgoulis G, Kirmanidis M, et al. Spontaneous subclavian artery rupture in neurofibromatosis type I. Neurol Sci 2011;32:979–80.

UPPER EXTREMITY

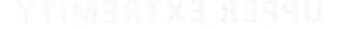
UPPER EXTREMITY

Preface
Upper Extremity

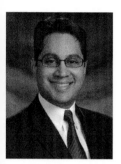

Asif M. Ilyas, MD
Editor

I am honored and excited to be a part of the new format of the *Orthopedic Clinics of North America*. Each issue will consist of cutting-edge and thorough reviews on the various subspecialties of orthopedics. I am charged with overseeing the upper extremity section, which focuses on the contemporary surgical issues involving the hand, wrist, elbow, and shoulder.

The first issue's section on the upper extremity will review some of our foremost controversies in upper extremity fracture management, including indications for reverse total shoulder arthroplasty, the management of radial nerve palsies following humeral shaft fractures, indications and outcomes for radial head arthroplasty, the management of complex posterior elbow wounds, and indications and outcomes for total elbow arthroplasty in the management of distal humerus fractures. Last, I would like to thank the authors for their sincere efforts and excellent work in presenting a coherent and concise review of these topics.

Asif M. Ilyas, MD
Thomas Jefferson University
Program Director of Hand Surgery
Rothman Institute
925 Chestnut Street
Philadelphia, PA 19107, USA

E-mail address:
asif.ilyas@rothmaninstitute.com

Orthop Clin N Am 44 (2013) xix
http://dx.doi.org/10.1016/j.ocl.2013.05.004
0030-5898/13/$ – see front matter © 2013 Published by Elsevier Inc.

orthopedic.theclinics.com

Current Indications and Outcomes of Total Wrist Arthroplasty

Shade Ogunro, MD, Irfan Ahmed, MD, Virak Tan, MD*

KEYWORDS

• Wrist • Arthroplasty • Replacement • Implant

KEY POINTS

- Total wrist arthroplasty, an alternative to wrist arthrodesis, is indicated in patients with painful, debilitating, panarthritis with or without progressive wrist deformity, and may be essential in patients with bilateral wrist and/or concomitant upper extremity disease.
- Though classically performed in the rheumatoid patient, advances have led present-day application of total wrist arthroplasty in patients with rheumatoid and nonrheumatoid inflammatory arthritis, osteoarthritis, and posttraumatic arthritis.
- Modern designs have significantly reduced rates of instability and prosthetic dislocations; however, carpal component loosening remains an obstacle to good and predictable long-term survival.
- Published outcomes are limited to early and/or midterm results for the 3 prostheses approved by the Food and Drug Administration.

Although Gluck performed the first total wrist arthroplasty (TWA) in 1890, it was not until the 1970s that interest in wrist arthroplasty gained momentum. In 1967, Swanson designed the first wrist implant with widespread commercial distribution. The Swanson double-stemmed, flexible-hinge, silicone implant functioned as a joint spacer, rather than a joint replacement. Despite early positive results, longer follow-up revealed implant subsidence and prosthetic fracture. Since this first design, TWA has undergone considerable improvements in material and design that have had a considerable impact on implant survival. Research in joint arthroplasty and, in particular, wrist arthroplasty has contributed to implant longevity, patient satisfaction, and improved clinical outcomes. This article reviews the current indications and clinical outcomes of TWA.

INDICATIONS AND CONTRAINDICATIONS

TWA is an alternative to wrist arthrodesis, and is indicated in patients with painful, debilitating, panarthritis with or without progressive deformity of the wrist. Its ideal candidate is the low-demand patient with painful, bilateral wrist disease and relatively good wrist alignment and motion despite arthritis. It is also ideal for patients with concomitant upper extremity arthritis. Where involvement of ipsilateral joints would complicate positioning of the hand in space, arthroplasty helps the patient compensate for lack of motion in neighboring joints. As with other joint replacements in the upper extremity, it is well described in patients afflicted with rheumatoid arthritis. As research in wrist arthroplasty has undergone expansion and refinement, so too have its indications. Such advances have led to its present-day application in

Disclosures pertaining to this article: None.
Department of Orthopaedics, UMDNJ-New Jersey Medical School, New Jersey Orthopaedic Institute, 140 Bergen Street, ACC D-Level, Newark, NJ 07103, USA
* Corresponding author.
E-mail address: tanvi@umdnj.edu

patients with rheumatoid and nonrheumatoid inflammatory arthritis, osteoarthritis, and posttraumatic arthritis. Wrist arthroplasty is also applicable in failed limited wrist fusion and in advanced avascular necrosis of the carpal bones.

As with other joint replacements, TWA is contraindicated in the nonfunctioning hand lacking neurologic function, as well as in high-demand patients, laborers, and those with a previous history of sepsis or deep local infection. Specific to TWA, it is also contraindicated in those that require regular use of walking aids for support during ambulation or transfers. Relative contraindications include those conditions with potentially inadequate carpal bone stock, such as a previous surgical complete fusion or a proximal row carpectomy.

Rheumatoid Arthritis

Earlier implant designs were uniquely reported in rheumatoid patients. As understanding of wrist arthroplasty improved, indications and contraindications within the rheumatoid population were further defined. The high rate of complications and failures associated with earlier implants led to its contraindication in rheumatoid patients with poor bone stock or severe osteopenia. In these patients, this could result in component loosening owing to inability to support the prosthetic components, especially the carpal component. Severe ligamentous laxity in the form of chronic or severe volar and ulnar subluxation is also contraindicated because of prosthesis instability and ultimate dislocation. Rheumatoid patients with highly active synovitis are prone to severe bony erosions and/or joint hyperlaxity, resulting in a higher risk of subsequent implant instability and loosening. In end-stage rheumatoid arthritis characterized by soft-tissue imbalance and volar subluxation of the wrist, ruptured or attenuated radial wrist extensors are also a contraindication for wrist replacement, and result in prosthesis instability and subluxation.

In treating the rheumatoid patient with multiple joint involvement, lower extremity replacements such as the hip and/or knee should be performed before wrist replacement, to avoid weight bearing on the wrist replacement during rehabilitation. By contrast, procedures on the digits should be performed after wrist arthroplasty to optimize joint alignment and tendon tension in the hand.

Nonrheumatoid Arthritis

With regard to nonrheumatoid inflammatory arthritides, systemic lupus erythematosus is a relative contraindication because of its predisposition to joint laxity. Although severely underpowered in the literature, early and midterm results after arthroplasty have been reported for the treatment of arthritis secondary to gout, psoriasis, lupus, undifferentiated spondyloarthropathy, and chondrocalcinosis.[1,2]

In a recent study, Nydick and colleagues[2] reported on early outcomes in 22 patients treated with the Maestro TWA system (Biomet, Warsaw, IN). In this study the etiology included scapholunate advanced collapse (n = 8), scaphoid nonunion advanced collapse (n = 5), primary osteoarthritis (n = 2), Kienböck disease (n = 2), and rheumatoid arthritis (n = 5). The data demonstrated efficacy for arthroplasty in nonrheumatoid conditions, likely attributable to better bone stock and better radiocarpal alignment, and potentially resulting in future low long-term failure rates. Patients with noninflammatory, nonrheumatoid arthritis tend to be healthier and have higher demands, theoretically leading to more rapid implant failure. With strict adherence to activity limitations, this patient population may be at a lower risk of implant loosening because they lack the bony erosions and/or joint hyperlaxity typically associated with synovitis.

ARTHROPLASTY VERSUS ARTHRODESIS

The main advantage of arthroplasty over arthrodesis is preservation or improvement of some degree of wrist mobility. Although arthrodesis effectively relieves pain and corrects deformity, the resulting lack of motion may significantly impair function, especially when the shoulder, elbow, and hand are also affected by arthritis.[3] At present, there are no prospective randomized trials comparing arthroplasty with arthrodesis. In a comparative, retrospective study of 51 operated wrists in 46 rheumatoid patients undergoing 24 arthrodeses and 27 arthroplasties, Murphy and colleagues[4] found no difference in Disability of the Arm, Shoulder, and Hand (DASH) or Patient-Related Wrist Evaluation (PRWE) scores, nor complications. Patients in the arthroplasty group did, however, report a trend toward greater ease with personal hygiene and fine dexterity requiring wrist flexion. The investigators concluded that although rheumatoid patients can and do accommodate arthrodesis, it should not be construed that these patients would prefer arthrodesis over arthroplasty or that they would not obtain greater benefit from arthroplasty.

In 2008, Cavaliere and Chung[5] performed a systematic review comparing 18 TWA studies representing approximately 500 procedures and 20 total wrist fusion studies, representing approximately 800 procedures. Based on their review of the existing literature, they reported more reliable pain relief with total wrist fusion, and higher complication and revision rates with TWA (30% arthroplasty group, 17% arthrodesis group). High satisfaction rates were seen in both groups. Of the 14 studies providing mean flexion, extension, and radial and ulnar deviations, only 3 studies showed an average active arc of motion within functional range as described by Palmer and colleagues.[6] From this systematic review, the investigators concluded that in the rheumatoid patient, outcomes for total wrist fusion were comparable and possibly better than those for TWA, and that current evidence did not support the widespread implementation of arthroplasty. The cases reviewed consisted of second-generation and early third-generation metal-polyethylene TWA prostheses, and did not include newer third-generation implants.

A subsequent study by Cavaliere and Chung[7] using a cost-utility analysis model showed that arthroplasty had only an incrementally higher cost in comparison with wrist fusion. Moreover, rheumatoid patients place emphasis on maintaining wrist motion, and for that reason would prefer arthroplasty to fusion and nonoperative management.[8]

OUTCOMES

From the double-stemmed silicone spacer to the more current anatomic metal-polyethylene implants, TWA implants have undergone considerable changes aimed at increasing implant survivorship. In long-term follow-up, the Swanson flexible-hinge, silicone joint spacer (first-generation implant) was complicated by implant subsidence and prosthetic fracture. Often considered the first true arthroplasty of the wrist, second-generation implants, consisting of an articulating metal-polyethylene design (Meuli and Volz) had an unacceptably high complication rate characterized by wrist imbalance and implant loosening. In a failed attempt to reduce wrist imbalance and distal component loosening, early third-generation implants (Biaxial, Trispherical, revised Meuli, and revised Volz) were designed to better reproduce normal wrist kinematics. Nowadays, third-generation metal-polyethylene implants are available. At present there are only 3 TWA designs approved by the US Food and Drug Administration (FDA): Universal 2 (KMI, San Diego, CA), ReMotion (SBI, Morrisville, PA), and Maestro (Biomet, Warsaw, IN).

Universal Total Wrist Arthroplasty

Although the Universal 2 TWA is FDA-approved, it is difficult to discuss the evolution of this implant without discussion of the Universal 1 TWA. Before the development of the Universal 1 TWA, third-generation metal-polyethylene implants were plagued with persistent implant loosening and wrist imbalance. Developed by Menon in the 1990s, the Universal 1 TWA introduced a new approach to distal fixation and the concept of anatomic components. A short central stem cemented into the capitate and 2 deep-threaded osteointegrative screws into the radial and ulnar aspects of the carpus were designed to provide superior distal fixation. Intercarpal fusion was also performed to provide long-term solid bony support. The radial component was inclined 20° to replicate the slope of the normal distal radius. The polyethylene insert, toroidal in shape, consisted of a broad articulation closely matching that of the proximal carpal row. Soft-tissue balancing was adjusted by variations in polyethylene size.

In 1998, Menon[9] published midterm results using the Universal 1 TWA implant. Thirty-seven procedures were performed in 31 patients, of whom 23 suffered from rheumatoid arthritis and the remaining 8 from osteoarthritis. The average follow-up was 6.7 years, ranging from 4 to 10 years. All patients were given the option to receive wrist fusion. Those without active wrist extension were not given the option of arthroplasty. After excluding 3 patients from the study, 34 were available for review. Of the 34 wrists, 88% (30 patients) were pain free while the remaining patients required periodic analgesics and occasionally wore a wrist brace for support. Although all ranges of motion increased postoperatively, only dorsiflexion and radial deviation increased to statistical significance. In this series the complication rate was 32%, occurring in 12 wrists. The most common complication was volar dislocation of the wrist, occurring in 5 wrists. No case demonstrated radiographic evidence of distal component loosening. However, radial component loosening was observed in 2 patients at 2 and 3 years postoperatively, requiring reoperation with extremely good results. Of the 3 patients eliminated from final review, 2 were converted to wrist fusion secondary to persistent flexion deformity interfering with activities of daily living and recurrent dislocation in a known alcoholic. The third patient received removal of hardware because of staphylococcal pyarthrosis of the wrist.

In a further follow-up study by Menon[10] that included 57 implants, carpal component loosening was not reported. Subsidence of the radial component was observed, but was not progressive or symptomatic. Pain relief and functional range of motion remained constant while dislocation occurred in 6 of the 57 patients, with 5 occurring in the first 37 cases. The initial higher incidence of dislocation was attributed to the lack of availability of different implant sizes and the thickness of polyethylene inserts at the time. Menon also criticized himself for excessive bone resection in his early cases.[10,11] Other investigators reported similar success with shorter follow-up, indicating that with a proper design, wrist replacement can provide suitable function and durability.[12]

In 2002, Divelbiss and colleagues[11] sought to duplicate Menon's results. In 22 rheumatoid wrists (19 patients), clinical results similar to those of Menon were achieved with regard to pain relief, range of motion, and complications. All ranges of motions improved postoperatively, although only extension, radial deviation, and supination increased to statistical significance. Average DASH scores improved from 46 points preoperatively to 32.1 points at 1-year follow-up, and continued to improve to 22.4 points at 2-year follow-up. The latter did not reach statistical significance given the lack of power (n = 8). Early volar dislocations were seen in 3 patients (14%) who were found to have highly active rheumatoid disease and marked joint laxity at the time of initial surgery. Of the dislocations only 1 patient was converted to wrist fusion for persistent instability, after failed revision of carpal baseplate and polyethylene exchange, followed by failed open reduction, capsule imbrication, and external fixation, followed by failed closed reduction and splinting. The patient suffered traumatic dislocations before her second and third revision surgeries. No cases demonstrated radiographic evidence of distal component loosening. Nonprogressive subsidence of the radial component was seen in 1 patient.

In a more recent study, Ward and colleagues[13] reviewed the long-term results associated with the Universal 1 TWA in 25 rheumatoid wrists (21 patients) with a minimum follow-up of 5 years. Clinical and radiographic review was available for 19 wrists (15 patients) with an average follow-up of 7.3 years (range 5–10.8 years). At a minimum of 5 years, the Universal 1 wrist prosthesis had a high failure rate of 50% (10 of 20 wrists). This failure rate includes revision of 1 patient who died before the minimum 5-year follow-up. In this patient, conversion to wrist fusion was performed secondary to recurrent implant instability at 2.2 years after the index procedure. Carpal component loosening was the most common cause of revisions, occurring in 45% of wrists (9 wrists in 8 patients). The mean time to revision

surgery for carpal component loosening was 5.5 years (range 2.7–9.34 years). Of the 9 wrists revised because of carpal loosening, only 5 had radiographic evidence of intercarpal union. An additional 2 patients had radiographic evidence of carpal component subsidence. Revision surgery revealed polyethylene wear, metallosis, and carpal component loosening in all wrists. There was no evidence of gross radial component loosening in any of these wrists.

At the time of latest follow-up, 10 wrists in 8 patients remained functional. Despite failures, those with a stable prosthesis did maintain a functional range of motion and had improvement in patient-reported outcome measures. In this group of patients, average DASH scores improved from 62 points preoperatively to 40 points postoperatively. All ranges of motion increased postoperatively. There was no significant change in wrist flexion or extension, radial deviation, ulnar deviation, and forearm supination. At the time of latest follow-up, intercarpal fusion was seen in all 10 functional wrists.

In this series, patients with carpal component loosening were less likely to have radiographic evidence of intercarpal fusion than those who had stable prostheses, although this difference did not reach significance. Also in this series, the failure rate was higher than previously reported for this prosthesis. Implant survival rates at 5 and 7 years for the original prosthetic components were 75% and 60%, respectively.

In an attempt to better understand the mechanical behavior of implant instability and the high rate of dislocations associated with the Universal 1 TWA, Grosland and colleagues[12] created a finite element analysis comparing toroidal and ellipsoidal carpal articulations. Using computer modeling and laboratory experiments, the elliptical distal articular surface provided consistent congruity and centralization of the contact area on the polyethylene over the entire range of prosthetic motion. This approach resulted in low stress and wear on the polyethylene and better articular stability without creating a fully constrained joint. The toroidal distal articulation maintained true congruency only during radial and ulnar deviations with the prosthesis in a neutral position.[12,14]

Pioneered by Adams, the next generation of the Universal TWA prosthesis made use of an ellipsoidal rather than a toroidal articulation. Improving on fixation, a beaded porous coating was applied to both radial and carpal components to allow for fixation by osseous integration. Radial and ulnar variable-angle screws allow compression between the carpal baseplate and the remaining carpus.

In a recent study, Ferreres and colleagues[1] reviewed midterm results using the Universal 2 TWA implant in 22 wrists (22 patients). Clinical and radiographic review was available for 21 wrists (21 patients) with average follow-up of 5.5 years (range 3–9 years). Although 2 wrists received the Universal 1 TWA implant and the remaining wrists the Universal 2 implant, the investigators did not exclude nor differentiate Universal 1 results from the final review. Fifteen patients had rheumatoid arthritis. Two patients had wrist destruction from grade IV Kienböck disease. The remaining 5 patients had nonrheumatoid inflammatory arthritis (lupus, psoriasis, undifferentiated spondyloarthropathy), chondrocalcinosis, and arthrosis. The PRWE score averaged 24 points, with an average of 11 points out of 50 for functional evaluation and 12 points out of 50 for pain. In terms of patient satisfaction, 10 patients were very satisfied with the procedure and 10 were satisfied. Only postoperative ranges of motion were available for review. The average range of flexion arc was 68°, with an average of 26° of extension and 42° of flexion. The average range of radial and ulnar deviation was 26°, with an average of 1° of radial deviation and 26° of ulnar deviation. Only average flexion and extension were within functional range of motion as described by Palmer.[6] Pain during activities of daily living was absent or slight in 17 patients. Where discomfort was present, it was attributable to neighboring diseased joints.

At the time of latest follow-up, 18 wrists showed no signs of radiolucency or loosening around the carpal component. Nonprogressive osteolysis was observed in 2 patients around the tip of the radial screw into the index finger metacarpal. Progressive carpal component subsidence and osteolysis was seen in 1 patient at 1 and 7 years' follow-up. The subsidence resulted in progressive radial inclination of the carpal component, yet the patient remained asymptomatic at the time of latest follow-up. Stress shielding of the radial styloid was also observed in 2 patients, with no signs of radial component loosening. In this series, there were no dislocations or surgical revisions of the components.

ReMotion TWA

The ReMotion TWA (SBI, Morrisville, PA) implant was designed to allow some degree of intercarpal rotation. The polyethylene ellipse snaps securely on a ball on the proximal side of the carpal plate, allowing 10° of relative rotation. Acting like a dampener, it avoids torque transmission to the carpal component. The relative axial motion

between the polyethylene and the carpal plate is believed to preserve the complex "dart thrower's" motion of the wrist.[15] Distal fixation is achieved by a central press-fit stem into the capitate and flanking variable-angle screws that allow compression between the carpal plate and remaining carpus. The radial component has 10° of palmar tilt and radioulnar inclination to approximate the native wrist (**Fig. 1**). Conferring further stability, bony resections are minimal, allowing preservation of the important ligaments of the wrist. Preservation of the rim of the distal radius is a key feature of the ReMotion implant.

In a prospective, nonrandomized series, Herzberg[16] reported early results using the ReMotion TWA. Although 22 procedures (21 patients) were performed between 2004 and 2010, only 20 wrists (19 patients) had a minimum 1-year follow-up (mean of 32 months) and were included in the study. In the rheumatoid group of 13 wrists, the postoperative flexion-extension arc decreased to 53° from 65° preoperatively (postoperative extension was 31° compared with 35°) while postoperative ulnar and radial deviations increased (ulnar deviation 17° postoperatively compared with 13°, and radial deviation 4° compared with 2°). Wrist scores in this study improved by an average of 41%, and grip strength by 57%. Subjectively, 11 patients were much better and 2 patients were better.

In the nonrheumatoid group of 7 wrists, TWA was indicated for osteoarthritis (n = 2), failed proximal row carpectomy (n = 1), failed SLAC reconstruction (n = 2), and failed wrist arthroplasty (n = 2). In this group, all ranges of motion improved postoperatively. Wrist scores and grip strength improved only by an average of 27% and 8%, respectively. Subjectively, 4 patients were much better and 3 patients were better. The series was too small to allow statistical comparison.

Loosening was observed in 2 rheumatoid patients. At 18 months' follow-up carpal loosening was observed in 1 patient, accompanied by carpal

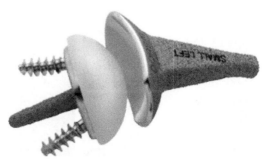

Fig. 1. ReMotion Total Wrist System (SBI, Morrisville, PA).

collapse and impaction across the carpometacarpal joints. This loosening remained relatively stable at 76 months' follow-up. At 12 months' follow-up radial component loosening was seen in the other patient, accompanied by impaction of the radial component into the distal radius without angulation of the implant. In both patients, the pain associated with loosening was not enough to necessitate surgical revision. No dislocations were noted in this series.

In a recent prospective, multicenter study, Herzberg[17] reported on early results using the ReMotion TWA in a larger cohort of patients. His review consisted of 129 rheumatoid and 86 nonrheumatoid patients with a minimum 2 years' follow-up. In the rheumatoid group, the quick-DASH score was 54 points and the postoperative flexion-extension arc was 58°. Grip strength improved by 40%, and periprosthetic osteolysis was seen 12% of rheumatoid patients. In the nonrheumatoid group the quick-DASH score was 21 points and the postoperative flexion-extension arc was 73°. Grip strength improved by 19%, and periprosthetic osteolysis was seen 18% of nonrheumatoid patients. At maximum follow-up, both groups had a survival rate of 92% for revisions. In the rheumatoid group 5% of cases had a complication requiring surgery, compared with 6% in the nonrheumatoid group. **Figs. 2–6** present radiographic and intraoperative images of a 47-year-old woman with rheumatoid arthritis undergoing TWA with the ReMotion TWA.

Maestro

The Maestro TWA (Biomet, Warsaw, IN) is the most recent FDA-approved implant. Its design mimics proximal row carpectomy and depends on replacement of the capitate head.[18] Joint articulation is achieved with a polyethylene proximal

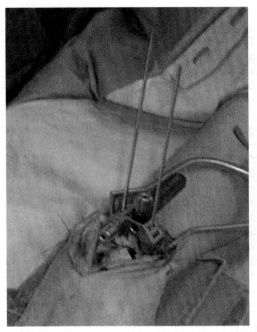

Fig. 3. Intraoperative imaging of the radial cutting block aligned with the dorsal surface of the radius with Kirschner wires using the ReMotion Total Wrist System (SBI, Morrisville, PA). (*Source from* Virak Tan, MD; with permission.)

component seated into the radius. Fixed and variable locking screws enhance distal component fixation. The Maestro TWA is highly modular, allowing for its use in total wrist and carpal hemiarthroplasties. Available for general use in 2004, clinical outcomes and complications are limited to early follow-up.

Nydick and colleagues[2] reported on 23 implants in 22 patients all receiving the Maestro TWA implant. All patients were available for review at an average follow-up of 28 months (range 4–55 months). All patients reported overall improvement in pain, with

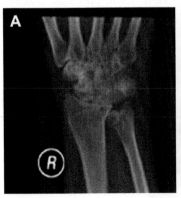
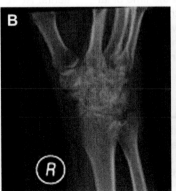
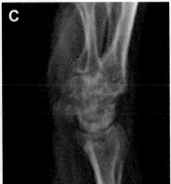

Fig. 2. (*A–C*) Posteroanterior, oblique, and lateral preoperative radiographs of a 47-year-old woman with severe painful rheumatoid arthritis of the wrist. (*Source from* Virak Tan, MD; with permission.)

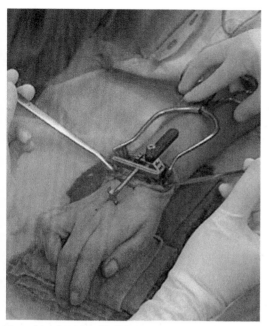

Fig. 4. Preparation of the carpal osteotomy with the saddle placed over the third metacarpal shaft. (*Source from* Virak Tan, MD; with permission.)

mean scores on the Visual Analog Scale for Pain improving from 8.0 to 2.2. All ranges of motion improved postoperatively with the exception of flexion, which slightly decreased postoperatively (45° preoperatively compared with 43° postoperatively). Only radial deviation improved to statistical significance. Grip strength averaged 60% of the contralateral side. The DASH and Mayo wrist scores were 31 and 54, respectively. Preoperative grip

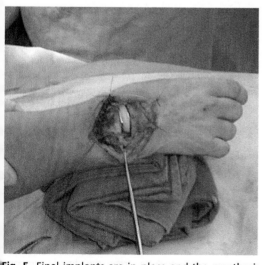

Fig. 5. Final implants are in place and the prosthesis has been reduced. (*Source from* Virak Tan, MD; with permission.)

strength and wrist scores were unavailable for review.

Radiographs at the latest follow-up visit revealed no evidence of prosthetic loosening. Complications occurred in 7 of 23 wrists (30%). Wrist contracture was the most common complication, occurring in 4 of 23 cases. Prosthetic failure caused by deep infection was seen in 1 patient with a prior history of intercarpal fusion. The remaining complications were due to synovitis and instability, in 1 patient each. Synovitis occurred secondary to a loose second metacarpal-carpal nonlocking screw in a patient with primary osteoarthritis. Volar wrist dislocation occurred in a patient with rheumatoid arthritis secondary to a fall shortly after surgery. After closed reduction and extension splinting, there was no recurrent instability.

This series reported not only on promising early results using the Maestro implant but also on promising results in nonrheumatoid patients. In this study, 18 of 23 implants were placed for nonrheumatoid arthritis, with the overwhelming majority placed for posttraumatic wrist arthritis secondary to SNAC (scapholunate advanced collapse) (n = 8) and SLAC (scaphoid nonunion advanced collapse) (n = 5) patterns of arthritis.

DISCUSSION

Although the wrist was among the first joints treated by prosthetic replacement, the evolution of TWA has lagged advancements made in large joint replacements because of the lower prevalence of symptomatic wrist arthritis and the ease and predictability of arthrodesis.[11] Since its first design, TWA has undergone considerable improvements in material, design, and surgical technique that have improved implant longevity. Although early and/or midterm results of newer third-generation implants are hopeful, it remains to be seen whether they can withstand the test of time with long-term follow-up. Numerous investigators have reported patient preference of wrist arthroplasty over arthrodesis. In the case of bilateral wrist and/or concomitant shoulder and elbow arthritis, advances in wrist arthroplasty are paramount for such patients wishing to continue to participate in activities of daily living. To help elucidate this debate, the future requires large, prospective, multicenter trials with long-term follow-up, identifying a durable and predictable prosthesis, followed by large prospective trials comparing replacement with fusion. Advances in implant design have accompanied the advances in surgical technique. Menon not only limited distal fixation to the carpus and the base of the

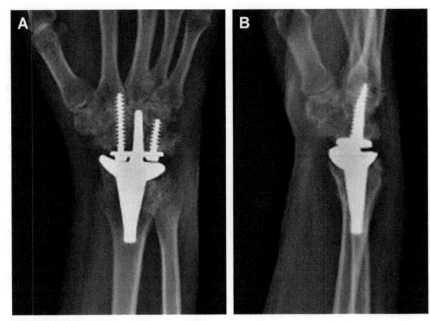

Fig. 6. (*A*) Anteroposterior and (*B*) lateral postoperative radiographs at 6 months' follow-up. (*Source from* Virak Tan, MD; with permission.)

metacarpals, he also introduced the concept of intercarpal fusion. Carpal fixation eliminated the longer lever arm associated with long stems extending into the metacarpal shafts. Intercarpal fusion provided a solid bony foundation for the carpal component. Both techniques have reduced early carpal component loosening and subsidence. In the future, it may be worth investigating the role of modern techniques in bone grafting and fusion with intercarpal arthrodesis. Furthermore, clinicians must await long-term results of wrist arthroplasty performed in nonrheumatoid conditions with better bone stock and radiocarpal alignment, yet higher demands. The future remains hopeful, and "as we continue to strive for improvements in design and [when] long-term results show these designs to work, indications for wrist arthrodesis will decrease and those for wrist arthroplasty will [continue to] increase."[15]

SUMMARY

TWA is an alternative to wrist arthrodesis in patients with painful, debilitating panarthritis of the wrist. In patients with bilateral wrist and/or concomitant upper extremity disease, it may be essential. Although challenges with wrist instability and prosthetic dislocations have largely been overcome, carpal component loosening remains an obstacle to good and predictable long-term survival. In reviewing the design rationales and recent outcomes of the 3 currently approved implants, only time will

tell if these implants will further the advances in wrist arthroplasty.

REFERENCES

1. Ferreres A, Lluch A, del Valle M. Universal total wrist arthroplasty: midterm follow-up study. J Hand Surg Am 2011;36:967–73.
2. Nydick JA, Greenberg SM, Stone JD, et al. Clinical outcomes of total wrist arthroplasty. J Hand Surg Am 2012;37(8):1580–4.
3. Adams BD. Total wrist arthroplasty. J Am Soc Surg Hand 2001;1(4):236–48.
4. Murphy DM, Khoury JG, Imbriglia JE, et al. Comparison of arthroplasty and arthrodesis for the rheumatoid wrist. J Hand Surg Am 2003;28:570–6.
5. Cavaliere CM, Chung KC. A systematic review of total wrist arthroplasty compared with total wrist arthrodesis for rheumatoid arthritis. Plast Reconstr Surg 2008;122:813–25.
6. Palmer AK, Werner FW, Murphy D, et al. Functional wrist motion: a biomechanical study. J Hand Surg Am 1985;10:39–46.
7. Cavaliere CM, Chung KC. A cost-utility analysis of non-operative management, total wrist arthroplasty, and total wrist fusion in rheumatoid arthritis. J Hand Surg Am 2010;35(3):379–91.
8. Cavaliere CM, Chung KC. Total wrist arthroplasty and total wrist arthrodesis in rheumatoid arthritis: a decision analysis from the hand surgeons perspective. J Hand Surg Am 2008;33(10): 1744–55.

9. Menon J. Universal total wrist implant: experience with a carpal component fixed with three screws. J Arthroplasty 1998;13(5):515–23.

10. Menon J. Total wrist arthroplasty for rheumatoid arthritis. In: Saffer P, Amadio PC, Foucher G, editors. Current practice in hand surgery. London: Martin Dunitz Ltd; 1997. p. 209–14.

11. Divelbiss BJ, Sollerman C, Adams BD. Early results of the Universal total wrist arthroplasty in rheumatoid arthritis. J Hand Surg Am 2002;27: 195–204.

12. Grosland NM, Rogge RD, Adams BD. Influence of articular geometry on prosthetic wrist stability. Clin Orthop Relat Res 2004;421:134–42.

13. Ward CM, Kuhl T, Adams BD. Five- to ten-year outcomes of the Universal total wrist arthroplasty in patients with rheumatoid arthritis. J Bone Joint Surg Am 2011;93(10):914–9.

14. Adams BD. Total wrist arthroplasty. Orthopedics 2004;27(3):278–84.

15. Gupta A. Total wrist arthroplasty. Am J Orthop 2008; 37(Suppl 8):12–6.

16. Herzberg G. Prospective study of a new total wrist arthroplasty: short term results. Chir Main 2011; 30(1):20–5.

17. Herzberg G. Promising preliminary results seen with last generation wrist arthroplasty implant. Orthopedics Today 2012;32(10):18.

18. Stanley J. Arthroplasty and arthrodesis of the wrist. In: Green D, Wolfe S, editors. Green's operative hand surgery. 6th edition. Philadelphia: Elsevier; 2011. p. 454–60.

Total Elbow Arthroplasty for Distal Humerus Fractures

Lori J. DeSimone, PA-C[a],
Joaquin Sanchez-Sotelo, MD, PhD[b],*

KEYWORDS

- Elbow • Arthroplasty • Joint replacement • Distal humerus fracture

KEY POINTS

- Total elbow arthroplasty provides a successful early outcome for most elderly patients with comminuted distal humerus fractures.
- The procedure typically involves resection of the fractured fragments, which allows implantation of the components without violation of the extensor mechanism.
- Life-long activity restrictions are recommended after elbow arthroplasty to minimize implant mechanical failure.
- Direct comparisons between internal fixation and arthroplasty for selected elderly patients with distal humerus fractures have shown better outcomes with arthroplasty.
- Mid-term and long-term studies do report several failures secondary to infection, loosening, and periprosthetic fractures.

INTRODUCTION

Fractures of the distal end of the humerus are serious injuries, with a high potential for a poor outcome and complications[1,2] due to a combination of confounding factors (**Box 1**). Internal fixation represents the standard of care for most distal humerus fractures.[2–4] However, total elbow arthroplasty has become increasingly popular for selected elderly patients when stable internal fixation is difficult to achieve due to osteopenia and comminution or to preexisting arthritic changes at the elbow.[3,5] Hemiarthroplasty of the distal humerus has also been contemplated for prosthetic replacement after distal humerus fractures.[3,6] However, the current published experience is limited, and the role of hemiarthroplasty is not covered in this article.

RATIONALE, PLUSES, AND MINUSES

Joint replacement is an accepted alternative for selected periarticular fractures, such as femoral neck, radial head, or proximal humerus fractures. As total elbow arthroplasty demonstrated a satisfactory track record for end-stage inflammatory arthritis, its indications were expanded to other conditions, including selected fractures of the distal humerus.[7]

Total elbow arthroplasty is indicated in elderly patients with distal humerus fractures with pre-existent symptomatic pathologic abnormality (ie,

Disclosures and Conflicts of Interest: The authors did not received payments or services, either directly or indirectly (ie, via their institution) from a third party in support of any aspect of this work. The authors' institution has had a financial relationship with entities in the biomedical arena (Zimmer and Tornier) that could be perceived to influence, or have the potential to influence, what is written in this work. The authors have had no other relationships or have engaged in no other activities that could be perceived to influence, or have the potential to influence, what is written in this work.

[a] Department of Orthopedic Surgery, Mayo Clinic, 200 First Street Southwest, Rochester, MN, USA; [b] Shoulder and Elbow Fellowship Program, Department of Orthopedic Surgery, Mayo Clinic, Gonda 14, 200 First Street Southwest, Rochester, MN 55905, USA
* Corresponding author.
E-mail address: sanchezsotelo.joaquin@mayo.edu

Orthop Clin N Am 44 (2013) 381–387
http://dx.doi.org/10.1016/j.ocl.2013.03.009
0030-5898/13/$ – see front matter © 2013 Elsevier Inc. All rights reserved.

Box 1
Challenges associated with fractures of the distal humerus

- Complex geometry of the distal humerus
- Involvement of the articular cartilage
- Comminution
- Osteopenia
- Exposure through the extensor mechanism
- Risk of ulnar neuropathy
- Risk of heterotopic ossification

a fractured rheumatoid elbow), low comminuted fractures with underlying osteopenia, and severe damage to the articular surface. It is contraindicated in fractures amenable to stable internal fixation, open fractures, and patients with anticipated high physical demands. The relative advantages and disadvantages of internal fixation and arthroplasty are summarized in **Table 1**.[3]

SURGICAL TECHNIQUE

The management of the fractured fragments at the time of total elbow arthroplasty has been a matter

Table 1
Advantages and disadvantages of internal fixation versus total elbow arthroplasty for distal humerus fractures

	Internal Fixation	Total Elbow Arthroplasty
Advantages	Durable No restrictions No prosthetic-related complications	Bone union not needed Quick return to ADLs Easier recovery Avoids nonunion/DJD
Disadvantages	Risk of nonunion Risk of posttraumatic DJD Risk of stiffness Requires intensive physical therapy	Mechanical failure Restrictions Higher infection rate

Abbreviations: ADLs, activities of daily living; DJD, degenerative joint disease.

of controversy in the past. The origin of the medial and lateral collateral ligament complexes is typically located in the fractured condyles. Implants that depend on the collateral ligaments for stability, or the condylar bone for implant fixation, may need to combine the arthroplasty with internal fixation of the fractured columns. However, this strategy requires more exposure, increases the complexity of the procedure, and requires fracture union for success.

Dr Bernard Morrey pioneered a completely different surgical strategy: the fractured fragments are resected and elbow stability is reestablished by using a linked implant designed so that humeral fixation does not require the integrity of the condyles (**Fig. 1**A).[7] The working space created by removing the fractured distal humerus provides enough exposure to prepare the humerus and ulna, and to implant the prosthetic components. Interestingly, removal of the origin of the forearm muscles both medially and laterally has not been demonstrated to impact grip, forearm strength, or elbow strength substantially. McKee and colleagues[8] compared 16 elbow replacements with preservation and 16 with resection of the condyles and found no differences in motion or strength. Because the extensor mechanism is not violated, the implants are cemented and linked, and bone union does not need to happen, patients can return to activities of daily living quickly, a major benefit in an elderly patient population that can hasten a quicker return to function and independence.

Exposure

The authors favor the use of a sterile tourniquet to avoid contamination of the surgical field if proximal extension of the skin incision is required. In the authors' practice, the ulnar nerve is routinely transposed in an anterior subcutaneous pocket. The posterior aspect of the joint is exposed under the triceps. The medial fractured fragments are resected subperiosteally, taking care to protect the integrity of the origin of the common flexor-pronator group (see **Fig. 1**A). The lateral fractured fragments are resected subperiosteally as well through Kocher interval. Most of the time, it is easier to deliver the humeral shaft through the medial window.

Component Implantation

Preparation of the humeral canal is straightforward using the instrumentation system of choice (see **Fig. 1**B). Ulnar preparation is more difficult with the triceps still attached to the olecranon, which is partly due to the bulk of the extensor mechanism

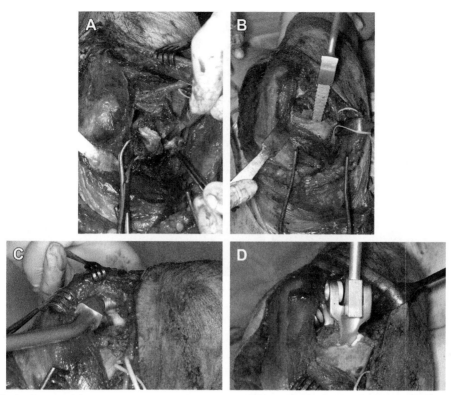

Fig. 1. (*A*) The fractured fragments are resected subperiosteally on each side of the triceps. (*B*) Humeral preparation is easy to complete through the medial paratricipital window. (*C*) Ulnar preparation can be more difficult unless a limited reflection of the medial edge of the triceps is performed. (*D*) The components can be implanted and linked leaving the triceps on.

and partly to the difficulty in rotating the forearm to provide exposure (see **Fig. 1**C). A helpful trick consists of raising subperiosteally off the olecranon approximately 20% of the triceps tendon from medial to lateral; by rolling the medial edge of the triceps laterally, the ulna is easier to rotate, and the integrity of the extensor mechanism is not markedly compromised.

Careful attention should be paid to component implantation in terms of both depth of insertion and rotation. On the ulnar side, the depth of insertion is easy to determine because the tip of the olecranon and the coronoid provides a very accurate reference; the component is inserted such that the center of rotation is equidistant from these 2 points. Rotationally, the ulnar component needs to be placed parallel to the flat dorsal aspect of the olecranon.[9]

On the humeral side, depth of insertion may be referenced off the roof of the olecranon fossa, but should be confirmed with intraoperative trials to assess soft tissue tension. With the trials in place and the elbow in 90° of flexion, moderate distraction can be applied by pulling up on the forearm, and the resting position of the humeral

trial may be recorded. The elbow should then be confirmed to extend fully, but without hyperextension. Humeral component rotation can be based off the posterior cortex, although there may be a difference of approximately 15°.[9]

The authors favor adding antibiotics and a catatonic dye to the bone cement used for fixation (1 g of vancomycin and 1 mL of methylene blue per batch of cement). Both canals are occluded with cement restrictors or a bone fragment, and the components are cemented in the desired position (see **Fig. 1**D). Once the cement has hardened, the implants are linked; the Kocher interval is repaired, and the common flexor-pronator group is carefully repaired to the medial triceps in an attempt to seal the joint fully (**Fig. 2**).

Postoperative Management

After surgery, the elbow is placed in a compressive dressing and kept in extension with an anterior plaster splint. The elbow is elevated using multiple pillows or hanging the arm. The arm should be brought down every couple of hours to avoid neurovascular complications. Patients start active and

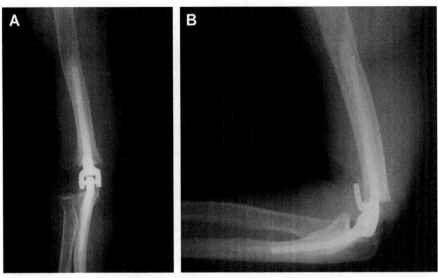

Fig. 2. Anteroposterior (*A*) and lateral (*B*) radiographs after elbow arthroplasty for a distal humerus fracture. Note the absence of the resected fractured condyles.

active-assisted range of motion exercises as tolerated within the first 2 days. However, priority is given to wound healing over motion, because most patients recover a functional arc of motion. Because infection can be such a devastating complication, elbows with severely compromised soft tissues are kept completely still until wound healing is confirmed.

Once recovered from surgery, patients are placed on weight restrictions indefinitely. Empirically, they are restricted from lifting with the affected side more than 5 to 10 pounds at a single event, and no more than 1 to 2 pounds repetitively.

OUTCOME AND COMPLICATIONS

Several peer-reviewed articles have reported the outcome and complications of total elbow arthroplasty for distal humerus fractures. Earlier publications reported short-term results. Some studies have compared elbow arthroplasty versus internal fixation in a limited number of selected patients. Information is now available regarding the outcome of this procedure at mid-term and long-term follow-up.

Short-Term Results

Cobb and Morrey first reported on a series of 21 distal humerus fractures in elderly patients treated using a semi-constrained total elbow replacement.[7] Mean range of motion was from 25 to 130°, and overall results were graded as excellent in 15 cases and good in 5 cases. The only complication reported in this study was a fractured ulnar

component. **Table 2** summarizes the information of additional studies, including 3 with almost universal satisfactory results at short-term follow-up.[10–12]

Comparative Studies

Two separate studies have compared internal fixation and arthroplasty.[13,14] Frankle and colleagues[13] compared 24 fractures in women older than 65 years treated with either internal fixation or replacement. The total elbow arthroplasty group was found to have superior motion and overall results. The average operative time was 2.5 hours for internal fixation versus 90 minutes for arthroplasty. In the internal fixation group, the following results were achieved: 4 of the 12 elbows had fair or poor results; mean extension was 30° (range, 10°–50°); mean flexion was 110° (range, 80°–120°); and there was one deep infection and 3 elbows salvaged with an arthroplasty. In the arthroplasty group, the following results were achieved: all elbows were rated as excellent (11) or good (1); mean extension was 15° (range, 0°–30°); mean flexion was 125° (range, 110°–130°); 2 elbows required debridement; and one elbow failed secondary to uncoupling of the linking mechanism.

McKee and coworkers published the only prospective randomized study to date.[14] Forty distal humerus fractures in patients over the age of 65 were randomized, with 20 elbows assigned to internal fixation and 20 elbows assigned to arthroplasty. There were 5 intraoperative conversions from internal fixation to arthroplasty. Elbow arthroplasty was associated with a significant reduction

Table 2
Results of total elbow arthroplasty for selected patients with distal humerus fractures

Study	Cases	Mean Age	Follow-up	ROM	MEPS	Comments
Short-term follow-up studies						
Cobb & Morrey,[7] 1997	21	72	3.3 y	25°–130°	Excellent 15, Good 5	Ulnar component fracture (1)
Ray et al,[10] 2000	7	82	3 y	20°–103°	Excellent 5, Good 2	Superficial infection (1)
Gambirasio et al,[11] 2001	10	84	17.8 mo	23.5°–125°	94 (80–100)	No complications
Garcia et al,[12] 2002	16	73	3 y	24°–125°	93 (80–100)	No complications
Comparative studies						
Frankle et al,[13] 2003	12	72	3.75 y	15°–120°	Excellent 11, Good 1	Disengagement (1) Superficial infection (2)
McKee et al,[14] 2009	25	77	2 y	26°–133°	86	Reoperations for stiffness (2) and deep infection (1)
Mid-term and long-term follow-up studies						
Kamineni & Morrey,[5] 2004	43	67	7 y	24°–132°	93	Revision in 5 cases
Streubel et al	25	67	10 y	30°–133°	79.3	Revision in 7 elbows Deep infection in 4 elbows

Abbreviation: ROM, range of motion.

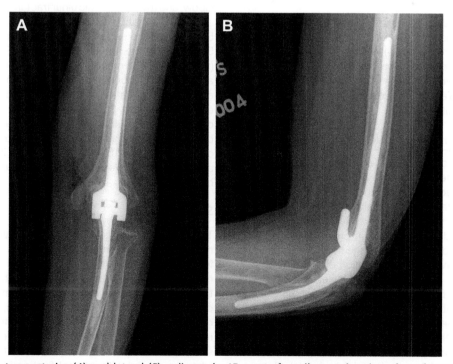

Fig. 3. Anteroposterior (*A*) and lateral (*B*) radiographs 15 years after elbow arthroplasty for a fracture of the articular surface of the distal humerus. The implants have remained well fixed.

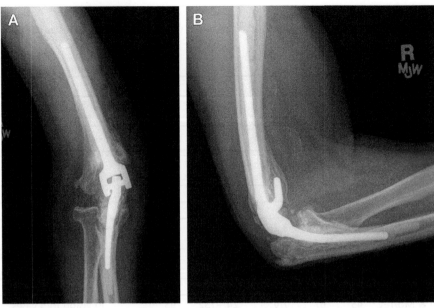

Fig. 4. Anteroposterior (*A*) and lateral (*B*) radiographs 5 years after elbow arthroplasty for a distal humerus fracture in an active male patient; note the presence of polyethylene wear.

in the operative time, better elbow scores (MEPS), and better early disability (DAHS) scores. There was a not statistically significant trend to better motion and less reoperations with arthroplasty as well. Three reoperations were required in the arthroplasty group for stiffness (2) and deep infection (1).

The results of these 2 studies seem to demonstrate that at short-term follow-up (3.75 and 2 years, respectively), elbow arthroplasty outperforms internal fixation in patients over the age of 65. However, these 2 studies fail to capture implant-related complications typically seen with longer follow-up.

Mid-term and Long-term Results

The Mayo Clinic experience, using a linked-semiconstrained total elbow arthroplasty for distal humerus fractures, has been updated twice. Kamineni and Morrey reported 43 elbows replaced at a mean age of 67 years and followed for a mean of 7 years.[5] The good clinical results in previous studies were confirmed, with an average MEPS of 93 points and an average arc of motion of 24° of extension and 132° of flexion (**Fig. 3**). However, revision surgery had been required in 5 elbows, and the overall complication rate was 29%.

Streubel and colleagues just updated the outcome of this procedure at the Mayo Clinic and specifically analyzed those elbows followed for a minimum of 5 years (unpublished data). Between 1982 and 2002, 43 consecutive linked semi-

constrained total elbow arthroplasties were performed for the treatment of a distal humerus fractures. In the first 5 postoperative years, 3 patients were lost to follow-up, 11 died with their implants in place, and 4 early failures occurred, including infection in 2 elbows, ulnar loosening in 1 elbow, and a periprosthetic ulnar fracture in 1 elbow.

For the 25 elbows followed for a minimum of 5 years (average follow-up, 9.7 years, range 5–15 years), the mean MEPS was 79.3 points (range, 35–100 points), and results were graded as excellent or good in 85% of the elbows. However, the complication rate was 38% and the reoperation rate was 31%. Complications included deep infection (4 elbows), aseptic loosening (5 elbows), and periprosthetic fractures (5 elbows). Reoperations included implant revision in 7 elbows, and irrigation and debridement or resection in 4 elbows (**Fig. 4**).

SUMMARY

Total elbow arthroplasty provides a relatively fast recovery and a predictable short-term outcome for elderly patients with a fracture of the distal humerus.[2,3,5,7,10–14] When performed through a triceps-on approach with fragment removal and cement fixation of a linked prosthesis, patients do not need much postoperative protection or rehabilitation. Comparative studies have demonstrated the superiority of elbow arthroplasty when compared with internal fixation in selected patients over the age of 65 followed for 2 to

4 years.[13,14] However, mid-term and long-term follow-up studies have documented an increasing number of failures over time. Infection seems to be the main complication in the first 5 years after arthroplasty, whereas aseptic loosening and peri-prosthetic fractures increase in frequency between 5 and 15 years after the procedure.[5]

Elbow arthroplasty will continue to play a role in the treatment of elderly patients with distal humerus fractures, especially for low-demand patients with severe osteopenia and/or preexistent elbow arthritis. However, improvements are required to continue to decrease the rates of infection and mechanical failure complicating this procedure. These improvements will likely require the use of implants with improved mechanical performance as well as refinement in the indications and postoperative care.

REFERENCES

1. Miller WE. Comminuted fractures of the distal end of the humerus in the adult. J Bone Joint Surg Am 1964;46:644–57.
2. Robinson CM, Hill RM, Jacobs N, et al. Adult distal humeral metaphyseal fractures: epidemiology and results of treatment. J Orthop Trauma 2003;17:38–47.
3. Sanchez-Sotelo J. Distal humeral fractures: role of internal fixation and elbow arthroplasty. J Bone Joint Surg Am 2012;94(6):555–68.
4. Sanchez-Sotelo J, Torchia ME, O'Driscoll SW. Complex distal humeral fractures: internal fixation with a principle-based parallel-plate technique. J Bone Joint Surg Am 2007;89(5):961–9.
5. Kamineni S, Morrey BF. Distal humeral fractures treated with noncustom total elbow replacement. J Bone Joint Surg Am 2004;86-A(5):940–7.
6. Burkhart KJ, Nijs S, Mattyasovszky SG, et al. Distal humerus hemiarthroplasty of the elbow for comminuted distal humeral fractures in the elderly patient. J Trauma 2011;71(3):635–42.
7. Cobb TK, Morrey BF. Total elbow arthroplasty as primary treatment for distal humeral fractures in elderly patients. J Bone Joint Surg Am 1997; 79(6):826–32.
8. McKee MD, Pugh DM, Richards RR, et al. Effect of humeral condylar resection on strength and functional outcome after semiconstrained total elbow arthroplasty. J Bone Joint Surg Am 2003;85-A(5): 802–7.
9. Sanchez-Sotelo J, Ramsey ML, King GJ, et al. Elbow arthroplasty: lessons learned from the past and directions for the future. Instr Course Lect 2011;60: 157–69.
10. Ray PS, Kakarlapudi K, Rajsekhar C, et al. Total elbow arthroplasty as primary treatment for distal humeral fractures in elderly patients. Injury 2000; 31(9):687–92.
11. Gambirasio R, Riand N, Stern R, et al. Total elbow replacement for complex fractures of the distal humerus: an option for the elderly patient. J Bone Joint Surg Br 2001;83:974–8.
12. Garcia JA, Mykula R, Stanley D. Complex fractures of the distal humerus in the elderly: the role of total elbow replacement as primary treatment. J Bone Joint Surg Br 2002;84:812–6.
13. Frankle MA, Herscovici D Jr, DiPasquale TG, et al. A comparison of open reduction and internal fixation and primary total elbow arthroplasty in the treatment of intraarticular distal humerus fractures in women older than age 65. J Orthop Trauma 2003;17(7): 473–80.
14. McKee MD, Veillette CJ, Hall JA, et al. A multicenter, prospective, randomized, controlled trial of open reduction–internal fixation versus total elbow arthroplasty for displaced intra-articular distal humeral fractures in elderly patients. J Shoulder Elbow Surg 2009;18(1):3–12.

years.[?] However, mid-term and long-term follow-up studies have documented an increasing number of these loose implant inserts to be the most common[?] with that 5 years after arthroplasty will ensue despite loosening and periprosthetic fractures increase in frequency between 4 and 5 years after the procedure.[?]

Elbow arthroplasty will continue to play a role in the treatment of distal humerus with distal humerus fractures, especially for low-demand patients with severe comminution and/or preexisting elbow arthritis. However, improvements are required to continue to decrease the rates of infection and mechanical failure complicating this procedure. These improvements will likely require the use of implants with improved mechanical performance as well as refinement to the indications and techniques.[?]

REFERENCES

1. [illegible reference text]
2. [illegible reference text]
3. [illegible reference text]

Reverse Shoulder Arthroplasty

Claudius D. Jarrett, MD[a,b], Brandon T. Brown, BS[c],
Christopher C. Schmidt, MD[d,*]

KEYWORDS

- Reverse shoulder arthroplasty • Implant designs • Cuff tear arthropathy • Shoulder arthritis
- Rheumatoid arthritis • Revision shoulder arthroplasty • Cuff deficient shoulder
- Proximal humerus fractures

KEY POINTS

- The reverse shoulder replacement changes the position of the normal shoulder joint by placing a sphere on the glenoid that articulates with a humeral socket.
- The reverse prosthesis provides a medial and distal fixed axis of rotation that improves deltoid function.
- Inferior glenosphere placement with inferior tilt, lateralizing the center of rotation, and a more varus humeral component may improve impingement, free range of motion, and minimize scapula notching.
- Appropriate deltoid tensioning decreases the risk for postoperative instability, nerve palsy, or acromial stress fractures.
- Focusing the postoperative rehabilitation on strengthening the anterior deltoid and pectoralis major can increase arm flexion, whereas strengthening the posterior deltoid in abduction increases external rotation.

INTRODUCTION

The reverse shoulder arthroplasty (RSA) has revolutionized reconstructive shoulder surgery. Secondary to promising clinical results, the reverse shoulder prosthesis has generated a great deal of enthusiasm in a relatively short period of time.[1–5] Initially recommended for patients with rotator cuff arthropathy, surgeons have expanded its application to massive cuff tears without arthritis, fracture care, rheumatoid arthritis, and failed prior surgery replacements with a high level of success.[6–16] An RSA flips the normal shoulder ball and socket anatomy. The design of the reverse prosthesis places the ball in the socket position and conversely positions the socket in the ball position. This stabilization design results in a semiconstrained prosthesis that stabilizes the glenohumeral center of rotation analogous to a functioning rotator cuff (**Fig. 1A–C**).[17] This effectively prevents superior migration of the humerus on the glenoid and thereby maintains the deltoid muscle's resting length (see **Fig. 1C**). The deltoid muscle, now restored to its anatomic resting length, can compensate for the rotator cuff deficiency. The RSA commonly provides rotator cuff patients with significant improvement in forward elevation and decrease in pain. Several clinical studies have reported considerable enhancement in activity and quality of life following a successful

Disclaimers: None.
[a] Upper Extremity Reconstructive Surgery, The Emory Orthopaedic Center, Emory University School of Medicine, 59 Executive Park South, Suite 2000, Atlanta, GA 30329, USA; [b] Department of Orthopaedic Surgery, The Emory Orthopaedic Center, Emory University School of Medicine, 59 Executive Park South, Suite 2000, Atlanta, GA 30329, USA; [c] Department of Orthopaedic Surgery, Swanson School of Mechanical Engineering and Material Science, University of Pittsburgh, 637 Benedum Hall, 3700 O'Hara Street, Pittsburgh, PA 15261, USA; [d] Orthopedic Specialist, UPMC, 9104 Babcock Boulevard, Suite 5113, Pittsburgh, PA 15237, USA
* Corresponding author.
E-mail address: cschmidthand@comcast.net

Orthop Clin N Am 44 (2013) 389–408
http://dx.doi.org/10.1016/j.ocl.2013.03.010
0030-5898/13/$ – see front matter © 2013 Elsevier Inc. All rights reserved.

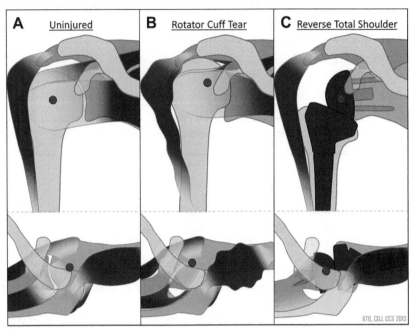

Fig. 1. (*A*) Normal functioning rotator cuff preserving the native shoulder center of rotation (*red dot*). (*B*) Rotator cuff–deficient shoulder with pathologic proximal migration of the center of rotation, top (*red dot*). Notice the pathologic anterior humeral head position, bottom (*red dot*). In this setting, the deltoid loses its mechanical advantage and is unable to successfully elevate the arm. (*C*) The RSA medially and distally placing a fixed center of rotation (*red dot*), which restores the deltoid's resting length, decreases its workload, and improves its function.

RSA.[1–5,18] In fact, patients following an RSA resume an activity level similar to patients' activity level after a traditional hemiarthroplasty or total shoulder replacement.[19] The commonly reported activities starting from low and progressing to high demand included cooking, baking, driving, gardening, leaf raking, lawn mowing, snow shoveling, wheelbarrow use, and shoveling dirt.[19] Although extensive long-term data are not available, short to intermediate outcome studies suggest that the survivorship of the reverse shoulder implant is comparable with hemiarthroplasty and total shoulder replacements.[3–5,20–25]

CAN AN RSA REPLACE THE ROTATOR CUFF?

The minimally constrained nature of the native shoulder joint allows a nearly limitless possible array of arm positions. The rotator cuff muscles play a key role in accomplishing this balance between mobility and stability. For most day-to-day activities, patients typically need the ability to elevate their arm approximately 120° in front of their body as well as 120° out to the side (**Fig. 2**).[26] Internal and external rotation of the shoulder are also required for many activities of daily living (ADLs). Most ADLs require approximately 60° of shoulder external rotation,

particularly when the elbow is away from the body, like washing ones hair, and 100° degrees of internal rotation when the arm is by one's side, such as putting on a belt, fastening a bra, or reaching to one's back pocket.[26]

When the rotator cuff is no longer functional, patients can lose this ability to actively elevate their shoulders to 90°; this loss of motion has been coined *pseudoparesis* (**Fig. 3**A). Following a reverse shoulder replacement, most patients regain the ability to elevate their shoulder again with minimal discomfort (see **Fig. 3**B, C). Postoperatively, studies have shown that patients can anticipate approximately 120° to 150° of active shoulder forward flexion and abduction with restoration of many ADLs.[1–5,18] In contrast to shoulder elevation, improvement of shoulder external and internal rotation can be limited following an RSA. Studies have shown minimal improvement in shoulder external rotation (as little as 2° to up to 31° postoperatively). Thus, the RSA cannot completely replace the native functional rotator cuff.[27–31]

HOW DOES IT WORK?

In the normal shoulder, the rotator cuff muscles provide a dynamic balanced force couple that

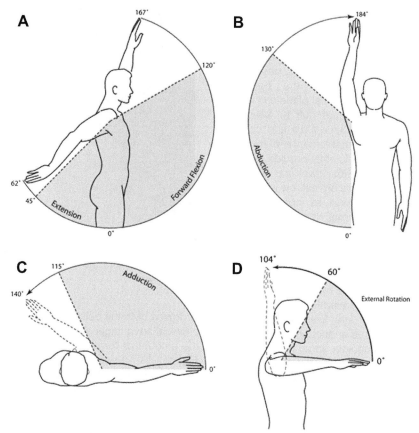

Fig. 2. Functional range of shoulder motion (*shaded*) compared with the normal anatomic range of motion in (*A*) flexion and extension, (*B*) abduction, (*C*) cross-body adduction, and (*D*) external rotation with the arm abducted at 90°. (*From* Namdari S, Yagnik G, Ebaugh DD, et al. Defining functional shoulder range of motion for activities of daily living. J Shoulder Elbow Surg 2012;21:1177–83; with permission.)

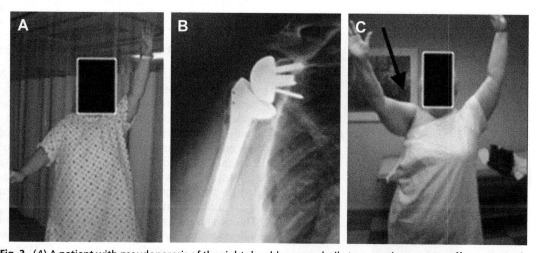

Fig. 3. (*A*) A patient with pseudoparesis of the right shoulder secondarily to a massive rotator cuff tear. Notice her inability to elevate the shoulder pass 90°. (*B*) A radiograph showing her RSA. (*C*) A postoperative picture depicting significant improvement in right shoulder elevation following surgery. Notice pseudoparesis is absent (*arrow*).

keeps the humeral head centered on the glenoid socket throughout all ranges of motion (see **Fig. 1**A). The glenohumeral joint is balanced in the axial plane by the subscapularis, anteriorly, and the infraspinatus and teres minor, posteriorly. The supraspinatus completes the balanced compressive force in the coronal place and counteracts the deltoid vector of pull to keep the humeral head center.[32] These axial and coronal force couples maintain a stable center of rotation, allowing the deltoid to efficiently provide a rotary force to elevate the arm with power and direction. The rotator cuff also plays a pivotal role in initiating shoulder abduction as well as controlling the needed internal and external rotation to position the hand in space.[33] When the rotator cuff function is compromised, such as with a massive tear, this normal balanced compressive force is lost. In this scenario, the deltoid losses its mechanical advantage and ability to provide a rotation torque to the arm (see **Fig. 1**B). Consequentially when patients attempt to elevate their arm, the deltoid pulls the humerus proximally, rather than rotating it, and leads to the classic shoulder shrug (**Fig. 4**). Overtime, this eccentric load across the shoulder joint results in superior glenohumeral instability, pathologic articulation of the humeral head with the acromion, and arthritis (**Fig. 5**).

The RSA directly addresses the altered kinematics of the rotator cuff deficient shoulder. The reverse ball and socket is a semi-constrained implant that provides a new fixed center of rotation.[34] Most modern reverse shoulder replacements medialize and distally place the center of rotation to a certain degree.[35] This modification

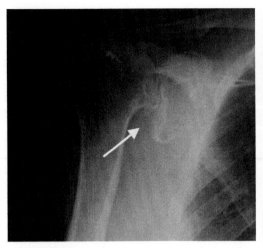

Fig. 5. Radiograph showing anterior superior migration of the humeral head (*arrow*) in relation to the glenoid fossa.

improves both the deltoid's moment arm (the mechanical advantage) and tension while decreasing the amount of force required for abduction (see **Fig. 1**C).[36–38] Research has shown that the RSA decreased the force required for abduction by approximately 30%.[38] Additionally, the change in the deltoid's vector of pull allows it to recruit more anterior and posterior fibers for flexion and abduction.[36–38] These changes significantly improve the deltoid's ability to raise the arm.[37,38] This biomechanical effect is also particularly important during the initiation phase of arm elevation. In the native shoulder, the rotator cuff supraspinatus tendon plays a key role in initiating shoulder elevation.[33] Following the RSA, the deltoid is now better suited to initiate shoulder abduction even without a functional supraspinatus.[36–38]

DESIGN FEATURES THAT IMPACT OUTCOME

The reverse shoulder replacement consists of 3 main components: the baseplate, the glenosphere, and the humeral socket (**Fig. 6**A–F). The baseplate is a metal-backed plate that directly contacts the glenoid. Varying design options of the baseplate include a flat or convex radius of curvature. The convex baseplate improves bony contact, whereas a more flat baseplate, depending on the design, may actually preserve more bone stock during reaming and implantation.[39] The convex baseplate design may also transmit a more compressive force (as opposed to a shear force) at the baseplate-bone interface.[40] Modern baseplates are secured to the glenoid with cementless fixation but are coated on the backside to allow bony ingrowth. The baseplate is typically

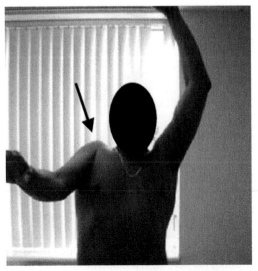

Fig. 4. A patient with a typical shoulder shrug (*arrow*) because of loss of the axial and coronal force couples.

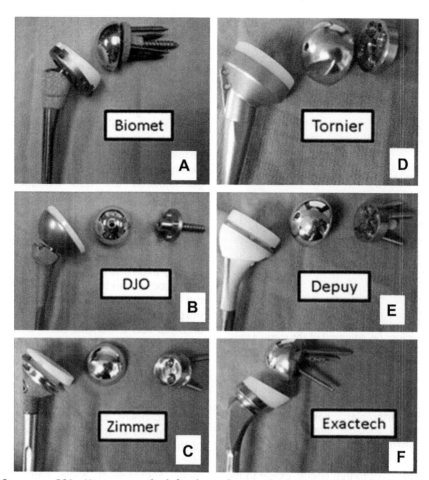

Fig. 6. The 6 common RSAs. Humerus on the left, glenosphere in the center, and baseplate on the right.

stabilized to the glenoid via a press-fit central post, keel, or central screw. Depending on the implant design chosen, up to 6 peripheral nonlocking or locking screws can be used for added compressive fixation strength, which has been shown to minimize the baseplate-glenoid micromotion and encourages bony ingrowth.[41] This modern baseplate design has minimized the risk for premature baseplate failure.[5] Some implants allow the peripheral baseplate screws to be freely redirected to locations within the scapula of increased bone stock. If variable angle screws are used, the screws should be directed to 1 of 3 columns: the base of the coracoid, the scapula spine, and/or down the lateral scapula pillar (**Fig. 7**).[42] The Tornier Aequalis (Tornier, Inc Bloomington, MN), the Depuy Delta XTEND (Depuy, Inc Warsaw, IN) and the Trabecular Metal Reverse (Zimmer, Warsaw, IN) systems all provide baseplates with a central post (see **Fig. 6**A–F). All 3 systems allow multiple peripheral screws to augment fixation. The Reverse Shoulder Prosthesis (DJO, LLC, Vista, CA) has a baseplate with a central 6.5 mm

cancellous screw. The technique allows bicortical fixation of the central screw when directed to exit along the medial anterior cortex of the scapula. In this system, 4 additional peripheral locking screws promote secure fixation of the baseplate. The Exactech Equinoxe Reverse Shoulder's baseplate (Exactech, Inc Gainesville, FL) provides a unique central post cage that secures in the glenoid vault and encourages bony ingrowth, whereas the Comprehensive (Biomet, Inc, Warsaw, IN) has a central boss that accepts a 6.5 modular central screw. There is no clear clinical data that compares the durability of the different baseplate designs. It is the authors' opinion that they are all very similar, and the patients' scapular anatomy and the surgeon's comfort level should decide whether one design should be used over another.

The glenosphere (see **Fig. 6**A–F) secures into the baseplate and becomes the new articulating ball. Glenosphere options vary in shape and design. Depending on the design chosen, they can place the new center of rotation directly on

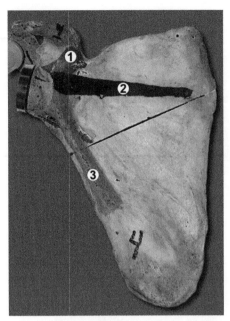

Fig. 7. Three regions (ie, columns) of the scapula most suitable for achieving strong screw purchase for optimal baseplate fixation: (1) the base of the coracoid, (2) the spine of the scapula, and (3) the scapular pillar. (*From* Humphrey CS, Kelly JD 2nd, Norris TR. Optimizing glenosphere position and fixation in reverse shoulder arthroplasty, part two: the three-column concept. J Shoulder Elbow Surg 2008;17: 595–601; with permission.)

the glenoid surface or further lateral, closer to the native shoulder. The Tornier Aequalis, Exactech Equinoxe, and Depuy Delta XTEND place the center of rotation at the surface of the glenoid. The DJO Reverse, Biomet Comprehensive, and Zimmer Trabecular Metal reverse implants allow the surgeon the option of shifting the center of rotation further lateral away from the glenoid with a built-in offset. The further away the center of rotation is placed from the glenoid surface, the higher the shear force at the glenoid/baseplate interface.[43] Studies have shown that with modern fixation techniques, the increase in micromotion is minimal even when the center of rotation is placed up to 10 mm away from the glenoid surface.[43] Although the Exactech Equinoxe places the center of rotation at the glenoid surface, it lateralizes the humerus instead via a larger glenosphere and offset humeral socket, which, in theory, improves the deltoid's moment arm while allowing more room for impingement-free range of motion. Eccentric glenospheres are also available that allow controlled distal placement of the center axis without compromising the location of bone fixation.[44]

The humeral socket (see **Fig. 6A–F**) is the opposing articulating surface for the glenosphere. Varying thickness and offset options for the humeral socket can be used as needed to elongate the deltoid, lateralize the humerus, and achieve the desired soft tissue tension. The humeral socket engages into a humeral stem that can be cemented or press fit into the humeral canal. Secondary to the medialized center of rotation, semiconstrained design, and limited space available for motion, the humeral socket is at risk of impinging with the scapula as it articulates with the glenosphere. If the humeral socket is allowed to repetitively abut the scapula neck with the use of the artificial shoulder, bony erosion can take place (ie, scapula notching) (**Fig. 8A**).[7,45] The humeral socket-shaft angle can vary between approximately 130° to more than 150° depending on the implant chosen. The more valgus (~150°–155°) humeral socket increases the deltoid tension by lengthening the acromion-humeral distance, which has been shown to improve active forward flexion and implant stability.[46,47] The more varus (~130°–140°) humeral socket more closely matches the native anatomic head neck angle. This varus angle seems to better minimize scapula

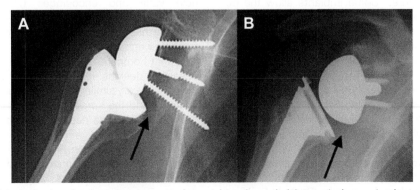

Fig. 8. (*A*) A typical valgus implant showing scapular notching (*arrow*). (*B*) A typical varus implant without scapular notching (*arrow*).

notching (see **Fig. 8**B).[46,48] The Tornier and Depuy reverse implants have a more valgus humeral socket-shaft angle, whereas the DJO, Zimmer, Biomet, and Exactech reverse implants have a more varus humeral socket-shaft angle.

SURGICAL TECHNIQUES THAT IMPACT OUTCOME

The current designs of the RSA are unable to completely compensate for all function lost in the rotator cuff–deficient shoulder. Following an RSA, improvement in external rotation of the shoulder varies considerably from patient to patient and depends on how much of the infraspinatus and teres minor (ie, external rotators) remain intact.[49] The medialization of the center of rotation, although improves elevation, limits the ability of the anterior and posterior deltoid fibers to contribute to internal and external rotation.[36–38,49] Researchers recently found that the RSA results in a considerable decrease in the ability of the deltoid and the remaining intact rotator cuff to contribute to shoulder external rotation.[49,50] Some current surgical techniques and implant designs attempt to offset this effect by minimizing the amount of medialization that occurs.[2,31,50] A lateralized center can be performed by either building out the glenoid with a bone graft or using a prosthesis with a built-in lateral center of rotation.[2,31,46,50] In theory, this allows the anterior and posterior deltoid fibers as well as the remaining intact rotator cuff to preserve their internal and external rotary line of pull.[2,3,31,50] Clinical results seem to support this concept by showing improved patient shoulder external rotation following the placement of a reverse prosthesis with surgical techniques that push the center of rotation further lateral.[2,3,31] However, lateralizing the center of rotation may not necessarily increase the activity level or variety of activities patients perform after an RSA.[19] Clear conclusive evidence on the benefit of lateralization is still somewhat elusive.

Preservation of the remaining rotator cuff, tendon transfers, and changing humeral version are other techniques to increase rotational motion and strength. The surgeon should attempt to preserve as much of the remaining posterior cuff as possible during reconstruction.[49] Researchers recently found that following a reverse total shoulder arthroplasty, the posterior deltoid may actually lose its external rotation function.[49] As a result, only the remaining teres minor and infraspinatus can provide any external rotation tasks during abduction postoperatively.[49] In the authors' hands as well as others, concomitant latissimus transfers

can significantly improve postoperative external rotation in patients with complete structural and functional loss of their infraspinatus and teres minor confirmed by magnetic resonance imaging.[51,52] Although patients can experience encouraging improvement in external rotation, achieving the level of rotation necessary for most ADLs continues to be difficult to achieve with this approach alone.[51,52]

Significant scapula notching has been associated with decreased clinical outcomes and premature baseplate failure and should be avoided if possible (see **Fig. 8**A).[7,45] To optimize results, the surgeon must focus on placing the glenoid baseplate and glenosphere in a position to maximize the impingement-free arc of motion. Several basic science studies have shown that placing the baseplate inferiorly on the glenoid with 15° to 30° of inferior tilt minimizes inferior scapular impingement.[46,53] Seeing that the scapula is a 3-dimensional structure, the effect of glenosphere positioning on anterior and posterior scapula impingement that occurs during internal and external rotation has also recently garnered attention. Li and colleagues[53] found that only inferior placement, inferior tilt, and lateralization best allowed impingement-free motion during internal and external rotation. Interestingly, a recent clinical study found that inferiorly tilting the glenosphere might not considerably impact the risk of inferior notching.[54] Fifty-two consecutive patients were randomized to undergo an RSA with or without an inferior tilt to the glenosphere. The severity of notching was graded at a minimum of 1 year postoperatively based on anteroposterior radiographs.[54] The investigators did not find a difference in the incidence of inferior notching between the two cohorts.[54] However, the effect of inferior glenosphere tilt on mechanical impingement and notching in other planes of motion (anterior or posterior) was not evaluated, thus preventing a true comparison. It also remains unclear how longer-term follow-up would impact their findings.[54] Although inferior tilt of the glenosphere may not avoid complete scapula impingement, it does have other added benefits. Slight inferior tilt seems to improve the compressive force at the baseplate/bone interface, assists in tensioning the deltoid, and, most importantly, prevent incidental superior tilt.

Much debate remains on whether a neutral version or a more retroversion is appropriate for the humeral socket. The native humeral version usually centers around 30° of retroversion. Limited clinical data suggest improved outcomes with a more neutral version.[55] Basic science investigations have found that version may not necessarily increase the internal and external impingement-free arc of motion but shifts an established range in the sagittal plane.[56,57] Increased retroversion seems to allow better external shoulder rotation at the expense of internal rotation.[56,57] Some investigators have proposed that for some patients this improvement in external rotation activities (eg, using the phone, washing hair, and so forth) is worthwhile, and the effect on most internal rotation activities would be negligible.[57] Humeral sockets positioned with a more neutral version have been shown to allow increased shoulder internal rotation but loss of external rotation, particularly with the shoulder adducted.[56,57] However, neutral version does not significantly impact shoulder external rotation in the more important abducted position.[56] A more neutral version may allow improvement of internal rotation activities that require positioning the hand in front or behind the body (ie, personal hygiene) without sacrificing external rotation activities that occur with the arm abducted (eg, using a phone, washing hair, and so forth).[56]

INDICATIONS
Rotator Cuff Disease With and Without Arthritis

Cuff tear arthropathy (CTA) and massive cuff tears with pseudoparalysis remain the most common and best indications for a reverse shoulder replacement. CTA entails a constellation of findings, including rotator cuff dysfunction, proximal and anterior escape of the humeral head, end-stage arthritis, and pseudoparalysis (**Fig. 9**A). Older patients may also present with massive irreparable rotator cuff tears and loss of active arm elevation (pseudoparalysis) without end-stage arthritis. The RSA can provide considerable improvement in function and quality of life in these patients (see **Fig. 9**B). However, the treating

surgeon must remain attentive of critical technical concepts to maximize results.

In the setting of CTA, significant superior glenoid wear can occur, and this bone loss places the surgeon at an increased risk for inadvertent superior tilt positioning of the glenosphere.[58] Superior tilt has been shown to result in decreased arc of motion, increased medial scapular impingement, instability, and higher failure rates.[20,29,45,59] Detailed preoperative planning and assessment of the native glenoid wear pattern should heighten the surgeon's awareness. Preoperatively, radiographs and a 3-dimensional computed tomography scan will often reveal superior glenoid wear. Current glenoid drill guides may be unable to accommodate for significant glenoid superior wear and other techniques anatomic landmarks should be used to assist in appropriate positioning.[58] Intraoperatively, if patients are positioned in a complete upright position, the alignment drill bit should at least be placed parallel to the floor. A simple technique that the surgeon may use intraoperatively is appreciating the inferior smiley face that results following appropriate eccentric reaming. To avoid medialization of the baseplate by excessive reaming, bone graft from the humeral head can be inserted superiorly between the glenoid and baseplate. The authors have found the aforementioned technique very useful.

Numerous outcome studies following the result of the modern reverse shoulder replacement for patients with CTA report reproducible improvement in pain, active elevation, overhead function, and objective outcome scores.[1–5,18] In a large series, Wall and colleagues[1] reported greater than 90% satisfaction rate with an average postoperative active forward flexion of approximately 135°. After a minimum of a 5-year follow-up, Cuff and colleagues[5] found a significant improvement in American Shoulder and Elbow Society (ASES)

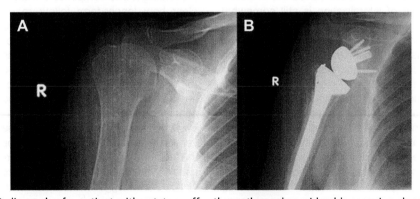

Fig. 9. (A) Radiograph of a patient with rotator cuff arthropathy and considerable superior glenoid wear. (B) Postoperative radiograph.

scores (from 31 to 77). The patients' ability to elevate their arms also significantly improved from 70° preoperatively to 150° at the final follow-up. Similar success has also been shown for elderly patients with massive irreparable rotator cuff tears without arthritis.[60] Caution should remain on implementing the reverse shoulder prosthesis, if pseudoparalysis is not present, because patients could risk losing the active elevation and rotation they had preoperatively.[60]

Rheumatoid Arthritis

The traditional unconstrained shoulder replacement in patients with rheumatoid arthritis leads to gradual superior migration of the humeral head secondary to a physiologically insufficient rotary cuff.[61] Betts and colleagues[61] reported a 100% occurrence of proximal of the artificial humeral head regardless of the index status of the rotator cuff. This progressive instability tends to correlate with a deterioration of function. This observation has fueled some to offer patients an RSA as a treatment alternative.[28,39,42,62,63]

Several studies have reported consistent improvement in objective measured outcomes and high patient satisfaction when using the RSA for rheumatoid arthritis.[10–14] With an average follow-up of nearly 4 years, Young and colleagues[10] reported improvement in active shoulder flexion from an average of 77° preoperatively to approximately 140° postoperatively, with a 94% patient satisfaction rate. Others have also reported similar success. Ekelund and Nyberg[11] found statistical improvement in both range of motion and pain in 23 patients with rheumatoid arthritis who underwent an RSA. Patients, on average, experienced improvement in active shoulder flexion of approximately 80° and a reduction in pain from an 8 to 1 on based the visual analog scale.[11] They reported a low risk for infection (~4%) despite their immune compromised cause.[11] Holcomb and colleagues[13] also found that postoperative shoulder elevation improved reliably from 52° to 126°, with an 86% success rate when they followed their patients for a minimum of 2 years.

Primary Glenohumeral Arthritis with Static Posterior Subluxation

Recently, investigators have highlighted the concerning results of using the traditional total shoulder replacement in the presence of primary shoulder arthritis with severe posterior glenoid erosion and static posterior glenohumeral subluxation.[64] Higher rates of postoperative posterior instability and premature glenoid failure were found in patients with considerable glenoid intermediate retroversion (>30°) or biconcave (type B2 glenoid)[64] "neo" glenoid retroversion (>27°).[64] These findings have caused some to propose using the reverse total shoulder replacement (TSR) as a more reliable surgical option for this subset of patients.[64]

Failed Shoulder Arthroplasty

The reverse shoulder prosthesis is now considered to be a viable alternative for patients with a failed prior shoulder replacement (**Fig. 10**A, B).[1,15,16,18,65,66] However, the lack of adequate humeral and glenoid bone stock as well as the absence of a functional rotator cuff, frequently encountered in the revision setting, adds a layer of added complexity. Improvements in both pain and function can be anticipated, but several important surgical concepts and techniques are often needed.[1,18]

In the revision setting, the surgeon may need to remove a well-fixed humeral component to implant an RSA. This task can be a daunting task that requires preservation of as much bone stock as feasibly possible that will support a new prosthesis. A useful technique that the authors find helpful involves using a vertical split osteotomy to facilitate component removal (**Fig. 11**A–C).[67] A longitudinal humeral unicortical osteotomy is started in the proximal edge of the bicipital groove with an osteotome down to the implant (see **Fig. 11**B). Multiple osteotomes are then used to twist, wedge, and "open book" the canal while preserving the medial cortex. This approach, although described for a cemented stem, can also be implemented for a press fit in the growth stem. This unicortical window allows access to the failed implant while creating a relatively small defect in the already compromised humerus.[67] The osteotomy is then closed with wires before cementing the implant (see **Fig. 11**C). Convertible implants are available in some systems that allow modular transformation of a hemiarthroplasty or traditional shoulder replacement into a reverse prosthesis (**Fig. 12**A, B).

Secondary to the frequent presence of a deficient proximal humeral bone stock, several technical options exist to augment native bone and improve fixation for the revised humeral stem. Tibial-strut allograft can be used to improve the stability and quality of the proximal humerus (**Fig. 13**).[15,68] In extreme cases of severe proximal humeral bone loss that also compromises the deltoid insertion, the authors' preference is to reconstruct using an allograft-prosthesis composite secured with cables and possibly a locking plate (**Fig. 14**).[15] Wires can be wrapped around the

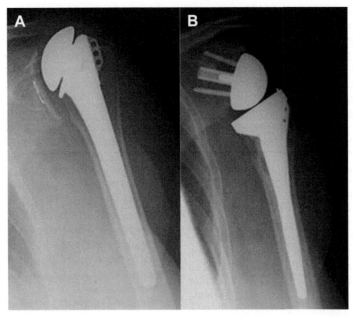

Fig. 10. (*A*) A radiograph of a loose glenoid and superior position of the humeral stem. (*B*) Revision with an RSA. Notice the glenoid defect was grafted with allograft femoral head and the baseplate post was driven into the native coracoid bone column.

distal aspect of the deltoid and provide the ability to repair the deltoid insertion to the allograft strut.[15] However, this more complex technique does come with the added cost of the graft, risk for infection, added operative time, and failure of allograft incorporation. Other researchers have found that allograft augmentation may not be necessary if the revision stem can be well secured in the remaining humeral shaft (see **Fig. 11**C).[69] Budge and colleagues[69] followed 15 patients with significant humeral bone loss that underwent a revision reverse TSA for a failed arthroplasty.

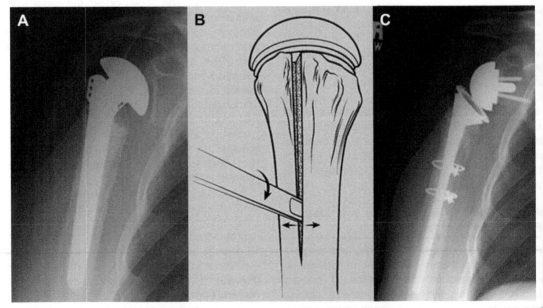

Fig. 11. (*A*) Well-cemented, painful hemiarthroplasty. (*B*) Vertical split open-book osteotomy allows removal of prior humeral component while preserving proximal bone stock. (*C*) Revision with RSA. Notice the cerclage wires closing the osteotomy. ([*B*] *From* Johnston PS, Creighton RA, Romeo AA. Humeral component revision arthroplasty: outcomes of a split osteotomy technique. J Shoulder Elbow Surg 2012;21:502–6; with permission.)

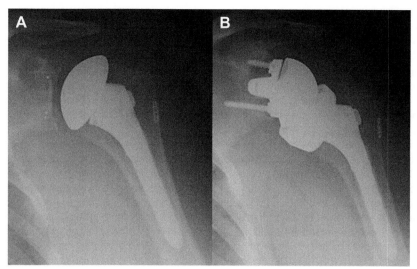

Fig. 12. (*A*) A painful total shoulder arthroplasty (TSA) secondary to loss of subscapularis function. (*B*) The use of a convertible humeral platform to revise the TSA to an RSA.

After a minimum of 2 years of follow-up, none of the patients showed evidence of humeral component subsidence or loosening. One patient did develop a prosthetic fracture of their modular humeral stem.[69] The authors encourage the use of a monoblock humeral component, if this approach is used, to mitigate the risk of implant failures and fractures.[69]

If insufficient glenoid bone stock is encountered, the surgeon may be at risk for overmedializing the baseplate, which increases the lateral force vector of the deltoid and may predispose the implant to dislocation. The coracoid can be used as an intraoperative landmark to avoid placing the baseplate too medial. If the residual glenoid bone stock has eroded near the coracoid, structural bone grafting

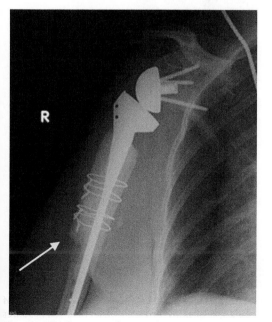

Fig. 13. Tibial-strut graft is used to improve proximal humeral bone stock.

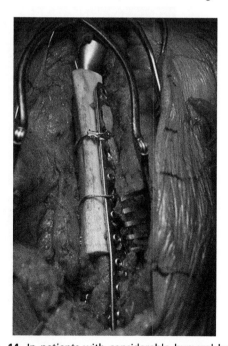

Fig. 14. In patients with considerable humeral bone loss, strut allograft–humeral component composite can be used to reconstruct the proximal humerus and stabilized with cerclage wiring, plate, and screws. (*From* Kelly JD 2nd, Zhao JX, Hobgood ER, et al. Clinical results of revision shoulder arthroplasty using the reverse prosthesis. J Shoulder Elbow Surg 2012; 21:1516–25; with permission.)

or using a lateralizing implant may be required to push the center of rotation further away from the midline. Norris and colleagues[70] and Boileau and colleagues[27] described a very useful technique of implementing a structural bone graft–baseplate composite to restore appropriate lateral offset in cases when greater than a centimeter of medialization has occurred secondary to severe glenoid erosion (**Fig. 15**). The baseplate with its central post and peripheral screws allows immediate stability of the structural graft to the scapula. In return, the structural graft improves the center of rotation and the deltoid tension.[70]

The surgeon must also appropriately focus on restoring adequate soft tissue tension to minimize the risk for postoperative instability, which can be particularly difficult to do in the revision setting.[71,72] The direction of instability is often described as occurring anteriorly.[73] However, considerably less force is required for lateral dislocation than anterior dislocation. Henninger and colleagues[36] found that it took 60% less force for lateral implant dislocation in comparison with anterior dislocation. Surgeons should assess for lateral instability in addition to other directions,

particularly with the arm at the side.[36,47] The treating surgeon has several technical options available to minimize the risk for instability. Research studies have found that lateralizing the center of rotation, increasing the acromion-humeral distance, or using a more valgus humeral socket has been shown to improve the deltoid tension, increase stability, and elevate the force required for dislocation.[36,46,47] During revision surgery, the restoration of appropriate arm length is a critical step in balancing the deltoid tension and preventing instability. However, this can be a difficult task to gauge secondary to significant humeral bone loss and lack of normal anatomic landmarks. Although subtle lengthening of the arm can be an effective tool for soft tissue balancing and stability, it should be conducted judiciously. Overlengthening can lead to complications, including acromial fatigue fractures, stiffness, and neurologic injury.[62,74] The authors have found that comparing full-length radiographs of the ipsilateral to the contralateral humerus can be a helpful guide in choosing the appropriate deltoid tension.[62,74]

Improvements in both function and quality of life have been reported when the RSA is used in the

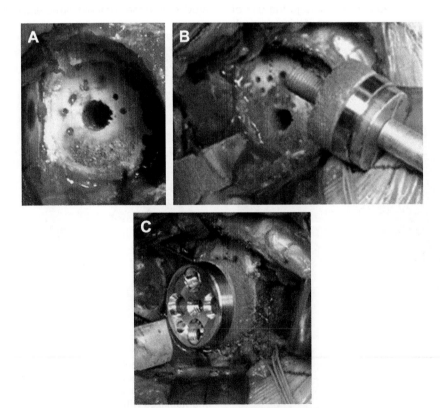

Fig. 15. A reamed glenoid (*A*), bone graft–baseplate composite (*B*), and implanted baseplate (*C*) now lateralized as a result of structural graft. (*From* Boileau P, Moineau G, Roussanne Y, et al. Bony increased-offset reversed shoulder arthroplasty: minimizing scapular impingement while maximizing glenoid fixation. Clin Orthop Relat Res 2011;469:2558–67; with permission.)

revision setting.[18] Boileau and colleagues[18] found improvement in arm elevation from an average of 55° preoperatively to 113° postoperatively. Objective outcome Constant scores also improved a statistical 32 points following a revision RSA.[18] Others have a reported a similar 60° improvement in active elevation postoperatively.[15,16] Patel and colleagues[16] reported a statistical improvement in all outcome measures at an average follow-up of approximately 40 months. In general, results following revision surgery are not as good as other indications, but patient-reported satisfaction rates are still quite gratifying. Kelly and colleagues[15] reported an 80% success rate in their series of revision surgery.

Acute Proximal Humerus Fracture and Fracture Sequelae

Early outcomes of applying the RSA for proximal humerus fractures in the elderly have garnered much enthusiasm.[6–9,75] The RSA in the acute setting can provide reproducible success rates and early recommencement of activity for the appropriate candidate (**Fig. 16**A, B).[6–9,75] Some of the major benefits of the RSA for proximal humerus fractures are that lack of tuberosity healing does not lead to functional disaster, as seen with hemiarthroplasty, and less restraints are needed during the early postoperative period.[8,9,76]

To optimize outcomes, several technical concepts should be remembered during reconstruction. Luckily in the fracture setting, the glenoid can be readily exposed to allow appropriate placement of the baseplate and glenosphere. However, more time and effort is often required on the

humeral side. The authors typically elbow flexed to 90° and use the forearm as a gauge of the epicondylar axis. The authors' goal is to retrovert the humerus between 0° and 30°. Next, the height of the humeral component can be properly set by reducing the medial calcar (humeral neck) and cementing the implant on top of the calcar. On rare situations whereby the medial calcar cannot be reduced, the authors position the height of the prosthesis so that the proximal lateral corner of the implant sits 5.6 cm above the superior border of the pectoralis major tendon.[77]

Although not obligatory to restore arm elevation, anatomic tuberosity healing does improve postoperative shoulder rotation.[8,9] The authors always attempt to anatomically repair the greater and lesser tuberosities to the humeral shaft analogous to a hemiarthroplasty (see **Fig. 16**B).[3,76] The cancellous portion of the fractured humeral head is an easily attainable source of autogenous bone grafting that can be placed at the tuberosity-metaphysis interface. To increase the bony surface area for tuberosity healing, a wedge-shaped portion of the native head can also be harvested and placed around the proximal implant as a horseshoe graft.[78] Further, balance should be found between appropriately lengthening the deltoid and positioning the humeral metaphysis proximal enough to allow anatomic reduction of the lesser and greater tuberosities. The authors typically leave the supraspinatus attached to the greater tuberosity as opposed to removing it, but this is controversial.[79]

The RSA for proximal humerus fractures has been shown to provide reliable, satisfactory results. Although an RSA may not achieve a level

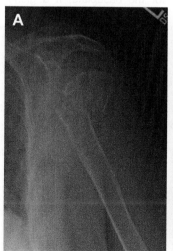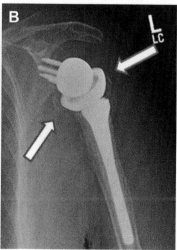

Fig. 16. Elderly osteoporotic patient with a 3-part proximal humerus fracture (A) after extensive consultation treated with a reverse shoulder replacement (B). Both greater and lesser tuberosities (*arrows*) are reduced and stabilized in attempts to improve active postoperative rotation.

of function as some hemiarthroplasties for fractures, it provides more predictable results and avoids catastrophic failures.[79,80] Patients can often anticipate a mean active elevation of approximately 90° to 120° with a high satisfaction rate.[7,9,75,78,80–84] Only a few studies provide direct comparison between hemiarthroplasty and the RSA for proximal humerus fractures.[80,82–84] Although some investigators did not find a significant difference between the two cohorts with a short-term (<2 years) follow-up,[80,83] others appreciated significantly better outcomes at a longer-term follow-up (>3 years) for the patients that underwent an RSA in comparison with a hemiarthroplasty.[82,84]

Treating patients with proximal humerus fracture malunions and nonunions continues to be a challenge with limited treatment options. The reverse shoulder prosthesis is now considered a welcomed alternative (**Fig. 17A, B**). Similar to the acute fracture, if the tuberosities can be easily mobilized, preserved, and restored to an anatomic position, attempts should be made to do so. Investigators have published reasonable satisfaction rates when applying the reverse shoulder in these scenarios.[1,18,85] Functional improvements were substantial but less significant in comparison with other diagnoses.[1,18] Martinez and colleagues[85] reported on a group of 18 patients who underwent an RSA for proximal humerus nonunions. They found that their patients experienced an average improvement in elevation from 35° to 90° postoperatively with a satisfaction rate just more than 75%.[85] The same group published a larger series of 44 patients treated with an RSA for sequelae of proximal humerus fractures and found similar results.[63] Shoulder abduction and forward elevation improved, on average, approximately 55° and 60°, respectively.[63] Thirty-eight of their 44 patients were either very satisfied or satisfied with their results.[63]

COMPLICATIONS

Some but not all complications include fractures, infections, instability, and nerve injuries.

Acromial fractures can present either early in the postoperative period or even more than a year from the index surgery.[86–89] Patients typically report an abrupt onset of intense lateral shoulder pain and a decline in function.[86–89] The diagnosis can be initially missed if radiographs are not specifically scrutinized for signs of cortical irregularity along the superior border of the acromion.[86–89] One should avoid overtensioning the deltoid and producing a tight shoulder to minimize the risk for acromial fractures in patients with weak bone. Most acromial stress fractures are minimally displaced and can be managed with immobilization in an abduction splint for 6 weeks. Significantly displaced or unstable acromial base fractures may warrant open reduction with internal fixation, but the literature is unclear with regard to the ultimate outcome.[86–89]

Periprosthetic fractures are of particular concern in patients with osteoporotic bone such as frequently encountered in rheumatoid arthritis. Both intraoperative fractures and postoperative fractures can occur at an elevated rate. The risk for intraoperative glenoid and humeral fractures can be decreases by placing close attention to surgical technique. Overzealous glenoid reaming should be avoided to preserve adequate fixation for the baseplate. If a glenoid fracture occurs,

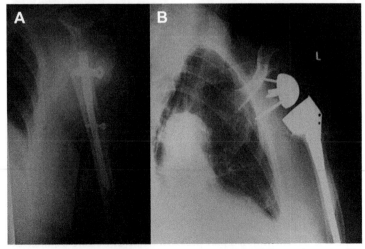

Fig. 17. (*A*) Patient with significant pain and loss of function secondary malunited proximal humerus fracture. (*B*) Patient underwent successful revision to RSA.

fragment-specific fixation or redirecting the baseplate and screws may allow for a sufficiently strong construct for bony ingrowth.[73] Minimizing extreme arm positioning while preparing the proximal humerus can prevent humeral fractures. Avoid forceful external rotation because this can easily result in a humeral shaft fracture (**Fig. 18**A). If fracture occurs before humeral implantation, then stabilization of the fracture with cerclage wiring or plate and screws should be performed before stem placement.[73] A longer stem may be necessary to bypass the fracture and ensure stable fixation distally. If fracture occurs after humeral seating and the implant is stable, the authors typically repair the fracture with plate, screws, and cerclage wires (see **Fig. 18**B).

The risk for postoperative infections remains a concern in RSA, particularly in patients that are immunocompromised or have undergone prior surgery.[90] The overall incidence of postoperative infection following an RSA ranges from approximately 1% to 12%.[6–16,75,90] The 2 more commonly cultured organisms are Staph species and *Propionibacterium acnes* (*P acne*).[90] A clear formal recommendation is not available; the authors currently chose to give either clindamycin or vancomycin for preoperative antibiotic prophylaxis instead of cefazolin sodium (Ancef) to more appropriately cover both common bacteria.[90–92] For patients at risk, the authors recommend the use of antibiotic cement when implanting the humeral stem. Studies have shown a statistically

decreased infection rate with the use of antibiotic cement in this scenario.[93] When an infection does occur, appropriate treatment can be a daunting task. Traditional general recommendations for a staged resection arthroplasty can lead to considerable bone and soft tissue loss, making a future reimplantation difficult and sometimes not feasible. Although limited, current data do support that if the baseplate and humeral stem are stable and patients are relatively healthy, retaining the major components may be possible regardless of the chronicity of the infection.[90] Zavala and colleagues[90] successfully treated 6 out of 8 infected RSPs using this approach. This approach should include a thorough debridement, liner/glenosphere exchange, and appropriate intravenous antibiotics.[90]

However, if the major components are loose or the patients' medical comorbidities decrease their ability to eradicate an infection, a more aggressive a 1- or 2-staged complete revision approach may be warranted. Beekman and colleagues[94] reported successfully eradicating infected RSA with a 1-staged revision, thus, preventing the need to expose patients to multiple anesthesias and surgical procedures. The authors currently prefer to perform a 2-staged revision with temporary placement of an antibiotic spacer (**Fig. 19**A–C). Multiple intraoperative cultures should be acquired to dictate appropriate antibiotic coverage. Cultures should be held for a minimum of 14 days to increase the accuracy of detecting *P acne*.[91,92]

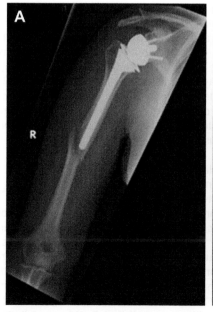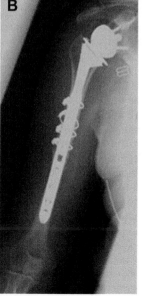

Fig. 18. (*A*) Periprosthetic humeral shaft fracture from excessive external rotation. (*B*) The fracture was stabilized with a hybrid locking plate–cerclage wiring construct and healed uneventfully.

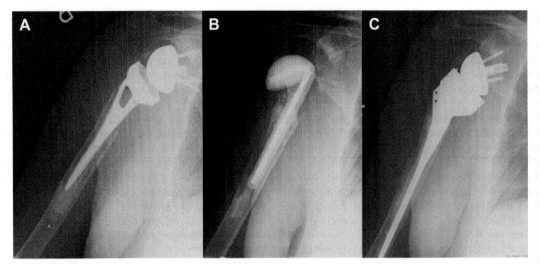

Fig. 19. (*A*) Radiographs showing gross humeral stem loosening caused by an infection. (*B*) First-stage revision with a temporary antibiotic spacer, (*C*) then later revised to a long-stem reverse shoulder replacement after the infection was successfully eradicated.

Resection arthroplasty tends to produce poor functional results and should be reserved for persistent infections or bone stock unsuitable to support a new prosthesis.[90,94]

Instability remains a vexing issue best avoided. Some investigators contribute the risk of instability to the status of the subscapularis.[54] Edwards and colleagues[54] found higher rates of implant instability with a compromised subscapularis. This finding may be a result of the compressive force couple that occurs to the subscapularis following implantation of a reverse shoulder prosthesis.[37] Ackland and colleagues[37] found that, after an RSA, the superior region of the subscapularis becomes an abductor, whereas the inferior and middle regions function as adductors. This co-contraction can generate a compressive at the joint surface and may improve shoulder stability.[37] However, other investigators have been unable to find a similar clinical correlation.[71] Clark and colleagues[71] reported that their incidence of postoperative instability was unaffected by the status of the subscapularis. This study matches the authors' clinical experience. Their results highlight the importance of appropriate deltoid tensioning over subscapularis repair for implant stability.[71] Another avenue the surgeon could consider to improve stability include implanting a more constrained humeral socket.[47]

Neurologic injury as a result of an RSA is thought to be a relatively underappreciated phenomenon.[18,95,96] Clinically evident symptoms have been reported to occur only in approximately 2% of cases, an incidence similar to that seen with the traditional total shoulder replacement.[18,97–99]

However, subclinical neuropathy has been shown to occur significantly more frequently following an RSA in comparison with a total shoulder replacement.[95] Nerve injury can occur during surgery as a result of surgical dissection, exuberant retraction, or arm positioning, particularly if a significant amount of preoperative soft tissue contractures exist.[96] Neurologic complaints can also occur as a result of lengthening the arm as the center of rotation is distally placed stretching traversing nerve axons.[95] This stretching may lead to symptoms in patients with occult preexisting peripheral nerve compression syndromes or occult cervical radiculopathy.[95] A thorough review of systems and physical examination may help in filtering out patients at risk. Most nerve injuries are thought to be partial brachial plexopathy and not an injury to a specific nerve.[18,95] Although intraoperative neuromonitoring has been reported, it has yet to decrease the incidence of postoperative neurologic injury.[96] Luckily, most neurologic complaints are transient and resolve with observation alone.[18,95,96]

POSTOPERATIVE REHABILITATION

With a well-positioned implant, a modest physician-directed home-therapy program is all that is needed for many patients and provides predictable results. Depending on the surrounding soft tissue and integrity of the subscapularis, some surgeons prefer a temporary period of immobilizing that ranges from 2 to 6 weeks. However, if the shoulder is well balanced intraoperatively, the senior author often successfully allows patients to wean out of their sling and initiate immediate active range of motion of their shoulder as pain allows.

Recent basic science work has reoriented the rehabilitation focus during the postoperative period. Following an RSA, the anterior deltoid and superior pectoralis major develop larger flexion moment arms during early flexion than they possessed in the native shoulder.[37] Interestingly, the superior subregion of the pectoralis major seems to become the most dominant shoulder flexor throughout flexion.[37] Emphasis on strengthening these muscles postoperatively may impart substantial shoulder flexion torque and improve patients' final active motion.[49]

Improving active shoulder external rotation continues to be an area of interest following the RSA. Most current designs considerably decrease the ability of the posterior deltoid to contribute with external rotation. Ackland and colleagues[37] found that the posterior deltoid subregion only participated in external rotation when the shoulder was in abduction. Rehabilitation focusing on strengthening active external rotation with the shoulder abduction may be more suited to maximize results.[49]

SUMMARY

The RSA provides substantial improvement in pain and overhead function in most patients. Although initially designed for the rotator cuff–deficient arthritic shoulder, its indications have broadened with promising results. Adhering to sound surgical techniques and remembering critical concepts allow the surgeon to maximize patient outcomes while minimizing complications. More long-term follow-up studies and basic science research are still needed because applications and surgical technique continue to evolve.

REFERENCES

1. Wall B, Nove-Josserand L, O'Connor DP, et al. Reverse total shoulder arthroplasty: a review of results according to etiology. J Bone Joint Surg Am 2007;89:1476–85.
2. Cuff D, Pupello D, Virani N, et al. Reverse shoulder arthroplasty for the treatment of rotator cuff deficiency. J Bone Joint Surg Am 2008;90:1244–51.
3. Frankle M, Siegal S, Pupello D, et al. The Reverse shoulder prosthesis for glenohumeral arthritis associated with severe rotator cuff deficiency. A minimum two-year follow-up study of sixty patients. J Bone Joint Surg Am 2005;87:1697–705.
4. Werner CM, Steinmann PA, Gilbart M, et al. Treatment of painful pseudoparesis due to irreparable rotator cuff dysfunction with the Delta III reverse-ball-and-socket total shoulder prosthesis. J Bone Joint Surg Am 2005;87:1476–86.
5. Cuff D, Clark R, Pupello D, et al. Reverse shoulder arthroplasty for the treatment of rotator cuff deficiency: a concise follow-up, at a minimum of five years, of a previous report. J Bone Joint Surg Am 2012;94:1996–2000.
6. Wall B, Walch G. Reverse shoulder arthroplasty for the treatment of proximal humeral fractures. Hand Clin 2007;23:425–30, v–vi.
7. Cazeneuve JF, Cristofari DJ. The reverse shoulder prosthesis in the treatment of fractures of the proximal humerus in the elderly. J Bone Joint Surg Br 2010;92:535–9.
8. Gallinet D, Adam A, Gasse N, et al. Improvement in shoulder rotation in complex shoulder fractures treated by reverse shoulder arthroplasty. J Shoulder Elbow Surg 2013;22:38–44.
9. Valenti P, Katz D, Kilinc A, et al. Mid-term outcome of reverse shoulder prostheses in complex proximal humeral fractures. Acta Orthop Belg 2012;78:442–9.
10. Young AA, Smith MM, Bacle G, et al. Early results of reverse shoulder arthroplasty in patients with rheumatoid arthritis. J Bone Joint Surg Am 2011; 93:1915–23.
11. Ekelund A, Nyberg R. Can reverse shoulder arthroplasty be used with few complications in rheumatoid arthritis? Clin Orthop Relat Res 2011;469: 2483–8.
12. Hattrup SJ, Sanchez-Sotelo J, Sperling JW, et al. Reverse shoulder replacement for patients with inflammatory arthritis. J Hand Surg Am 2012;37: 1888–94.
13. Holcomb JO, Hebert DJ, Mighell MA, et al. Reverse shoulder arthroplasty in patients with rheumatoid arthritis. J Shoulder Elbow Surg 2010;19:1076–84.
14. Sperling JW, Cofield RH, Schleck CD, et al. Total shoulder arthroplasty versus hemiarthroplasty for rheumatoid arthritis of the shoulder: results of 303 consecutive cases. J Shoulder Elbow Surg 2007; 16:683–90.
15. Kelly JD 2nd, Zhao JX, Hobgood ER, et al. Clinical results of revision shoulder arthroplasty using the reverse prosthesis. J Shoulder Elbow Surg 2012; 21:1516–25.
16. Patel DN, Young B, Onyekwelu I, et al. Reverse total shoulder arthroplasty for failed shoulder arthroplasty. J Shoulder Elbow Surg 2012;21:1478–83.
17. Grammont PM, Baulot E. Delta shoulder prosthesis for rotator cuff rupture. Orthopedics 1993; 16:65–8.
18. Boileau P, Watkinson D, Hatzidakis AM, et al. Neer Award 2005: the Grammont reverse shoulder prosthesis: results in cuff tear arthritis, fracture sequelae, and revision arthroplasty. J Shoulder Elbow Surg 2006;15:527–40.

19. Lawrence TM, Ahmadi S, Sanchez-Sotelo J, et al. Patient reported activities after reverse shoulder arthroplasty: part II. J Shoulder Elbow Surg 2012;21: 1464–9.

20. Favard L, Levigne C, Nerot C, et al. Reverse prostheses in arthropathies with cuff tear: are survivorship and function maintained over time? Clin Orthop Relat Res 2011;469:2469–75.

21. Raiss P, Schmitt M, Bruckner T, et al. Results of cemented total shoulder replacement with a minimum follow-up of ten years. J Bone Joint Surg Am 2012; 94:e17:11-10.

22. Singh JA, Sperling JW, Schleck C, et al. Periprosthetic infections after total shoulder arthroplasty: a 33-year perspective. J Shoulder Elbow Surg 2012; 21:1534–41.

23. Singh JA, Sperling JW, Schleck C, et al. Periprosthetic infections after shoulder hemiarthroplasty. J Shoulder Elbow Surg 2012;21:1304–9.

24. Singh JA, Sperling JW, Cofield RH. Revision surgery following total shoulder arthroplasty: analysis of 2588 shoulders over three decades (1976 to 2008). J Bone Joint Surg Br 2011;93:1513–7.

25. Bartelt R, Sperling JW, Schleck CD, et al. Shoulder arthroplasty in patients aged fifty-five years or younger with osteoarthritis. J Shoulder Elbow Surg 2011;20:123–30.

26. Namdari S, Yagnik G, Ebaugh DD, et al. Defining functional shoulder range of motion for activities of daily living. J Shoulder Elbow Surg 2012;21:1177–83.

27. Boileau P, Moineau G, Roussanne Y, et al. Bony increased-offset reversed shoulder arthroplasty: minimizing scapular impingement while maximizing glenoid fixation. Clin Orthop Relat Res 2011;469: 2558–67.

28. Frankle M, Levy JC, Pupello D, et al. The reverse shoulder prosthesis for glenohumeral arthritis associated with severe rotator cuff deficiency. A minimum two-year follow-up study of sixty patients surgical technique. J Bone Joint Surg Am 2006; 88(Suppl 1 Pt 2):178–90.

29. Levigne C, Boileau P, Favard L, et al. Scapular notching in reverse shoulder arthroplasty. J Shoulder Elbow Surg 2008;17:925–35.

30. Sirveaux F, Favard L, Oudet D, et al. Grammont inverted total shoulder arthroplasty in the treatment of glenohumeral osteoarthritis with massive rupture of the cuff. J Bone Joint Surg 2004;86: 388–95.

31. Valenti P, Sauzieres P, Katz D, et al. Do less medialized reverse shoulder prostheses increase motion and reduce notching? Clin Orthop Relat Res 2011;469:2550–7.

32. Zeman CA, Arcand MA, Cantrell JS, et al. The rotator cuff-deficient arthritic shoulder: diagnosis and surgical management. J Am Acad Orthop Surg 1998;6:337–48.

33. Howell SM, Imobersteg AM, Seger DH, et al. Clarification of the role of the supraspinatus muscle in shoulder function. J Bone Joint Surg Am 1986;68: 398–404.

34. Baulot E, Sirveaux F, Boileau P. Grammont's idea: the story of Paul Grammont's functional surgery concept and the development of the reverse principle. Clin Orthop Relat Res 2011;469:2425–31.

35. Hsu SH, Greiwe RM, Saifi C, et al. Reverse total shoulder arthroplasty—biomechanics and rationale. Operat Tech Orthop 2011;21:52–9.

36. Henninger HB, Barg A, Anderson AE, et al. Effect of lateral offset center of rotation in reverse total shoulder arthroplasty: a biomechanical study. J Shoulder Elbow Surg 2012;21:1128–35.

37. Ackland DC, Roshan-Zamir S, Richardson M, et al. Moment arms of the shoulder musculature after reverse total shoulder arthroplasty. J Bone Joint Surg Am 2010;92:1221–30.

38. Henninger HB, Barg A, Anderson AE, et al. Effect of deltoid tension and humeral version in reverse total shoulder arthroplasty: a biomechanical study. J Shoulder Elbow Surg 2012;21:483–90.

39. James J, Huffman KR, Werner FW, et al. Does glenoid baseplate geometry affect its fixation in reverse shoulder arthroplasty? J Shoulder Elbow Surg 2012;21:917–24.

40. Anglin C, Wyss UP, Pichora DR. Mechanical testing of shoulder prostheses and recommendations for glenoid design. J Shoulder Elbow Surg 2000;9:323–31.

41. Harman M, Frankle M, Vasey M, et al. Initial glenoid component fixation in "reverse" total shoulder arthroplasty: a biomechanical evaluation. J Shoulder Elbow Surg 2005;14:162S–7S.

42. Humphrey CS, Kelly JD 2nd, Norris TR. Optimizing glenosphere position and fixation in reverse shoulder arthroplasty, Part Two: the three-column concept. J Shoulder Elbow Surg 2008;17:595–601.

43. Virani NA, Harman M, Li K, et al. In vitro and finite element analysis of glenoid bone/baseplate interaction in the reverse shoulder design. J Shoulder Elbow Surg 2008;17:509–21.

44. Chou J, Malak SF, Anderson IA, et al. Biomechanical evaluation of different designs of glenospheres in the SMR reverse total shoulder prosthesis: range of motion and risk of scapular notching. J Shoulder Elbow Surg 2009;18:354–9.

45. Simovitch RW, Zumstein MA, Lohri E, et al. Predictors of scapular notching in patients managed with the Delta III reverse total shoulder replacement. J Bone Joint Surg Am 2007;89:588–600.

46. Virani NA, Cabezas A, Gutierrez S, et al. Reverse shoulder arthroplasty components and surgical techniques that restore glenohumeral motion. J Shoulder Elbow Surg 2013;22(2):179–87.

47. Clouthier AL, Hetzler MA, Fedorak G, et al. Factors affecting the stability of reverse shoulder

arthroplasty: a biomechanical study. J Shoulder Elbow Surg 2013;22(4):439–44.

48. Kempton LB, Balasubramaniam M, Ankerson E, et al. A radiographic analysis of the effects of glenosphere position on scapular notching following reverse total shoulder arthroplasty. J Shoulder Elbow Surg 2011;20:968–74.

49. Ackland DC, Richardson M, Pandy MG. Axial rotation moment arms of the shoulder musculature after reverse total shoulder arthroplasty. J Bone Joint Surg Am 2012;94:1886–95.

50. Greiner S, Schmidt C, Konig C, et al. Lateralized reverse shoulder arthroplasty maintains rotational function of the remaining rotator cuff. Clin Orthop Relat Res 2013;471(3):940–6.

51. Boileau P, Chuinard C, Roussanne Y, et al. Reverse shoulder arthroplasty combined with a modified latissimus dorsi and teres major tendon transfer for shoulder pseudoparalysis associated with dropping arm. Clin Orthop Relat Res 2008; 466:584–93.

52. Boileau P, Rumian AP, Zumstein MA. Reversed shoulder arthroplasty with modified L'Episcopo for combined loss of active elevation and external rotation. J Shoulder Elbow Surg 2010;19:20–30.

53. Li X, Knutson Z, Choi D, et al. Effects of glenosphere positioning on impingement-free internal and external rotation after reverse total shoulder arthroplasty. J Shoulder Elbow Surg 2012. [Epub ahead of print].

54. Edwards TB, Trappey GJ, Riley C, et al. Inferior tilt of the glenoid component does not decrease scapular notching in reverse shoulder arthroplasty: results of a prospective randomized study. J Shoulder Elbow Surg 2012;21:641–6.

55. Mole D, Favard L. Excentered scapulohumeral osteoarthritis. Rev Chir Orthop Reparatrice Appar Mot 2007;93:37–94 [in French].

56. Gulotta LV, Choi D, Marinello P, et al. Humeral component retroversion in reverse total shoulder arthroplasty: a biomechanical study. J Shoulder Elbow Surg 2012;21:1121–7.

57. Stephenson DR, Oh JH, McGarry MH, et al. Effect of humeral component version on impingement in reverse total shoulder arthroplasty. J Shoulder Elbow Surg 2011;20:652–8.

58. Bries AD, Pill SG, Wade Krause FR, et al. Accuracy of obtaining optimal base plate declination in reverse shoulder arthroplasty. J Shoulder Elbow Surg 2012;21:1770–5.

59. Cazeneuve JF, Cristofari DJ. Delta III reverse shoulder arthroplasty: radiological outcome for acute complex fractures of the proximal humerus in elderly patients. Orthop Traumatol Surg Res 2009; 95:325–9.

60. Mulieri P, Dunning P, Klein S, et al. Reverse shoulder arthroplasty for the treatment of irreparable rotator cuff tear without glenohumeral arthritis. J Bone Joint Surg Am 2010;92:2544–56.

61. Betts HM, Abu-Rajab R, Nunn T, et al. Total shoulder replacement in rheumatoid disease: a 16- to 23-year follow-up. J Bone Joint Surg Br 2009;91: 1197–200.

62. Ladermann A, Walch G, Lubbeke A, et al. Influence of arm lengthening in reverse shoulder arthroplasty. J Shoulder Elbow Surg 2012;21:336–41.

63. Martinez AA, Calvo A, Bejarano C, et al. The use of the Lima reverse shoulder arthroplasty for the treatment of fracture sequelae of the proximal humerus. J Orthop Sci 2012;17:141–7.

64. Walch G, Moraga C, Young A, et al. Results of anatomic nonconstrained prosthesis in primary osteoarthritis with biconcave glenoid. J Shoulder Elbow Surg 2012;21:1526–33.

65. Levy J, Frankle M, Mighell M, et al. The use of the reverse shoulder prosthesis for the treatment of failed hemiarthroplasty for proximal humeral fracture. J Bone Joint Surg Am 2007;89:292–300.

66. Walker M, Willis MP, Brooks JP, et al. The use of the reverse shoulder arthroplasty for treatment of failed total shoulder arthroplasty. J Shoulder Elbow Surg 2012;21:514–22.

67. Johnston PS, Creighton RA, Romeo AA. Humeral component revision arthroplasty: outcomes of a split osteotomy technique. J Shoulder Elbow Surg 2012;21:502–6.

68. Chacon A, Virani N, Shannon R, et al. Revision arthroplasty with use of a reverse shoulder prosthesis-allograft composite. J Bone Joint Surg Am 2009;91:119–27.

69. Budge MD, Moravek JE, Zimel MN, et al. Reverse total shoulder arthroplasty for the management of failed shoulder arthroplasty with proximal humeral bone loss: is allograft augmentation necessary? J Shoulder Elbow Surg 2012. [Epub ahead of print].

70. Norris TR, Kelly JD, Humphrey CS. Management of glenoid bone defects in revision shoulder arthroplasty. Tech Shoulder Elbow Surg 2007;8:37–46.

71. Clark JC, Ritchie J, Song FS, et al. Complication rates, dislocation, pain, and postoperative range of motion after reverse shoulder arthroplasty in patients with and without repair of the subscapularis. J Shoulder Elbow Surg 2012;21:36–41.

72. Trappey GJt, O'Connor DP, Edwards TB. What are the instability and infection rates after reverse shoulder arthroplasty? Clin Orthop Relat Res 2011;469:2505–11.

73. Cheung E, Willis M, Walker M, et al. Complications in reverse total shoulder arthroplasty. J Am Acad Orthop Surg 2011;19:439–49.

74. Ladermann A, Williams MD, Melis B, et al. Objective evaluation of lengthening in reverse shoulder arthroplasty. J Shoulder Elbow Surg 2009;18: 588–95.

75. Bufquin T, Hersan A, Hubert L, et al. Reverse shoulder arthroplasty for the treatment of three- and four-part fractures of the proximal humerus in the elderly: a prospective review of 43 cases with a short-term follow-up. J Bone Joint Surg Br 2007; 89:516–20.

76. Boileau P. Tuberosity malposition and migration: reasons for poor outcomes after hemiarthroplasty for displaced fractures of the proximal humerus. J Shoulder Elbow Surg 2002;11:401–12.

77. Murachovsky J, Ikemoto RY, Nascimento LG, et al. Pectoralis major tendon reference (PMT): a new method for accurate restoration of humeral length with hemiarthroplasty for fracture. J Shoulder Elbow Surg 2006;15:675–8.

78. Levy JC, Badman B. Reverse shoulder prosthesis for acute four-part fracture: tuberosity fixation using a horseshoe graft. J Orthop Trauma 2011;25:318–24.

79. Sirveaux F, Roche O, Mole D. Shoulder arthroplasty for acute proximal humerus fracture. Orthop Traumatol Surg Res 2010;96:683–94.

80. Gallinet D, Clappaz P, Garbuio P, et al. Three or four parts complex proximal humerus fractures: hemiarthroplasty versus reverse prosthesis: a comparative study of 40 cases. Orthop Traumatol Surg Res 2009;95:48–55.

81. Klein M, Juschka M, Hinkenjann B, et al. Treatment of comminuted fractures of the proximal humerus in elderly patients with the Delta III reverse shoulder prosthesis. J Orthop Trauma 2008;22:698–704.

82. Boyle MJ, Youn SM, Frampton CM, et al. Functional outcomes of reverse shoulder arthroplasty compared with hemiarthroplasty for acute proximal humeral fractures. J Shoulder Elbow Surg 2013;22:32–7.

83. Young SW, Segal BS, Turner PC, et al. Comparison of functional outcomes of reverse shoulder arthroplasty versus hemiarthroplasty in the primary treatment of acute proximal humerus fracture. ANZ J Surg 2010;80:789–93.

84. Garrigues GE, Johnston PS, Pepe MD, et al. Hemiarthroplasty versus reverse total shoulder arthroplasty for acute proximal humerus fractures in elderly patients. Orthopedics 2012;35:e703–8.

85. Martinez AA, Bejarano C, Carbonel I, et al. The treatment of proximal humerus nonunions in older patients with the reverse shoulder arthroplasty. Injury 2012. [Epub ahead of print].

86. Walch G, Mottier F, Wall B, et al. Acromial insufficiency in reverse shoulder arthroplasties. J Shoulder Elbow Surg 2009;18:495–502.

87. Hattrup SJ. The influence of postoperative acromial and scapular spine fractures on the results of reverse shoulder arthroplasty. Orthopedics 2010;33.

88. Wahlquist TC, Hunt AF, Braman JP. Acromial base fractures after reverse total shoulder arthroplasty: report of five cases. J Shoulder Elbow Surg 2011;20:1178–83.

89. Crosby LA, Hamilton A, Twiss T. Scapula fractures after reverse total shoulder arthroplasty: classification and treatment. Clin Orthop Relat Res 2011;469:2544–9.

90. Zavala JA, Clark JC, Kissenberth MJ, et al. Management of deep infection after reverse total shoulder arthroplasty: a case series. J Shoulder Elbow Surg 2012;21:1310–5.

91. Dodson CC, Craig EV, Cordasco FA, et al. Propionibacterium acnes infection after shoulder arthroplasty: a diagnostic challenge. J Shoulder Elbow Surg 2010;19:303–7.

92. Patel A, Calfee RP, Plante M, et al. Propionibacterium acnes colonization of the human shoulder. J Shoulder Elbow Surg 2009;18:897–902.

93. Nowinski RJ, Gillespie RJ, Shishani Y, et al. Antibiotic-loaded bone cement reduces deep infection rates for primary reverse total shoulder arthroplasty: a retrospective, cohort study of 501 shoulders. J Shoulder Elbow Surg 2012;21:324–8.

94. Beekman PD, Katusic D, Berghs BM, et al. One-stage revision for patients with a chronically infected reverse total shoulder replacement. J Bone Joint Surg Br 2010;92:817–22.

95. Ladermann A, Lubbeke A, Melis B, et al. Prevalence of neurologic lesions after total shoulder arthroplasty. J Bone Joint Surg Am 2011;93:1288–93.

96. Nagda SH, Rogers KJ, Sestokas AK, et al. Neer Award 2005: peripheral nerve function during shoulder arthroplasty using intraoperative nerve monitoring. J Shoulder Elbow Surg 2007;16:S2–8.

97. Bohsali KI, Wirth MA, Rockwood CA Jr. Complications of total shoulder arthroplasty. J Bone Joint Surg Am 2006;88:2279–92.

98. Boardman ND 3rd, Cofield RH. Neurologic complications of shoulder surgery. Clin Orthop Relat Res 1999;(368):44–53.

99. Lynch NM, Cofield RH, Silbert PL, et al. Neurologic complications after total shoulder arthroplasty. J Shoulder Elbow Surg 1996;5:53–61.

Posterior Elbow Wounds
Soft Tissue Coverage Options and Techniques

Ketan M. Patel, MD, James P. Higgins, MD*

KEYWORDS

- Posterior elbow wounds • Olecranon wounds • Elbow reconstruction • Flaps
- Upper extremity flaps

KEY POINTS

- Aggressive wound preparation is crucial to ensure success with reconstructive techniques.
- Early considerations for protection of the ulnar nerve may prevent injury with repeat surgery.
- A Doppler Allen examination before radial forearm flap harvest will help minimize donor site morbidity following flap harvest.
- The reversed lateral arm flap provides versatile and reliable soft tissue coverage for the posterior elbow region.
- Local perforator-based propeller flap options can be successfully used with limited donor site morbidity.

INTRODUCTION

Advances in upper extremity soft tissue reconstruction have been paralleled by the precise description and characterization of soft tissue vascular anatomy. The number and variety of wound management and coverage options have increased, allowing surgeons to tailor their treatment plans to the requirements of each clinical scenario.

Reconstructive Principles

The soft tissue envelope of the posterior elbow is a common site of wound complications because of a confluence of issues. Its location and prominence make it an area at risk in high-energy trauma. Surgical treatment of complex elbow fractures commonly uses the posterior approach for extensile access to the medial and lateral aspects of the joint, leaving the olecranon at risk for wound dehiscence and potential hardware exposure. Infectious or inflammatory olecranon bursitis also risk tissue breakdown in this difficult location. Finally, the anatomic location of this tissue over the apex of a joint capable of more than 130° of flexion exposes these wounds to tension and motion, further inhibiting healing and risking dehiscence. The reasons that put this location at risk of chronic wound development also make the prospect of success with local wound care unlikely. Local debridement and dressing changes may commonly succeed in decreasing the size of the wound but may fail to achieve final and stable closure.

Failure of local wound care is followed by consideration given to local skin flap advancement or rotation flaps. In assessing areas adjacent to a wound, mobility and pliability are often related to the chronicity of the wound. Long-standing wounds have varying degrees of inflammation

Financial Disclosure: All authors have no conflicts of interest or financial disclosures. No funding was used for the preparation of this article.
Curtis National Hand Center, MedStar Union Memorial Hospital, 3333 North Calvert Street, Baltimore, MD 21218, USA
* Corresponding author. 3333 North Calvert Street, Baltimore, MD 21218.
E-mail address: jameshiggins10@hotmail.com

Orthop Clin N Am 44 (2013) 409–417
http://dx.doi.org/10.1016/j.ocl.2013.03.011
0030-5898/13/$ – see front matter © 2013 Elsevier Inc. All rights reserved.

and loss of tissue elasticity. These conditions make local tissue rearrangement and local flap options less feasible. Attempts at local skin advancement are performed with postoperative extension splinting to minimize tissue tension. These efforts are limited by the concern for creation or exacerbation of elbow stiffness with prolonged immobilization. If these conservative measures fail, more involved flap coverage is considered.

With pedicled transfer options, understanding the type and extent of previous surgeries/injuries may limit available flap options. A prior lateral approach to a humerus fracture, for example, will compromise vascular supply to the lateral arm flap and eliminate this option for reconstruction. Similarly, radial artery damage can compromise the vascularity for a pedicled radial forearm flap. The need for evaluation of the integrity of the superficial arch of the hand is heightened in the setting of concomitant more distal injury to the hand if radial forearm flap harvest is being considered.

Preoperative Considerations

Preoperative considerations before olecranon coverage are many and are related to the complexity and extent of the wound.

The status of the underlying bone will alter surgical plans significantly. In the setting of chronic atraumatic olecranon wounds, superficial osteomyelitis is anticipated and saucerization of the exposed and contaminated bone is required before flap elevation and closure. Posterior elbow wounds encountered after fracture management are more complex. Consideration must be given to removal of exposed hardware and debridement of exposed fractures. This can be considerably complicated if the fracture is not yet healed and current fixation is considered ideal or irreplaceable. In these settings, contaminated hardware may be preserved after debridement and irrigation in pursuit of delaying hardware removal until fracture union is achieved. In these difficult settings, the risk of loss of fracture fixation must be weighed against the risks of temporary preservation of contaminated implants.

The complexity and intra-articular involvement of underlying fractures may make the anticipation of stiffness a near certainty, and should alert the reconstructive surgeon to the possibility of future surgeries in the same field. Elbow capsulectomy, for example, may be significantly easier if performed through a matured fasciocutaneous flap than a less pliable and mobile muscle flap.

The ulnar nerve should always be given consideration in preoperative planning for posterior elbow coverage. If the nerve has not been previously transposed, the surgeon should consider transposition if the wound debridement or flap elevation will expose the nerve and leave the cubital tunnel at risk for scarring or compression. If a future capsulectomy requiring medial column dissection is anticipated, ulnar nerve transposition may also be helpful in avoiding future nerve injury.

The vascular status of the various flaps described herein is not routinely assessed with preoperative studies with the exception of the radial forearm flap. If the radial forearm flap is planned as the primary or backup procedure, a careful Allen test is performed to ensure that the perfusion to the hand would not be compromised with absence of the radial artery inflow. The authors perform this in the office with the use of a surface Doppler probe. This does not provide quantitative measurements and must be interpreted critically to determine if radial forearm flap harvest is safe. The authors require that the quality and intensity of the Doppler signal audible on the volar pads of the digits (with particular attention given to the thumb) remain unchanged after manual compression of the radial artery at the wrist.

Finally, consideration should be given to the size and location of the wound anticipated after debridement with the elbow in full flexion. A fibrotic infected wound assessed before debridement with the elbow extended may greatly underestimate the size and location of tissue required.

Flap Options and Techniques

Various muscle, fasciocutaneous, and cutaneous flaps have been described as coverage options for posterior elbow wounds. The most common flaps used for this area include the reversed lateral arm, latissimus dorsi, brachioradialis, flexor carpi ulnaris, radial forearm, and local perforator-based cutaneous flaps. These flap types are discussed and advantages and limitations of each type of flap are highlighted.

Lateral arm flap

Anatomy The lateral arm flap is a versatile flap used for pedicled transfer to the posterior elbow region. The vascular anatomy permits this flap to be used as an antegrade or retrograde ("reversed") pedicled flap. This septofasciocutaneous flap is based on the posterior branch of the radial collateral artery (PRCA), which arises from the profunda brachial artery. This vessel courses along the periosteum of the lateral column of the humerus and is elevated with the lateral intermuscular septum and overlying skin.

The cutaneous vessels originating from the PRCA are focused in the distal lateral arm, where 2 to 5 branches supply the lateral arm skin. An antegrade flap will provide perfusion distal to the lateral epicondyle, permitting the "extended lateral arm flap" harvest to include the proximal dorsal forearm skin (**Fig. 1**).

The PRCA communicates with the radial recurrent artery of the proximal forearm as well as with the recurrent branch of the posterior interosseous system. These interconnections permit retrograde harvest of the same angiosome. This retrograde configuration is the most commonly used flap design for coverage of olecranon wounds.

Technique Retrograde lateral arm flaps are designed by drawing a line between the deltoid insertion and the lateral epicondyle, indicating the location of the lateral intermuscular septum. A longitudinal ellipse is drawn with its proximal apex at the spiral groove. Distally the surgeon has 2 choices. The ellipse may be completed at the level of the lateral epicondyle, creating an island flap based on the septum and wide subcutaneous leash of vessels coursing proximally. If this option is selected, the flap may be tunneled subcutaneously into the wound (**Figs. 2** and **3**). Alternatively, the surgeon may choose to incompletely incise the proximal ellipse to preserve a skin bridge to the proximal forearm. In this setting, the lateral arm skin is serving as a rotation flap on this vascular

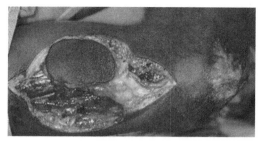

Fig. 2. A reversed lateral arm flap is shown elevated. A subcutaneous tissue leash is created to ensure appropriate vascularity.

pedicle. These rotation flaps should be purposefully designed to incorporate the lateral wound edge as the posterior margin of the flap to permit insetting of the adjacent skin (**Fig. 4**). With either of these retrograde flap designs, the proximal PRCA is ligated at the spiral groove to allow mobilization of the distally based pedicle and skin. Flap width and length are variable, but a width of approximately 6 cm will allow for primary closure of the donor site and obviate the need for skin grafting.

Less commonly, the lateral arm flap may be used as an antegrade flap, which is the "extended" design incorporating the proximal dorsal forearm skin. This may be attempted if the wound does not extend significantly distal to the olecranon and the wound margin is used as the posterior margin of the flap. Because the forearm skin envelope is not as redundant as the brachium, a skin graft may be needed for closure of a portion of the donor site.

Outcomes Tung and colleagues[1] evaluated 7 patients who underwent reversed lateral arm flap for posterior elbow defects and found that complete healing with restoration of full range of motion occurred in all patients. They found that nearly half of patients had forearm parasthesias

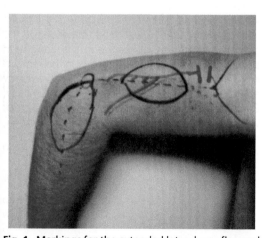

Fig. 1. Markings for the extended lateral arm flap and the reversed lateral arm flap are shown. The arterial supply (PRCA) is shown in red. Proximal division of this artery will allow for the reversed flap based on collateral flow. An antegrade extended lateral arm flap is based on distal random pattern perfusion over the proximal forearm. The radial nerve is indicated in green and should be visualized and protected when isolating the vascular pedicle.

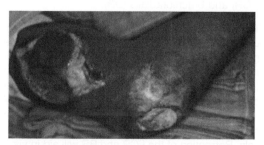

Fig. 3. Posterior elbow wound is shown. Subcutaneous tunneling of the flap into the defect can allow for single-stage reconstruction. Adequate room for tunneling is necessary to avoid compression or kinking of the pedicle.

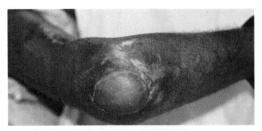

Fig. 4. The flap is shown well-healed 3 months postoperatively.

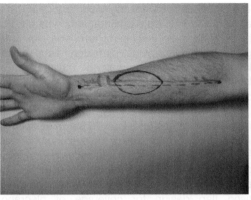

Fig. 5. The axis of the radial artery is shown. Two clusters of skin perforators are located proximally and distally. Flap design is centered on the axis. Careful attention to the position of the flap design will ensure adequate length for tunneling to the defect.

or scarring issues. Similarly, Prantl and colleagues[2] evaluated 8 patients who had a distally based lateral arm flap. All flaps survived; one complication related to wound breakdown occurred. Hamdi and Coessens[3] evaluated the donor site morbidity of patients who underwent lateral arm and extended lateral arm flaps. They found that subjective patient satisfaction was rated as high and minimal elbow functional change from the contralateral side occurred. In addition, they found an average area of decreased sensation of 45 cm[2] in the posterior lateral aspect of the forearm.

Radial forearm flap

Anatomy Radial forearm flaps have been used for a wide array of reconstructive procedures as pedicled and as free tissue transfers. The popularity of this flap is based on its ease of dissection, long pedicle, and thin, pliable skin segment. The axis of this flap runs along the length of the radial artery, from the middle of the antecubital fossa to the radial styloid. In the forearm, the radial artery delivers 2 clusters of skin perforators: one in the proximal forearm, and the other in the distal forearm, with the largest skin perforators located within 2 cm of the radial styloid (**Fig. 5**).[4] This septocutaneous flap has large-caliber vessels, allowing for a robust blood supply with skin perforators in the septum between the flexor carpi radialis (FCR) and brachioradialis (BR).

Technique The skin paddle taken with this flap is centered on the axis of the radial artery. One must ensure that the pedicle length is adequate to allow for tunneling and rotation of the flap to the posterior elbow area. The axis of rotation is as proximal as the midpoint of the antecubital fossa. Flap elevation begins on either the ulnar or radial side with dissection toward the radial vessels. Retraction of the FCR and BR will aid in visualization and inclusion of the intermuscular septum and the main vascular pedicle within the flap. Great care should be taken to ensure that the dissection is in the subfascial plane of the BR

and FCR muscles to ensure preservation of the septal vessels. During dissection of the radial side of the flap, great care should be taken to preserve and protect the dorsal sensory branch of the radial nerve (DSBRN), as it emerges from the dorsal margin of the BR and branches distally.

As an antegrade pedicled flap, division of the radial artery is mandatory to allow for rotation. Once this is performed, proximal pedicle dissection proceeds until sufficient pedicle length is achieved. The donor site usually requires a skin graft for closure (**Figs. 6** and **7**).

Outcomes The clinical consequence of a single-vessel hand as a result of radial artery harvest has recently been questioned because of the potential long-term consequences.[5] Long-term studies indicate that flow dynamics in the remaining ulnar artery following radial artery harvest may accelerate atherosclerotic changes.[6,7] Similarly, Suominen and colleagues[8] found increased peak velocity in the remaining ulnar artery. In addition,

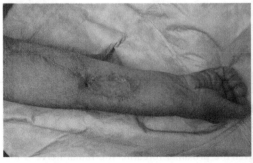

Fig. 6. A healed radial forearm donor site is shown following a pedicled flap transfer.

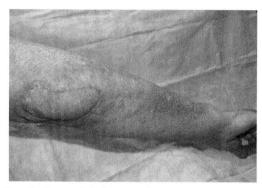

Fig. 7. The radial forearm flap inset and healed following a posterior elbow wound. A thin, pliable flap can be harvested using this technique.

they found an 11.9% decrease in grip strength and an impaired thermoregulatory system of the donor hand.[9] While the clinical relevance of these findings are debated, the radial forearm flap remains a commonly used flap for posterior elbow wound coverage.

Jones and colleagues[10] evaluated outcomes following elbow coverage with pedicled radial forearm flaps. On evaluating the donor site of 56 patients, the study described 100% split-thickness skin graft take for donor site closure. In addition, there were no complaints of cold intolerance, dissatisfaction of the appearance, or dysesthesias. Key steps mentioned to improve donor site morbidity include limiting radial extension of the flap to the radial border of the forearm to minimize exposure of the radial sensory branch, advancing skin flaps to close the wound slightly to decrease the amount of skin graft needed, and using nonmeshed skin graft with few fenestrations.

Brachioradialis flap

Anatomy The BR muscle aids in forearm flexion with an origin of attachment on the lateral supracondylar ridge of the humerus and an insertion on the styloid process of the radius. The dominant blood supply to this muscle is the radial recurrent artery arriving in the proximal portion of the muscle as a proximal branch of the radial artery, or it can have direct connections from the radial artery or brachial artery.[11] The radial nerve is in close proximity to the arterial supply on the underside of the muscle.

Technique To isolate this muscle, an incision is designed over the proximal radial forearm. The distal tendon is divided at the musculotendinous junction, taking great care to identify and protect the DSBRN. Division of the tendon will allow for expeditious dissection proximally to the level of the dominant pedicle. The dominant vascular pedicle marks the pivot point of the muscle flap. Tunneling the muscle toward the posterior elbow will allow the flap to reach the upper elbow and posterior elbow regions. Skin grafting over the muscle is necessary to complete the wound closure. Negative pressure wound therapy is usually initiated over the grafted area to ensure graft take and limit shearing forces.

Outcomes BR transfer for posterior elbow wounds allows for an additional advantage of distal tendon transfer. This component can allow for collateral ligament and/or joint stabilization. But, when muscle flaps are disinserted, there is potential for some degree of functional loss. Few studies have reported the donor site morbidity of BR harvest. A recent functional study indicates that the BR primary function is to serve as an elbow stabilizer during elbow flexion tasks. In addition, secondary function was found in pronation activity.[12] When harvested, some loss of pronation may be expected when moving from full supination, but limited morbidity when the forearm is in neutral positions.[13]

A cutaneous portion can be included with this muscle flap.[14,15] Leversedge and colleagues[14] found that consistent perfusion was located in the cutaneous portion directly above the muscle belly. They found that no cutaneous perfusion was found 1 cm distal to the musculotendinous junction. Including a cutaneous portion may eliminate the need for skin grafting.

Flexor carpi ulnaris

Anatomy The flexor carpi ulnaris (FCU) is located superficially on the ulnar aspect of the forearm. Two proximal heads (ulnar and humeral) are separated by the ulnar nerve and posterior ulnar recurrent artery. This muscle functions to flex and ulnar-deviate the wrist with attachment at the pisiform. The dominant blood supply is the posterior ulnar recurrent artery and arrives on the deep surface of the muscle close to the origin. Deep along the length of the muscle courses the ulnar neurovascular bundle.

Technique The incision for harvesting of this flap lies along the axis of a line drawn from the medial epicondyle and the pisiform. The muscle is the most superficial and ulnar of the forearm muscles and the musculotendinous junction is approximately 7 cm from the wrist. Division at this level will allow for quick proximal dissection to the level of the dominant pedicle, which is located approximately 6 cm distal to the olecranon tip and provides the most reliable perfusion to the muscle belly (**Figs. 8–11**).[16]

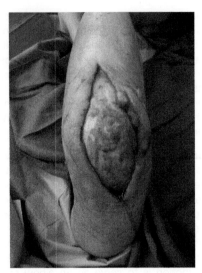

Fig. 8. A resultant wound following excision of an infected olecranon bursa is shown.

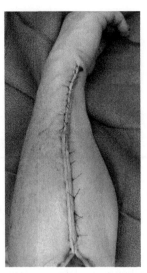

Fig. 10. The access incision can be seen extending down the forearm along the ulnar border.

Outcomes Several variations of the FCU flap exist. As a musculocutaneous flap, durable cutaneous paddle can contribute to durability over the olecranon.[17,18] Skin perfusion is appreciated along the entire aspect of the muscle. An ellipse of skin can be harvested centered over the muscle. In addition, donor site functional deficits can be minimized with the use of a split FCU flap. The 2 proximal heads of the FCU can be differentially split using a flap based on the ulnar head for wound coverage. This portion of the muscle contributes to 75% of the width of the entire muscle.[19,20] Using this method, limited donor site morbidity results because a large portion of the muscle is left intact.

Latissimus flap

Anatomy The latissimus muscle is a large, flat muscle extending from the humerus to multiple attachments along the posterior aspect of the thorax and abdomen. The muscle is responsible for adduction, extension, and medial rotation of the humerus. The thoracodorsal vessels, the main blood supply to this flap, are located in an optimal position for pedicled transfer to the chest, arm, and elbow regions. This muscle flap can be taken with a cutaneous paddle centered over the anterior aspect of the muscle, where the abundance of skin perforators exists. This skin segment may

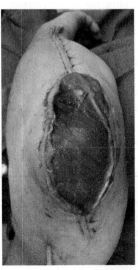

Fig. 9. FCU muscle flap inset into the defect is shown.

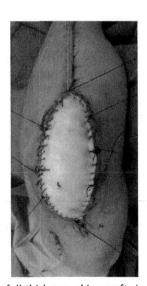

Fig. 11. A full-thickness skin graft is placed for completion of wound coverage.

be helpful if the wound extends to the posterior brachium. The skin paddle will not reach the olecranon region reliably.

Technique For muscle flap harvest, a curvilinear incision centered on the oblique axis in line with the humerus attachment provides ample exposure to all aspects of the muscle. Rapid dissection of the muscle from distal to proximal must ensure that the lumbar fascia remains intact and the rhomboids are not accidentally harvested with the muscle. Once in the axilla, care is taken to avoid injury to the thoracodorsal vessels. Subcutaneous tunneling permits this muscle flap to reach the elbow region. Skin grafting is required for coverage of the muscle at the olecranon level.

Outcomes The wide, large dimensions of this muscle allow for its use in larger defects of the posterior elbow. Donor site morbidity associated with latissimus harvest has been reported to be tolerably low with compensation by other shoulder girdle muscles in short-term evaluation.[21–23] A recent long-term study suggests joint instability and decreased strength in an average follow-up period of 92 months.[24]

In clinical use, Sajjad and colleagues[25] evaluated 28 patients who underwent pedicled latissimus flaps for extensive soft tissue defects around the elbow. Of the patients, 10% had partial flap loss, but all patients went on to heal completely. Stevanovic and colleagues[26] evaluated 16 patients who underwent latissimus flaps for elbow defects of 100 cm². Three patients had partial flap necrosis. The study recommended cautious use of the latissimus flap for wounds 8 cm distal to the olecranon to ensure successful reconstruction.

These caveats were echoed by Choudry and colleagues[27] in a review of 99 cases of soft tissue coverage of posterior elbow wounds. The use of the latissimus dorsi pedicled flap was prone to complication, particularly when the wound extended distal to the olecranon.

Local fasciocutaneous flaps

Anatomy The precise characterization of perforator anatomy in the area of the elbow has allowed design of cutaneous and fasciocutaneous flaps that can provide adequate soft tissue coverage of posterior elbow wounds. Skin-perforating vessels emerging from the radial artery allow for design of cutaneous flaps. In the distal arm, the radial collateral artery forms a vascular network with the posterior and anterior radial collateral arteries. In the same manner and location of the lateral arm flap, propeller-based flaps can be

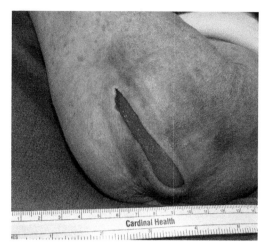

Fig. 12. A chronic posterior elbow wound is shown.

designed and pivoted off of single skin perforators. A thorough understanding of the vascular connections in the distal arm is necessary to design these flaps. In addition, a handheld Doppler is crucial to isolating these perforating vessels.[28]

Distally, the radial artery has a proximal cluster of skin perforators located in the proximal one-third of the forearm.[4] Located on an axis of the radial artery from the mid-antecubital fossa to the radial styloid, this proximal cluster of vessels serves as potential pedicles for propeller-type flaps. In addition, subcutaneous linking vessels to nearby skin perfusing vessels allow large cutaneous skin paddles to survive off single isolated perforators.

The posterior interosseous artery (PIA) can provide perfusion to a forearm-based fasciocutaneous flap that can be used for soft tissue coverage of the elbow. The PIA emerges from the ulnar artery and lies between the extensor carpi ulnaris and extensor digiti minimi. Cutaneous perforators are found in the middle-third of the forearm.

Technique Propeller flaps based on the proximal cluster of radial artery perforators are carefully designed because the pivot point may have variability depending on the location of the dominant

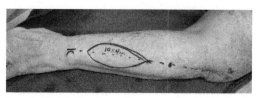

Fig. 13. The axis and design of a posterior interosseous artery flap are shown.

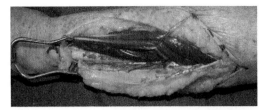

Fig. 14. The arterial pedicle is appreciated traveling within the space between the extensor carpi ulnaris and extensor digiti minimi.

perforator. A long and narrow cutaneous island design can allow for primary closure of the defect site.

Elevation begins distally and proceeds proximally with examination of each radial artery perforator. Subfascial or suprafascial dissection can be performed as linking vessels travel within the subcutaneous tissues. During proximal dissection, adequate size perforators are kept until a comparison with neighboring perforators can be performed. Once an adequate sized perforator is selected, the flap is "islandized" completely. This will allow for rotation radially toward the posterior elbow region. Inset is complete by either de-epithelializing the flap and tunneling or excising intervening skin to allow for inset. The donor site can be closed if the resulting defect is narrow enough to allow for tension-free closure.

The PIA flap is centered on a line from the lateral epicondyle of the humerus to the distal radial ulnar joint. The middle and distal thirds of this line form the transverse axis of this flap (**Figs. 12** and **13**). Care must be taken to avoid injury to the dorsal branch of the ulnar nerve distally and the posterior interosseous nerve proximally (**Figs. 14–16**).[29]

Outcomes Limited studies have evaluated these perforator-based type flaps for posterior elbow wounds. Clinically, these thin flaps can be used with minimal donor site morbidity because no major axial extremity vasculature is ligated. In

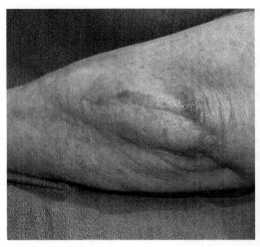

Fig. 16. The flap is shown 6 months after surgery. Good contour with a close match to adjacent tissue is appreciated.

addition, primary donor site closure can occur if flap width is limited to 4 to 6 cm.

SUMMARY

There are a myriad of options for soft tissue reconstruction of the posterior elbow region. In analyzing these defects, understanding the role of certain flap options for specific wound types will help ensure successful outcomes. Considerations for donor site morbidity are more appreciated when muscle flaps are chosen, given the potential for loss of function. Skin grafting is commonly used when muscle flaps are used without cutaneous skin paddles. Cutaneous and fasciocutaneous flaps can be designed in several regions around the elbow without sacrificing major axial vessels of the extremity. Tension-free inset with immobilization in the postoperative period can eliminate potential flap loss or other complications.

REFERENCES

1. Tung TC, Wang KC, Fang CM, et al. Reverse pedicled lateral arm flap for reconstruction of posterior soft-tissue defects of the elbow. Ann Plast Surg 1997;38:635–41.
2. Prantl L, Schreml S, Schwarze H, et al. A safe and simple technique using the distal pedicled reversed upper arm flap to cover large elbow defects. J Plast Reconstr Aesthet Surg 2008;61:546–51.
3. Hamdi M, Coessens BC. Evaluation of the donor site morbidity after lateral arm flap with skin paddle extending over the elbow joint. Br J Plast Surg 2000; 53:215–9.

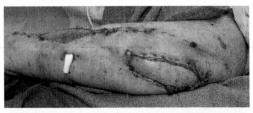

Fig. 15. The flap is shown inset into the posterior elbow defect. The donor site has been skin grafted over top of the exposed muscle.

4. Saint-Cyr M, Mujadzic M, Wong C, et al. The radial artery pedicle perforator flap: vascular analysis and clinical implications. Plast Reconstr Surg 2010; 125:1469–78.

5. Higgins JP. A reassessment of the role of the radial forearm flap in upper extremity reconstruction. J Hand Surg Am 2011;36:1237–40.

6. Gaudino M, Serricchio M, Tondi P, et al. Chronic compensatory increase in ulnar flow and accelerated atherosclerosis after radial artery removal for coronary artery bypass. J Thorac Cardiovasc Surg 2005;130:9–12.

7. Gaudino M, Anselmi A, Serricchio M, et al. Late haemodynamic and functional consequences of radial artery removal on the forearm circulation. Int J Cardiol 2008;129:255–8.

8. Suominen S, Ahovuo J, Asko-Seljavaara S. Donor site morbidity of radial forearm flaps. A clinical and ultrasonographic evaluation. Scand J Plast Reconstr Surg Hand Surg 1996;30:57–61.

9. Suominen S, Asko-Seljavaara S. Thermography of hands after a radial forearm flap has been raised. Scand J Plast Reconstr Surg Hand Surg 1996;30: 307–14.

10. Jones NF, Jarrahy R, Kaufman MR. Pedicled and free radial forearm flaps for reconstruction of the elbow, wrist, and hand. Plast Reconstr Surg 2008;121: 887–98.

11. Sanger JR, Ye Z, Yousif NJ, et al. The brachioradialis forearm flap: anatomy and clinical application. Plast Reconstr Surg 1994;94:667–74.

12. Boland MR, Spigelman T, Uhl TL. The function of brachioradialis. J Hand Surg Am 2008;33:1853–9.

13. Bekler HI, Ozkan T. Biomechanical assessment of brachioradialis pronatorplasty. Acta Orthop Traumatol Turc 2011;45:109–14.

14. Leversedge FJ, Casey PJ, Payne SH, et al. Vascular anatomy of the brachioradialis rotational musculocutaneous flap. J Hand Surg Am 2001;26:711–21.

15. Lalikos JF, Fudem GM. Brachioradialis musculocutaneous flap closure of the elbow utilizing a distal skin island: a case report. Ann Plast Surg 1997;39:201–4.

16. Payne DE, Kaufman AM, Wysocki RW, et al. Vascular perfusion of a flexor carpi ulnaris muscle turnover pedicle flap for posterior elbow soft tissue reconstruction: a cadaveric study. J Hand Surg Am 2011;36:246–51.

17. Shen S, Pang J, Seneviratne S, et al. A comparative anatomical study of brachioradialis and flexor carpi ulnaris muscles: implications for total tongue reconstruction. Plast Reconstr Surg 2008;121: 816–29.

18. Roukoz S. Musculocutaneous flexor carpi ulnaris flap for reconstruction of posterior cutaneotricipital defects of the elbow. Plast Reconstr Surg 2003; 111:330–5.

19. Lingaraj K, Lim AY, Puhaindran ME, et al. Case report: the split flexor carpi ulnaris as a local muscle flap. Clin Orthop Relat Res 2007;455:262–6.

20. Wysocki RW, Gray RL, Fernandez JJ, et al. Posterior elbow coverage using whole and split flexor carpi ulnaris flaps: a cadaveric study. J Hand Surg Am 2008;33:1807–12.

21. Russell RC, Pribaz J, Zook EG, et al. Functional evaluation of latissimus dorsi donor site. Plast Reconstr Surg 1986;78:336–44.

22. Spear SL, Hess CL. A review of the biomechanical and functional changes in the shoulder following transfer of the latissimus dorsi muscles. Plast Reconstr Surg 2005;115:2070–3.

23. Brumback RJ, McBride MS, Ortolani NC. Functional evaluation of the shoulder after transfer of the vascularized latissimus dorsi muscle. J Bone Joint Surg Am 1992;74:377–82.

24. Giordano S, Kääriäinen K, Alavaikko J, et al. Latissimus dorsi free flap harvesting may affect the shoulder joint in long run. Scand J Surg 2011;100: 202–7.

25. Sajjad Y, Hameed A, Gill NA, et al. Use of a pedicled flap for reconstruction of extensive soft tissue defects around elbow. J Coll Physicians Surg Pak 2010;20:47–50.

26. Stevanovic M, Sharpe F, Thommen VD, et al. Latissimus dorsi pedicle flap for coverage of soft tissue defects about the elbow. J Shoulder Elbow Surg 1999; 8:634–43.

27. Choudry UH, Moran SL, Li S, et al. Soft-tissue coverage of the elbow: an outcome analysis and reconstructive algorithm. Plast Reconstr Surg 2007; 119:1852–7.

28. Murakami M, Ono S, Ishii N, et al. Reconstruction of elbow region defects using radial collateral artery perforator (RCAP)-based propeller flaps. J Plast Reconstr Aesthet Surg 2012;65:1418–21.

29. Penteado CV, Masquelet AC, Chevrel JP. The anatomic basis of the fascio-cutaneous flap of the posterior interosseous artery. Surg Radiol Anat 1986;8:209–15.

Management of Radial Nerve Palsy Following Fractures of the Humerus

Genghis E. Niver, MD, Asif M. Ilyas, MD*

KEYWORDS

- Radial nerve • Humerus fracture • Holstein-Lewis fracture

KEY POINTS

- A radial nerve palsy is the most common peripheral nerve injury following a humerus fracture, occurring in up to 2% to 17% of cases.
- Surgical exploration is recommended in cases with open or complex fractures, particularly those associated with penetrating trauma.
- Radial nerve palsies associated with closed fractures of the humerus have traditionally been recommended to be treated with observation, with late exploration restricted to cases without spontaneous nerve recovery at 3 to 6 months.
- Advocates for early exploration believe that late exploration can result in increased muscular atrophy, motor endplate loss, compromised nerve recovery on delayed repair, and significant interval loss of patient function and livelihood.
- Early exploration can hasten nerve injury characterization and repair, as well as facilitate early fracture stabilization and rehabilitation.

BACKGROUND

In the United States, more than 237,000 humerus fractures occur each year. Humeral shaft fractures represent between 1% and 5% of all fractures.[1,2] Initial retrospective studies by Mast and colleagues[3] described humeral shaft fractures as being most common among male patients younger than 35 involved in high-energy trauma.[2] However, more recent studies have described a bimodal incidence with women older than 50 years suffering these fractures from low-energy injuries, such as falls from a standing height.[4,5]

Complicating these fractures are radial nerve injuries, which are the most common peripheral nerve injuries associated with humeral fractures.[6,7] The incidence of radial nerve injuries with humerus fractures has been documented between 2% and 17%.[8–10] A prospectively collected database of more than 5700 patients with polytrauma revealed the radial nerve to be the most frequently injured peripheral nerve, seen in 9.5% of humeral fractures.[11] However, this polytrauma population also included open fractures. Controversy still exists in the treatment of humeral shaft fractures with associated radial nerve injuries. Algorithms have been proposed to provide recommendations with regard to management and treatment of these nerve injuries. However, pros and cons are associated with each of these algorithms.

All named authors hereby declare that they have no conflicts of interests to disclose related to the topic of this article.

Hand and Upper Extremity Surgery, Rothman Institute, Thomas Jefferson University, 925 Chestnut Street, Philadelphia, PA 19107, USA

* Corresponding author.

E-mail address: asif.ilyas@rothmaninstitute.com

Orthop Clin N Am 44 (2013) 419–424

http://dx.doi.org/10.1016/j.ocl.2013.03.012

ANATOMY

The humeral shaft is defined as the region "between the superior border of the pectoralis major insertion and the area immediately above the supracondylar ridge."[12]

Prior descriptions historically have placed the radial nerve and profunda brachial artery in the musculospiral groove and lateral intermuscular septum of the humerus.[9] However, the spiral groove is truly the origin of the brachialis muscle. Fibers of the medial head of the triceps and brachialis separate the radial nerve from the humeral cortex. Direct contact with the humerus typically most consistently occurs as the nerve approaches the lateral supracondylar ridge.[13]

Humeral shaft fractures can be described by their anatomic location by dividing the humeral shaft into thirds or fifths. The level of the fracture can provide the initial evidence of a radial nerve injury.[3] Holstein and Lewis described an association of a radial nerve injury with a spiral fracture of the distal third humeral shaft fracture, since referred to as a Holstein-Lewis fracture.[8] However, 1 to 5 cm of muscle separates the humerus and radial nerve at a level just proximal to the distal third of the humerus.[14] Due to the force of injury, the proximal segment moves distally, causing displacement of the intermuscular septum. The radial nerve, which runs through this septum, may subsequently get tethered and injured. The nerve may also get lacerated when the apex of the distal fragment moves radially and proximally.[8] Although this mechanism of radial nerve injury has been widely accepted, many recent studies dispute the constant relationship between the Holstein-Lewis fracture fragment and radial nerve injury.[9,14,15] Similarly, a study by Bono and colleagues[16] noted that the radial nerve has a more proximal decussation than previously reported. Their conclusion was that the nerve travels the distal half of the humerus along a superficial course.

In addition, the AO classification can be used to describe fractures and their associated patterns.[1] The AO classification divides diaphyseal humeral shaft fractures into 3 categories depending on the amount of contact between the major fracture fragments. Simple fractures with more than 90% contact between the main fracture fragments are known as AO Type A fractures. AO Type B fractures (wedge fractures) and AO Type C fractures (complex fractures) have little or no contact between major fragments. Subtypes also exist based on direction and fracture extent within the 3 major categories.

According to Tytherleigh-Strong and colleagues,[5] fractures of the middle third of the humeral shaft arise with an incidence of 64.2% and AO Type A fractures have a similar incidence of 63.3%. Researchers differ in their incidence of radial nerve injury with regard to location of the humeral shaft fracture. For instance, Bostman and colleagues[15] noted an equal incidence of radial nerve injuries in fractures of the middle and distal third humeral shaft. However, some have reported that a higher likelihood of neurovascular injuries occurs in middle third of humerus fractures,[9] whereas others have observed an increase in neurovascular injuries in distal third humeral shaft fractures.[17] Fracture pattern associated with radial nerve palsies is also variable; most occur in the presence of a spiral fracture, although transverse and oblique fractures can also result in a radial nerve injury.[9,15,17]

CLASSIFICATION/DIAGNOSIS

Radial nerve palsies can be classified as either partial or complete. To begin determining the type of palsy, one must perform a complete physical examination. A thorough baseline examination consists of sensory and motor evaluation of the median, ulnar, and radial nerves. Radial nerve sensation can be tested to light touch and pinprick on the dorsal hand at the level of the first web space. Radial nerve motor function can be determined by testing active extension of the wrist and of the fingers (including the thumb) at the metacarpophalangeal joints. In addition, the absence of brachioradialis or extensor carpi radialis longus firing may indicate a proximal injury at the level of the humeral shaft.[18]

After a thorough physical examination, complete motor loss has been noted to occur in 50% to 68% of radial nerve palsies.[9,17] Primary nerve palsies noted during the initial physical examination usually have occurred at the time of injury. Secondary nerve palsies may arise at any point during the active treatment of the fracture; these can represent up to 20% of all nerve palsies.[15,19] The Seddon or Sunderland classification system can be used in further defining the type of peripheral nerve injury.[20,21] The initial definition of a radial nerve injury as primary or secondary may be a prognostic factor in the ultimate recovery of the nerve. One study demonstrated 40% recovery in patients with a primary palsy and 100% recovery in patients with a secondary palsy after treatment of a humeral shaft fracture (closed or open reduction with internal fixation).[22] Other studies with primary radial nerve palsies have demonstrated spontaneous recovery in 85% after closed fractures of the humerus.[15]

Secondary nerve palsies after humeral shaft fractures may occur during closed treatment or after surgical fixation. Shah and Bhatti[23] reviewed 62 patients with radial nerve palsies and humeral shaft fractures, of which 17 patients developed a secondary nerve palsy. Of these 17 patients, 11 of them had true closed management of their fractures consisting of cast/splint treatment, with or without manipulation of their fracture; 4 patients were treated with olecranon pin traction. Eight of these 17 patients had surgical exploration of their nerves, with all of them demonstrating intact nerves; however, 3 patients had nerves impinging on fracture fragments and 1 patient had the radial nerve entrapped in scar. All 17 patients who had secondary nerve palsy demonstrated complete recovery of their radial nerve function. This study demonstrated that closed management of humeral shaft fractures can lead to secondary nerve palsies, all of which recovered.

Surgical management of humeral shaft fractures can also lead to secondary palsies of the radial nerve. The least invasive technique is intramedullary nailing; however, this is not recommended in radial nerve palsies associated with humeral shaft fractures, as potential entrapment of the nerve in the fracture site leaves it vulnerable to further damage. The incidence of radial nerve injury following this technique has been reported to be between 0% and 5%.[24] Other series examining radial nerve palsy following intramedullary nailing has identified that most palsies are temporary and resolve spontaneously.[25–27] Alternatively, open reduction with compression plating is the most common procedure for humeral shaft fracture fixation. This technique can lead to radial nerve injury in up to 10% of cases.[28,29] This approach allows for an anatomic reduction with the most predictable rate of fracture union.[30,31] Routine exploration of the radial nerve is recommended during compression plating of the humerus, particularly in cases with preoperative radial nerve palsies.[24]

MANAGEMENT/TREATMENT

To begin evaluating the status of a radial nerve injury and what type of treatment should be used, an electrodiagnostic study can be helpful. These studies are not useful in the acute setting, but may have a role in the subacute setting in determining the level and extent of nerve injury.[18] It can also be used to determine a baseline nerve function at the 3-week point to guide treatment during the observation period. These baseline electrodiagnostic studies may demonstrate "fibrillation potentials, positive sharp waves, and monophasic action potentials of short duration."[32] Most patients with spontaneous recovery begin to demonstrate recovery during the first few months;

however, an electrodiagnostic study may serve as an adjunct study for those lacking nerve recovery at the 6-week or 12-week point.[23,33,34] If a follow-up electrodiagnostic study at the 12-week point shows similar findings as the baseline, then exploration may be indicated. However, if the 12-week follow-up study shows "improved nerve function with larger polyphasic motor unit action potentials of longer duration," then some degree of spontaneous recovery may be expected.[32] However, the course of this subset of patients is not predictable.

Significant controversy persists with regard to the management of a radial nerve palsy associated with a humeral shaft fracture. Currently, noncontroversial and generally well-accepted indications for early exploration include open fractures, radial nerve palsy after closed reduction, associated vascular injuries, high-velocity gunshot wounds, penetrating injuries, severe soft tissue injuries, or any case with a high suspicion of a direct nerve laceration (**Box 1**).[8–10,17,29,35–39] Ring and colleagues[40] retrospectively reviewed patients with a high-energy humeral shaft fracture with an associated complete radial nerve palsy. All 6 patients with a transected radial nerve had a complex open fracture.

However, the management of a radial nerve palsy with a closed humerus fracture can be divided into 2 treatment camps:

1. Late exploration
2. Early exploration.

Late Exploration

Although early reports recommended surgical management with exploration for primary radial nerve palsies after humeral shaft fractures,[8,35] with time, investigators have leaned toward no immediate exploration of the radial nerve following closed fractures of the humerus because of a high rate of recovery (over 70%).[3,17,19,22,29,35,41] One study found an incidence of 87.3% functional recovery after primary radial nerve palsies

---

Box 1
Indications for early exploration of a radial nerve palsy following fracture of the humerus

- Radial nerve palsy after a closed reduction
- Open fracture
- Vascular injury
- High-velocity gunshot wound
- Associated severe soft tissue injury

managed with no immediate surgical exploration.[42] Similarly, many studies have noted that
the radial nerve is usually contused and does not
require immediate exploration.[9,15,19,22] During
routine exploration of radial nerve palsies associated with humeral shaft fractures, one study found
a transection rate of only 12%.[9] Another study, by
Sonneveld and colleagues,[43] reviewed 17 cases of
radial nerve palsies after humeral shaft fractures.
Fourteen fractures were explored, with 13 of the
radial nerves noted to be undamaged. Clinical recovery was seen in 12 of the 14 patients with nerve
exploration. In a systematic literature review of
radial nerve palsy associated with fractures of
the humeral shaft, Shao and colleagues[44] identified a spontaneous radial nerve recovery rate of
70.7% in patients treated nonoperatively, and an
overall recovery rate of 88.1% regardless of treatment and timing of intervention. Furthermore, they
did not find a difference in outcome among patients treated with early or late exploration.

In short, proponents of late exploration may
argue that delaying surgical exploration can
decrease the risk of the usual surgical complications, such as infection or scarring, in patients
who may otherwise recover radial nerve spontaneously anyway. Another potential advantage of delaying surgery is to permit thickening of the
neurilemmal sheath, making future nerve repair
easier.[18]

Early Exploration

Advocates of early exploration of a radial nerve
palsy may argue that a sufficient number of radial
nerve injuries requiring treatment after closed
humeral shaft fractures routinely exist, warranting
early exploration. Moreover, early exploration
and expedient repair of a radial nerve laceration
will result in a more superior outcome than a
delayed repair. Series with late exploration have
revealed nerve laceration or entrapment to be present 6% to 25% of the time.[9,19,20,22,35,45] Moreover, the systematic review performed by Shao
and colleagues[44] identified a spontaneous recovery rate of 70% but an overall recovery rate of
only 88%. In addition, Pollock and colleagues[9]
noted nerve lacerations in 20% to 42% of cases
after late exploration. They also noted poor results
clinically after late repair. Evidence has also been
shown that delays of more than 5 months can
result in poorer outcomes.[10] Delaying surgery
may result in irreversible nerve damage without motor endplate reinnervation within 12 to
18 months of injury for useful return of function.[18]
Similarly, if no improvement is seen after 7 months,
then spontaneous recovery is not likely to occur.[46]

Box 2
**Potential advantages of early exploration of a
radial nerve palsy following a closed fracture of
the humerus**

- Earlier nerve injury characterization and
  repair
- Immediate fracture stabilization and earlier
  rehabilitation
- Less muscular atrophy and endplate loss
- Earlier return to function

Subsequently, advocates for early exploration of
a radial nerve palsy with a simple closed humerus
fracture would argue that after consideration of the
plethora of available series, including a number of
series that have documented the risk of a nerve
laceration or incarceration with a closed fracture
of the humerus to be as high as 25%, that expec-
tant or delayed nerve exploration can compromise
ultimate recovery (**Box 2**). Prolonged observation
of cases with a lacerated or incarcerated radial
nerve will result in no radial nerve recovery, potential atrophy and motor endplate loss, compromised nerve recovery on late exploration and
repair, and significant interval loss of patient function and livelihood. In contrast, early exploration
and repair performed earlier can facilitate better
characterization of the nerve injury, quicker nerve
recovery on repair with less distal endplate loss,
less muscular atrophy, quicker return to function,
and peace of mind. Moreover, after fracture fixation and stabilization is achieved, a neurolysed
or repaired nerve will potentially benefit from a better environment for recovery with less tension,
motion, or callus formation to impede nerve
healing.[17,35]

SUMMARY

A radial nerve palsy is the most common peripheral nerve injury following a humerus fracture
occurring in up to 2% to 17% of cases.[8–10] These
injuries can be classified as either partial or complete, depending on the extent of physical examination findings, as well as primary or secondary
depending on the palsy's timing of presentation.
Surgical exploration is recommended in cases
with open or complex fractures, particularly those
associated with penetrating trauma. Radial nerve
palsies associated with closed fractures of the
humerus have traditionally been recommended
to be treated with observation, with late exploration restricted to cases without spontaneous nerve
recovery at 3 to 6 months. Advocates for early

exploration believe that late exploration can result in increased muscular atrophy, motor endplate loss, compromised nerve recovery on delayed repair, and significant interval loss of patient function and livelihood. In contrast, early exploration maximizes nerve injury characterization and repair as well as facilitates early fracture stabilization, which can avoid late nerve injury or incarceration. Moreover, early exploration yielding a nerve injury that is repaired can lead to quicker nerve recovery with less motor endplate loss, less muscular atrophy, and quicker return to function.

REFERENCES

1. Browner BD. 3rd edition. Skeletal trauma: basic science, management, and reconstruction, vol. 2. Philadelphia: Saunders; 2003. p. xxiii, 2626, xli.
2. Ekholm R, Adami J, Tidermark J, et al. Fractures of the shaft of the humerus. An epidemiological study of 401 fractures. J Bone Joint Surg Br 2006;88(11): 1469–73.
3. Mast JW, Spiegel PG, Harvey JP Jr, et al. Fractures of the humeral shaft: a retrospective study of 240 adult fractures. Clin Orthop Relat Res 1975;112: 254–62.
4. Rose SH, Melton LJ 3rd, Morrey BF, et al. Epidemiologic features of humeral fractures. Clin Orthop Relat Res 1982;168:24–30.
5. Tytherleigh-Strong G, Walls N, McQueen MM. The epidemiology of humeral shaft fractures. J Bone Joint Surg Br 1998;80(2):249–53.
6. Omer GE Jr. Results of untreated peripheral nerve injuries. Clin Orthop Relat Res 1982;163:15–9.
7. Samardzic M, Grujicic D, Milinkovic ZB. Radial nerve lesions associated with fractures of the humeral shaft. Injury 1990;21(4):220–2.
8. Holstein A, Lewis GM. Fractures of the humerus with radial-nerve paralysis. J Bone Joint Surg Am 1963; 45:1382–8.
9. Pollock FH, Drake D, Bovill EG, et al. Treatment of radial neuropathy associated with fractures of the humerus. J Bone Joint Surg Am 1981;63(2):239–43.
10. Amillo S, Barrios RH, Martínez-Peric R, et al. Surgical treatment of the radial nerve lesions associated with fractures of the humerus. J Orthop Trauma 1993;7(3):211–5.
11. Noble J, Munro CA, Prasad VS, et al. Analysis of upper and lower extremity peripheral nerve injuries in a population of patients with multiple injuries. J Trauma 1998;45(1):116–22.
12. DeFranco MJ, Lawton JN. Radial nerve injuries associated with humeral fractures. J Hand Surg Am 2006;31(4):655–63.
13. Whitson RO. Relation of the radial nerve to the shaft of the humerus. J Bone Joint Surg Am 1954;36(1): 85–8.
14. Rockwood CA, Green DP, Bucholz RW. Rockwood and Green's fractures in adults. 6th edition. Philadelphia: Lippincott Williams & Wilkins; 2006.
15. Böstman O, Bakalim G, Vainionpää S, et al. Radial palsy in shaft fracture of the humerus. Acta Orthop Scand 1986;57(4):316–9.
16. Bono CM, Grossman MG, Hochwald N, et al. Radial and axillary nerves. Anatomic considerations for humeral fixation. Clin Orthop Relat Res 2000;373:259–64.
17. Garcia A Jr, Maeck BH. Radial nerve injuries in fractures of the shaft of the humerus. Am J Surg 1960; 99:625–7.
18. Lowe JB 3rd, Sen SK, Mackinnon SE. Current approach to radial nerve paralysis. Plast Reconstr Surg 2002;110(4):1099–113.
19. Kettelkamp DB, Alexander H. Clinical review of radial nerve injury. J Trauma 1967;7(3):424–32.
20. Seddon HJ. Nerve lesions complicating certain closed bone injuries. J Am Med Assoc 1947;135(11):691–4.
21. Sunderland S. A classification of peripheral nerve injuries producing loss of function. Brain 1951;74(4): 491–516.
22. Shaw JL, Sakellarides H. Radial-nerve paralysis associated with fractures of the humerus. A review of forty-five cases. J Bone Joint Surg Am 1967; 49(5):899–902.
23. Shah JJ, Bhatti NA. Radial nerve paralysis associated with fractures of the humerus. A review of 62 cases. Clin Orthop Relat Res 1983;172:171–6.
24. Farragos AF, Schemitsch EH, McKee MD. Complications of intramedullary nailing for fractures of the humeral shaft: a review. J Orthop Trauma 1999;13(4): 258–67.
25. Crolla RM, de Vries LS, Clevers GJ. Locked intramedullary nailing of humeral fractures. Injury 1993; 24(6):403–6.
26. Ingman AM, Waters DA. Locked intramedullary nailing of humeral shaft fractures. Implant design, surgical technique, and clinical results. J Bone Joint Surg Br 1994;76(1):23–9.
27. Rommens PM, Verbruggen J, Broos PL. Retrograde locked nailing of humeral shaft fractures. A review of 39 patients. J Bone Joint Surg Br 1995;77(1):84–9.
28. Bell MJ, Beauchamp CG, Kellam JK, et al. The results of plating humeral shaft fractures in patients with multiple injuries. The Sunnybrook experience. J Bone Joint Surg Br 1985;67(2):293–6.
29. Dabezies EJ, Banta CJ 2nd, Murphy CP, et al. Plate fixation of the humeral shaft for acute fractures, with and without radial nerve injuries. J Orthop Trauma 1992;6(1):10–3.
30. Chapman JR, Henley MB, Agel J, et al. Randomized prospective study of humeral shaft fracture fixation: intramedullary nails versus plates. J Orthop Trauma 2000;14(3):162–6.
31. McCormack RG, Brien D, Buckley RE, et al. Fixation of fractures of the shaft of the humerus by dynamic

compression plate or intramedullary nail. A prospective, randomised trial. J Bone Joint Surg Br 2000; 82(3):336–9.

32. Mohler LR, Hanel DP. Closed fractures complicated by peripheral nerve injury. J Am Acad Orthop Surg 2006;14(1):32–7.

33. Robinson LR. Traumatic injury to peripheral nerves. Muscle Nerve 2000;23(6):863–73.

34. Robinson LR. Role of neurophysiologic evaluation in diagnosis. J Am Acad Orthop Surg 2000;8(3): 190–9.

35. Packer JW, Foster RR, Garcia A, et al. The humeral fracture with radial nerve palsy: is exploration warranted? Clin Orthop Relat Res 1972;88:34–8.

36. Vander Griend R, Tomasin J, Ward EF. Open reduction and internal fixation of humeral shaft fractures. Results using AO plating techniques. J Bone Joint Surg Am 1986;68(3):430–3.

37. Foster RJ, Swiontkowski MF, Bach AW, et al. Radial nerve palsy caused by open humeral shaft fractures. J Hand Surg Am 1993;18(1):121–4.

38. Modabber MR, Jupiter JB. Operative management of diaphyseal fractures of the humerus. Plate versus nail. Clin Orthop Relat Res 1998;347:93–104.

39. Bercik MJ, Kingsbery J, Ilyas AM. Peripheral nerve injuries following gunshot fracture of the humerus. Orthopedics 2012;35(3):e349–52.

40. Ring D, Chin K, Jupiter JB. Radial nerve palsy associated with high-energy humeral shaft fractures. J Hand Surg Am 2004;29(1):144–7.

41. Dameron TB Jr, Grubb SA. Humeral shaft fractures in adults. South Med J 1981;74(12):1461–7.

42. Heim D, Herkert F, Hess P, et al. Surgical treatment of humeral shaft fractures—the Basel experience. J Trauma 1993;35(2):226–32.

43. Sonneveld GJ, Patka P, van Mourik JC, et al. Treatment of fractures of the shaft of the humerus accompanied by paralysis of the radial nerve. Injury 1987; 18(6):404–6.

44. Shao YC, Harwood P, Grotz MR, et al. Radial nerve palsy associated with fractures of the shaft of the humerus: a systematic review. J Bone Joint Surg Br 2005;87(12):1647–52.

45. Klenerman L. Fractures of the shaft of the humerus. J Bone Joint Surg Br 1966;48(1):105–11.

46. Gelberman RH. Operative nerve repair and reconstruction, vol. 2. Philadelphia: Lippincott; 1991. p. xxix, 1625, 37.

Radial Head Fractures
Indications and Outcomes for Radial Head Arthroplasty

John R. Fowler, MD*, Robert J. Goitz, MD

KEYWORDS

- Radial head arthroplasty • Essex-Lopresti • Radial head fracture • Terrible triad • Elbow instability

KEY POINTS

- Radial head fractures without associated bony or ligamentous injury can be safely treated with internal fixation, if possible, or arthroplasty if unreconstructable.
- Radiocapitellar contact, through either repair or replacement of the radial head, is an essential aspect of proper management for radial head fractures with associated injuries.
- Excision of an unreconstructable radial head should be done with caution, as it can result in elbow or longitudinal forearm instability.
- The ability to generalize outcomes after radial head arthroplasty is limited by the heterogeneity of indications, injury severity, type of implant, and choice of outcome measurements.
- The treatment of radial head fractures with associated ligamentous and/or bony pathology using radial head arthroplasty has been reported to result in good or excellent outcomes in 76% to 94% at long-term follow-up.

INTRODUCTION

The treatment of comminuted radial head fractures remains controversial. Radial head excision can be successfully performed in isolated radial head injuries; however, radial head excision also has been noted to result in pain, instability, proximal migration of the radius, decreased strength, and osteoarthrosis in some cases.[1–3] These negative outcomes are related to the critical role the radial head plays in force transmission and stability of the elbow. The radial head transmits up to 90% of the force across the elbow[4] and functions as an important secondary stabilizer to valgus stress.[5] This critical role is emphasized when radial head fractures are associated with additional ligamentous and bony pathology, which is the case in nearly one-third of radial head fractures.[6] The likelihood of associated injuries strongly correlates with the severity of the radial head fracture, increasing from 20% in nondisplaced fractures to 80% in comminuted fractures.[6]

These findings have led some to believe that restoration of radiocapitellar contact, through either repair or replacement of the radial head, is an essential aspect of proper management.[7–9] Failure to address the radiocapitellar articulation may lead to valgus elbow instability, elbow stiffness, proximal radial migration, degenerative changes at the wrist and elbow, and chronic pain.[10] However, degenerative changes of the capitellum due to wear remains a concern with the use of implant arthroplasty.[10–12] Radial head fractures are a common injury, with an incidence of 30 per 100,000 persons per year.[13] Previous

Disclosures: None.
Division of Hand, Upper Extremity, and Microvascular Surgery, Department of Orthopaedic Surgery, University of Pittsburgh, Suite 1010, 3471 Fifth Avenue, Pittsburgh, PA 15213, USA
* Corresponding author.
E-mail address: johnfowler10@gmail.com

Orthop Clin N Am 44 (2013) 425–431
http://dx.doi.org/10.1016/j.ocl.2013.03.013

series found radial head fractures to account for 1% to 5% of all fractures and 33% to 75% of all elbow fractures.[1,13–15] Therefore, understanding the proper management of these fractures is essential.

Since Speed[16] performed the first documented radial head arthroplasty in 1941, implant materials have included acrylic,[17] silicone,[18–21] cobalt-chromium,[12,22–28] titanium,[10–12] and pyrocarbon.[29] The use of silicone implants has become less popular because of their inability to reconstitute normal biomechanics, resulting in suboptimal wear characteristics, particulate debris, implant failure, and elbow instability.[30] Metallic implants are now commonly used and published reports have documented promising results.[10–12,22,24,31] The specific type of implant used, however, is likely less important than adhering to proper indications and technique. The purpose of this article was to review the indications and outcomes of radial head arthroplasty.

CLASSIFICATION

The Mason classification is the most commonly used classification system for radial head fractures.[32] Type I fractures are nondisplaced, Type II fractures are displaced partial head fractures, and Type III fractures are displaced fractures that involve the entire radial head. Johnston[33] modified the Mason classification, by adding a fourth type, defined as a fracture of the radial head with associated elbow dislocation. Broberg and Morrey[34] further modified the Mason classification by defining the amount of fracture displacement. A Type I fracture is defined as less than 2 mm of displacement. A Type II fracture has 2 mm or more displacement and/or involves 30% or more of the joint surface. A Type III fracture is a comminuted fracture and a Type IV fracture is any of the previously mentioned types with a concomitant elbow dislocation.

In an attempt to better guide operative treatment, Hotchkiss[35] modified the Mason classification with respect to mechanical block to motion. Type I fractures are defined as nondisplaced fractures or minimally displaced marginal lip fractures (<2 mm displacement) that do not block motion and can be treated nonoperatively. Type II fractures are displaced fractures (usually >2 mm) that may have a mechanical block to motion or are incongruous but do not have severe comminution. Type II fractures are often amenable to open reduction and internal fixation. Type III fractures are comminuted fractures that are unable to be repaired and are excised or undergo radial head arthroplasty.

Although the Mason classification and its modifications are well accepted and commonly used, Ring[36] found that the radiographic parameters used to define displacement have been an unreliable indicator of instability. He noted that the presence of more than 3 fragments has a higher correlation with poor results following open reduction and internal fixation. Also, radial head fractures associated with elbow dislocations indicate a complex injury pattern and should alert the surgeon to associated fractures and ligamentous injuries that may also result in a less optimal outcome.[36]

INDICATIONS FOR RADIAL HEAD ARTHROPLASTY

Despite numerous studies and advances in technology, controversy still exists over the indications for open reduction and internal fixation versus radial head arthroplasty for comminuted radial head fractures. Historically, excision of the radial head was indicated in comminuted radial head fractures that were deemed unreconstructable. Reports of proximal radial migration associated with an interosseous membrane injury, an Essex-Lopresti lesion, have led surgeons to exercise caution when considering primary radial head excision for acute radial head fractures. Associated ligamentous and bony injuries around the elbow represent a contraindication to excision of the radial head because of role of the radial head as the primary stabilizer to valgus stress.[37]

Radial head arthroplasty is indicated in the following situations (**Box 1**): (1) an acute comminuted fracture in which satisfactory reduction and stable fixation cannot be obtained[7]; (2) complex elbow injuries that involve greater than 30% of the articular rim of the radial head, which cannot be reconstructed; (3) fractures with 3 or more fragments or significant comminution[7]; (4) instability of the elbow after radial head excision[11]; (5) patients who present in a delayed manner with persistent pain and instability from radial head primary resections, malunions, or after complex elbow fracture-dislocations involving the radial head[12,38]; (6) suspected Essex-Lopresti lesion[7,39]; (7) associated terrible triad injuries[7]; (8) unreconstructable radial head fractures with concomitant medial collateral ligament injury, interosseous membrane injury, or elbow dislocation.[40,41]

Contraindications to radial head arthroplasty include (1) nondisplaced or minimally displaced radial head fracture with no mechanical block to motion and no elbow instability, (2) active infection in or around the elbow joint, (3) neurologic injury preventing meaningful use of the elbow, (4) stable

Box 1
Indications for radial head arthroplasty

- Acute comminuted fracture in which satisfactory reduction and stable fixation cannot be obtained
- Complex elbow injuries that involve greater than 30% of the articular rim of the radial head, which cannot be reconstructed
- Fractures with 3 or more fragments or significant commination
- Instability of the elbow after radial head excision
- Pain and instability from radial head primary resections, malunions, or after complex elbow fracture-dislocations involving the radial head
- Suspected Essex-Lopresti lesion
- Associated terrible triad injuries
- Unreconstructable radial head fractures with concomitant medial collateral ligament injury, interosseous membrane injury, or elbow dislocation

elbow arthrodesis, and (5) congenital radial head dislocation.

OUTCOMES

The ability to generalize outcomes after radial head arthroplasty is limited by the heterogeneity of indications, injury severity, type of implant, and choice of outcome measurements. Most published series contain a heterogeneous patient population ranging from isolated fractures to comminuted fractures with associated elbow dislocations and/or terrible triad injuries.[10,12,22–24,31,42] The timing of radial head arthroplasty also varies in the literature, with some investigators performing surgery within a week of injury[10,22,40] and others in delayed fashion, even several years after the initial injury.[12,24,26,43]

Cobalt-chromium

The first radial head arthroplasty was performed in the 1940s using cobalt-chromium caps in a canine model, followed shortly thereafter by use in humans.[16] Ten years later, Carr and Howard[25] reported on the use of the cobalt-chromium cap in 12 cases of uncomplicated radial head fractures. Silastic and titanium implants temporarily supplanted cobalt-chromium as the material of choice in radial head implants, but most recent series have used cobalt-chromium implants.[10,12,22–24,28,31,43]

Two studies have reported mean follow-up of longer than 8 years. Popovic and colleagues[22] reviewed 51 patients with a comminuted fracture of the radial head treated with either monoblock or modular radial head replacement. The radial head fractures were associated with an elbow dislocation in 34 patients and a Monteggia fracture in 6. At an average follow-up of 8.4 years (range 4–13 years), the investigators reported an average Mayo Elbow Performance Score (MEPS) of 83 (range 59–95) with 39 (76%) good or excellent results. Radiographic assessment found 37 (73%) patients with progressive osteolysis around the implant. Reported mean arc of elbow flexion-extension was 115°. With respect to pain, 41 (80%) patients reported no pain or mild pain with activities. Burkhart and colleagues[31] retrospectively reviewed 17 patients with an average follow-up of 106 months (range 78–139 months). Acute radial head replacement was performed in 9 patients and delayed replacement was performed in 8 patients. The injury patterns were heterogeneous, with 4 patients having isolated nonreconstructable radial head fracture, 2 patients had associated elbow dislocations, 3 patients had a terrible triad, 6 patients had Monteggia fractures, and 1 patient had an Essex-Lopresti lesion. Despite the complex injury patterns, the average MEPS score was 90.8, with 16 (94%) good or excellent results. The investigators found no difference in outcomes between primary and delayed implantation. The mean DASH score was 9.8, mean flexion arc was 124° (range 110–150°), and extension deficit was 21° (range 0–40°). Heterotopic ossification developed in 12 patients. Complications occurred in 5 patients, prosthetic dislocation in 2, and capitellar erosion in 3.

Multiple studies have reported satisfactory outcomes at medium-term follow-up.[23,24,27] Judet and colleagues[24] reviewed 12 patients with mean follow-up of 49 months. Acute radial head replacement was performed in 5 patients and delayed replacement in 7 patients after failed excision. All patients who underwent acute reconstruction had good results, based on the Brodberg and Morrey Index, compared with no good or excellent results in the delayed reconstruction group. These results could be misleading, however, as the delayed reconstruction group had undergone between 2 and 4 procedures per patient before reconstruction. Flinkkila and colleagues[23] reviewed 35 patients, at mean follow-up of 53 months (range 12–106 months), with an acute radial head fracture and associated unstable elbow injury treated with a modular uncemented press-fit cobalt chromium radial head replacement. The associated elbow injury was a terrible triad in 19 patients. The average MEPS score was 86 (range 40–100), resulting in good or excellent results in 26 (74%) patients. The investigators removed 9 implants (26%), and 4 patients required excision of heterotopic ossification. Knight and colleagues[27] performed a retrospective review of 31 patients treated with a cobalt-chromium implant for comminuted fractures of the radial head. The radial head fracture was associated with an elbow dislocation in 21 patients. The investigators noted a successful result in 24 (77%) patients with mean follow-up of 4.5 years. Two of the implants required removal because of painful loosening and 7 cases were complicated by nonprogressive radiolucencies around the prostheses. Brinkman and colleagues[43] treated 11 patients who failed open reduction internal fixation or excision with delayed radial head arthroplasty at a mean of 8 years after initial injury. The investigators reported 100% good or excellent results at mean follow-up of 2 years (range 1–4 years).

Several studies have reported acceptable short-term outcomes. Grewal and colleagues[40] prospectively evaluated 26 patients in whom an unreconstructable radial head fracture had been treated with a modular radial head prosthesis. At 24-month follow-up, 16/26 (62%) patients were rated as good or excellent, with an overall average MEPS score of 83 points. Mean elbow flexion was 138° and average DASH 24.4 (±21.4). Radiographic lucency was present around 13 (50%) implants. Mild posttraumatic arthritis was evident in 5 (19%) and heterotopic ossification was present in 6 (23%). Chapman and colleagues[26] reviewed 16 patients, at an average follow-up of 33 months. Of this group, 8 patients underwent acute reconstruction and 8 patients underwent delayed reconstruction. In the acute group, the investigators found 3 patients with an excellent result and 5 patients with a good result. Despite 5 fracture-dislocations in the acute group compared with all ground-level falls and no fracture-dislocations in the chronic group, the acute group performed better on the Disabilities of the Arm, Shoulder and Hand questionnaire (DASH). Lim and Chan[28] reviewed 6 patients after radial head arthroplasty with a cemented cobalt-chromium prosthesis at an average follow-up of 30 months. Despite good pain relief with an average visual analog scale (VAS) score of 1.8, the average flexion arc was found to be 100° and 4/6 (67%) experienced a good or excellent result according to the Brodberg and Morrey Performance Index. Chien and colleagues[44] reviewed 13 patients who underwent radial head arthroplasty at mean follow-up of 38 months (range 20–70). The investigators found good to excellent results in 11 (85%) patients,

based on MEPS, with 2 patients undergoing implant removal. Doornberg and colleagues[45] retrospectively reviewed 27 patients treated with a modular prosthesis. The radial head fracture was associated with an elbow dislocation in 10 patients and a terrible triad in 13. At final follow-up, the average arc of motion was 111° (range 35–155°), 17 (68%) of 25 had radiographic evidence of lucency. The average MEPS score was 85 (range 30–100), resulting in 22 (81%) of 27 good or excellent results. The average DASH score was 17 (range 0–82). Radiographic evidence of lucency around the stem was present in 17 (68%) and radiographic evidence of arthritis was present in 12 (44%).

Silastic

Silicone implants were commonly used until concerns arose regarding suboptimal wear characteristics, particulate debris, and implant failure with repetitive compressive loads.[30] The compressibility of silicone makes it unable to adequately restore the biomechanics of the elbow and may result in progressive osteoporosis of the capitellum.[19,27] An early series by Mackay and colleagues[19] found satisfactory results in 17 (94%) of 18 patients, but noted hardware failure in 3 patients within 26 months. Less promising results were noted by Morrey and colleagues[20] and Swanson and colleagues.[21] Morrey and colleagues[20] reported 5 (29%) failures in 17 patients, finding that all of the failures occurred in patients who underwent delayed reconstruction, at an average of 24 months after radial head excision. Swanson and colleagues[21] compared 12 patients with delayed arthroplasty after radial head resection with 6 patients with acute arthroplasty and found consistent radial shortening with a correlation to decreased forearm supination in the delayed replacement group compared with no shortening in the acute group. The investigators found the best results when the implant was used primarily in fractures, to maintain the normal mechanical relationships. A recent series by Maghen and colleagues[18] retrospectively reviewed 23 patients with unreconstructable radial head fractures who were treated with silastic radial head arthroplasty and concomitant repair and/or reconstruction of the medial ulnar collateral ligament and/or lateral ulnar collateral ligament. At an average follow-up of 70 months (range 16–165), the investigators found an average arc of motion of 134°, an average DASH of 11.8 (range 0–56), and an average Mayo Elbow Performance Score (MEPS) of 88.9 (range 45–100). The investigators argued that silastic implants may still be a reasonable implant option if associated injuries are appropriately treated to minimize reliance on the implant for stability.[18]

Titanium

Harrington and Tountas[46] published one of the first series using titanium radial head prosthesis in 1981. The investigators reported good or excellent results in 14 (93%) of 15 patients at average follow-up of 6.9 years. In an update of their series, Harrington and colleagues[11] reported 16 (80%) of 20 good or excellent outcomes, based on the Mayo Clinic Functional Index, at mean follow-up of 12.1 years (range 6–29 years). The series included 13 patients with Mason IV injuries. Only 6 (30%) of 20 were completely pain free at final follow-up, but an additional 10 had pain only with continuous activity. The investigators note degenerative changes of the capitellum in 9 patients (45%). Shore and colleagues[12] studied 32 patients, with mean follow-up of 8 years (range 2–14 years), treated with delayed radial head arthroplasty an average of 2.4 years after the injury. The radial head fractures were associated with an elbow dislocation in 17 patients and terrible triad in 7 patients. The average MEPS score was 83, with 21 (66%) obtaining good or excellent results. Posttraumatic arthritis was observed in 74%. The MEPS score in 11 patients with moderate posttraumatic arthritis was 79 compared with 93 in 10 patients with mild arthritis. In contrast to other series, Shore and colleagues[12] did not remove any implants.

Moro and colleagues[10] retrospectively reviewed 25 patients with 10 Mason III and 15 Mason IV radial head fractures, treated with acute radial head arthroplasty using a noncemented titanium prosthesis. At mean follow-up of 39 months (range 26–58 months), the investigators noted 16 (64%) good or excellent results with 5 (20%) patients demonstrating radiographic evidence of posttraumatic arthritis. Heterotopic ossification was found in 8 (32%) patients. Ashwood and colleagues[42] studied outcomes in 16 patients treated with a titanium radial head prosthesis. The average MEPS score at final follow-up (average 2.8 years) was 87 (range 65–100) with 13 (81%) obtaining good or excellent results. The average VAS score was 1.7 (range 0–4.5) and 7 of 9 employed patients were able to return to work. On average, patients lost 15° of extension and 10° of flexion compared with the uninjured side.

Pyrocarbon

Pyrocarbon radial head prostheses have been introduced as an alternative to metallic implants.

Ricon and colleagues[29] performed a retrospective analysis of 28 patients with Mason III radial head fractures treated with a pyrocarbon radial head prosthesis. The radial head fracture was associated with an elbow dislocation in 23 patients. At an average follow-up of 23 months, patients had an average MEPS score of 92 (range 70–100). The mean flexion-extension arc was 105° (range 65–130). Although these outcomes are comparable to those achieved with cobalt-chromium and titanium prostheses, enthusiasm should be tempered until longer-term follow-up data are available.

SUMMARY

Radial head fractures without associated bony or ligamentous injury can be safely treated with internal fixation, if possible, or excision if unreconstructable. However, unreconstructable radial head fractures in association with elbow dislocation and/or ligamentous injury in the elbow or forearm represent a specific subset of injuries that require restoration of the radiocapitellar articulation for optimal function. The treatment of radial head fractures with associated ligamentous and/or bony pathology using radial head arthroplasty has been reported to result in good or excellent outcomes in 76% to 94% at long-term follow-up.[11,22,31] There does, however, appear to be a concern for development of posttraumatic arthritis and capitellar wear, with estimates ranging from 19% at short-term follow-up[40] to 74% at long-term follow-up.[12]

Multiple studies have found better results in acute radial head replacement compared with acute excision with delayed reconstruction.[20,21,24] The etiology of these findings is unclear, but it is likely a result of selection bias, as the patients with an unsuccessful excision undergo reconstruction whereas those with a successful outcome after radial head excision are not selected for the study. The decision to perform radial head arthroplasty rather than radial head excision must be made on an individualized basis, tailored to the patient's needs, expectations, and injury pattern. Radial head arthroplasty may result in persistent pain likely due to capitellar wear. Despite a high percentage of good or excellent outcomes in most patients in most series, there remains a significant number of patients who later require implant removal.[23,27,44]

Overall, the quality of evidence describing outcomes of radial head arthroplasty is poor. Most series consist of retrospective reviews of small numbers of patients with a heterogeneous injury pattern and time to surgery. Further prospective or randomized series will be needed to determine the true efficacy of radial head arthroplasty for unstable radial head fractures in both the acute and chronic settings.

REFERENCES

1. Herbertsson P, Josefsson PO, Hasserius R, et al. Fractures of the radial head and neck treated with radial head excision. J Bone Joint Surg Am 2004; 86(9):1925–30.

2. Ikeda M, Oka Y. Function after early radial head resection for fracture: a retrospective evaluation of 15 patients followed for 3–18 years. Acta Orthop Scand 2000;71(2):191–4.

3. Morrey BF, Tanaka S, An KN. Valgus stability of the elbow. A definition of primary and secondary constraints. Clin Orthop Relat Res 1991;(265): 187–95.

4. Morrey BF, An KN, Stormont TJ. Force transmission through the radial head. J Bone Joint Surg Am 1988;70(2):250–6.

5. Bryce CD, Armstrong AD. Anatomy and biomechanics of the elbow. Orthop Clin North Am 2008; 39(2):141–54, v.

6. van Riet RP, Morrey BF, O'Driscoll SW, et al. Associated injuries complicating radial head fractures: a demographic study. Clin Orthop Relat Res 2005; 441:351–5.

7. Ring D. Radial head fracture: open reduction-internal fixation or prosthetic replacement. J Shoulder Elbow Surg 2011;20(Suppl 2):S107–12.

8. Kaas L, Struijs PA, Ring D, et al. Treatment of mason type II radial head fractures without associated fractures or elbow dislocation: a systematic review. J Hand Surg 2012;37(7):1416–21.

9. Davidson PA, Moseley JB Jr, Tullos HS. Radial head fracture. A potentially complex injury. Clin Orthop Relat Res 1993;(297):224–30.

10. Moro JK, Werier J, MacDermid JC, et al. Arthroplasty with a metal radial head for unreconstructable fractures of the radial head. J Bone Joint Surg Am 2001;83(8):1201–11.

11. Harrington IJ, Sekyi-Otu A, Barrington TW, et al. The functional outcome with metallic radial head implants in the treatment of unstable elbow fractures: a long-term review. J Trauma 2001;50(1):46–52.

12. Shore BJ, Mozzon JB, MacDermid JC, et al. Chronic posttraumatic elbow disorders treated with metallic radial head arthroplasty. J Bone Joint Surg Am 2008;90(2):271–80.

13. Duckworth AD, Clement ND, Jenkins PJ, et al. The epidemiology of radial head and neck fractures. J Hand Surg 2012;37(1):112–9.

14. Rosenblatt Y, Athwal GS, Faber KJ. Current recommendations for the treatment of radial head fractures. Orthop Clin North Am 2008;39(2):173–85, vi.

15. Tejwani NC, Mehta H. Fractures of the radial head and neck: current concepts in management. J Am Acad Orthop Surg 2007;15(7):380–7.

16. Speed K. Ferrule caps for the head of the radius. Surg Gynecol Obstet 1941;73:845–80.

17. Cherry JC. Use of acrylic prosthesis in the treatment of fracture of the head of the radius. J Bone Joint Surg Br 1953;35(1):70–1.

18. Maghen Y, Leo AJ, Hsu JW, et al. Is a silastic radial head still a reasonable option? Clin Orthop Relat Res 2011;469(4):1061–70.

19. Mackay I, Fitzgerald B, Miller JH. Silastic replacement of the head of the radius in trauma. J Bone Joint Surg Br 1979;61(4):494–7.

20. Morrey BF, Askew L, Chao EY. Silastic prosthetic replacement for the radial head. J Bone Joint Surg Am 1981;63(3):454–8.

21. Swanson AB, Jaeger SH, La Rochelle D. Comminuted fractures of the radial head. The role of silicone-implant replacement arthroplasty. J Bone Joint Surg Am 1981;63(7):1039–49.

22. Popovic N, Lemaire R, Georis P, et al. Midterm results with a bipolar radial head prosthesis: radiographic evidence of loosening at the bone-cement interface. J Bone Joint Surg Am 2007;89(11):2469–76.

23. Flinkkila T, Kaisto T, Sirnio K, et al. Short- to mid-term results of metallic press-fit radial head arthroplasty in unstable injuries of the elbow. J Bone Joint Surg Br 2012;94(6):805–10.

24. Judet T, Garreau de Loubresse C, Piriou P, et al. A floating prosthesis for radial-head fractures. J Bone Joint Surg Br 1996;78(2):244–9.

25. Carr CR, Howard JW. Metallic cap replacement of radial head following fracture. West J Surg Obstet Gynecol 1951;59(10):539–46.

26. Chapman CB, Su BW, Sinicropi SM, et al. Vitallium radial head prosthesis for acute and chronic elbow fractures and fracture-dislocations involving the radial head. J Shoulder Elbow Surg 2006;15(4): 463–73.

27. Knight DJ, Rymaszewski LA, Amis AA, et al. Primary replacement of the fractured radial head with a metal prosthesis. J Bone Joint Surg Br 1993;75(4): 572–6.

28. Lim YJ, Chan BK. Short-term to medium-term outcomes of cemented Vitallium radial head prostheses after early excision for radial head fractures. J Shoulder Elbow Surg 2008;17(2):307–12.

29. Ricon FJ, Sanchez P, Lajara F, et al. Result of a pyrocarbon prosthesis after comminuted and unreconstructable radial head fractures. J Shoulder Elbow Surg 2012;21(1):82–91.

30. King GJ. Management of comminuted radial head fractures with replacement arthroplasty. Hand Clin 2004;20(4):429–41, vi.

31. Burkhart KJ, Mattyasovszky SG, Runkel M, et al. Mid- to long-term results after bipolar radial head

arthroplasty. J Shoulder Elbow Surg 2010;19(7): 965–72.

32. Mason ML. Some observations on fractures of the head of the radius with a review of one hundred cases. Br J Surg 1954;42(172):123–32.

33. Johnston GW. A follow-up of one hundred cases of fracture of the head of the radius with a review of the literature. Ulster Med J 1962;31:51–6.

34. Broberg MA, Morrey BF. Results of treatment of fracture-dislocations of the elbow. Clin Orthop Relat Res 1987;(216):109–19.

35. Hotchkiss RN. Displaced fractures of the radial head: internal fixation or excision? J Am Acad Orthop Surg 1997;5(1):1–10.

36. Ring D. Displaced, unstable fractures of the radial head: fixation vs. replacement—what is the evidence? Injury 2008;39(12):1329–37.

37. O'Driscoll SW, Jupiter JB, King GJ, et al. The unstable elbow. Instr Course Lect 2001;50:89–102.

38. Monica JT, Mudgal CS. Radial head arthroplasty. Hand Clin 2010;26(3):403–10, vii.

39. Edwards GE, Rostrup O. Radial head prosthesis in the management of radial head fractures. Can J Surg 1960;3:153–5.

40. Grewal R, MacDermid JC, Faber KJ, et al. Comminuted radial head fractures treated with a modular metallic radial head arthroplasty. Study of

outcomes. J Bone Joint Surg Am 2006;88(10): 2192–200.

41. Pfaeffle HJ, Stabile KJ, Li ZM, et al. Reconstruction of the interosseous ligament restores normal forearm compressive load transfer in cadavers. J Hand Surg 2005;30(2):319–25.

42. Ashwood N, Bain GI, Unni R. Management of Mason type-III radial head fractures with a titanium prosthesis, ligament repair, and early mobilization. J Bone Joint Surg Am 2004;86(2):274–80.

43. Brinkman JM, Rahusen FT, de Vos MJ, et al. Treatment of sequelae of radial head fractures with a bipolar radial head prosthesis: good outcome after 1–4 years follow-up in 11 patients. Acta Orthop 2005;76(6):867–72.

44. Chien HY, Chen AC, Huang JW, et al. Short- to medium-term outcomes of radial head replacement arthroplasty in posttraumatic unstable elbows: 20 to 70 months follow-up. Chang Gung Med J 2010; 33(6):668–78.

45. Doornberg JN, Parisien R, van Duijn PJ, et al. Radial head arthroplasty with a modular metal spacer to treat acute traumatic elbow instability. J Bone Joint Surg Am 2007;89(5):1075–80.

46. Harrington IJ, Tountas AA. Replacement of the radial head in the treatment of unstable elbow fractures. Injury 1981;12(5):405–12.

MUSCULOSKELETAL ONCOLOGY

Preface
Musculoskeletal Oncology

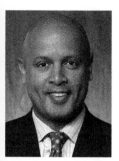

Felasfa Wodajo, MD
Editor

The exciting relaunch of *Orthopedic Clinics of North America* provides a fresh opportunity for presenting musculoskeletal oncology to our orthopedic community. Presently, most academic writing on musculoskeletal tumors is either narrowly focused new research appearing in peer-reviewed orthopedic and oncologic journals or, alternately, invited in-depth reviews of a single oncologic topic. It is possible that neither of these formats addresses well the needs of the non-oncologic orthopedic surgeon. We feel there remains an audience in the wider orthopedic community for writing that is up-to-date and relevant for topics in bone and soft tissue tumors.

As section editor for Musculoskeletal Oncology, my goal is to share writing that is accurate, interesting, and timely and that appeals to nononcologic orthopedists. In this first volume, we present part I of an article by Dr Mihir Thacker on benign pediatric soft tissue masses that an orthopedic surgeon may be asked to evaluate. Dr Thacker completed fellowship training in both pediatrics

and oncology and is on staff at the well-known Nemours/Alfred I. DuPont Children's Hospital in Wilmington, Delaware, giving him a unique vantage to diagnose and treat children with benign and malignant soft tissue masses. In future volumes, we will address management of metastatic lesions, bone lesions that can safely be observed, vascular malformations commonly encountered in orthopedics, as well as many other topics. I hope you enjoy these articles and very much encourage you to share your ideas and feedback in the comments.

Felasfa Wodajo, MD
Musculoskeletal Tumor Surgery
Virginia Hospital Center
Orthopedic Surgery
Georgetown University Hospital
VCU School of Medicine
Inova Campus, Virginia, USA

E-mail address:
wodajo@tumors.md

Orthop Clin N Am 44 (2013) xxi
http://dx.doi.org/10.1016/j.ocl.2013.05.006
0030-5898/13/$ – see front matter © 2013 Published by Elsevier Inc.

Benign Soft Tissue Tumors in Children

Mihir M. Thacker, MD

KEYWORDS

• Pediatric • Soft tissue tumor • Neoplasm • Soft tissue mass • Vascular malformation • Hamartoma

KEY POINTS

- Soft tissue masses in children are often benign or reactive processes.
- Transillumination is an easy clinical test to differentiate cystic from solid superficial masses.
- Unlike in bone tumors, imaging by itself is rarely diagnostic in soft tissue tumors.
- Vascular lesions are the most common soft tissue masses in children.

INTRODUCTION

Soft tissue masses in children are common and comprise a heterogeneous group of lesions, including inflammatory processes, reactive processes, hamartomas, and benign and malignant tumors (**Box 1**).[1] Reactive processes and hamartomas are fairly frequent, as are benign soft tissue tumors. Soft tissue sarcomas, especially those involving the extremities, are fairly uncommon in children and therefore not always placed high on the list of differential diagnoses. Also, unlike bone tumors, the imaging of soft tissue tumors can be nonspecific and can make the diagnosis challenging. The histopathologic appearance of some of the soft tissue masses can be fairly similar as well, and it is essential to put together the clinical picture along with the imaging and histologic appearance to make the appropriate diagnosis of soft tissue tumors.

CLINICAL PRESENTATION

A good history and physical examination are critical toward developing the appropriate differential diagnosis of soft tissue masses. Physical examination may occasionally be diagnostic, for example transillumination in a dorsal wrist mass suggests a ganglion, and a palpable or auscultable bruit suggests a high-flow vascular malformation. Imaging and pathology findings in isolation may result in an erroneous diagnosis in patients with soft tissue tumors, unless placed in the appropriate clinical setting. The age of the child, location of the tumor,[2,3] preexisting conditions, duration, rate of growth, consistency, transillumination, and associated symptoms will aid not only in formulation of an appropriate differential diagnosis but also to determine the best next step.

The role of transillumination of superficial masses cannot be overemphasized. This is a simple clinical test, which *appropriately done* for superficial lesions, helps differentiate a cystic lesion from a solid one, a key factor in determining further workup and eventually treatment. A thorough knowledge of these clinical entities and appropriate diagnostic workup in solid lesions help avoid performing an unplanned resection ("whoops procedure") in a patient with a malignant soft tissue tumor.

Financial Disclosure: No financial disclosure to declare from National Institutes of Health (NIH); Wellcome Trust; Howard Hughes Medical Institute (HHMI); and other(s).
Conflict of Interests: No conflict of interests to declare.
Department of Orthopedic Surgery, Nemours-Alfred I duPont Hospital for Children, 1600 Rockland Road, Wilmington, DE 19803, USA
E-mail address: mihir.thacker@nemours.org

orthopedic.theclinics.com

Box 1
World Health Organization classification of soft tissue tumors (abbreviated)

Adipocytic tumors

Benign: includes lipoma and its variants, lipomatosis, lipoblastoma, lipoblastomatosis

Intermediate: atypical lipomatous tumor/well-differentiated liposarcoma (LPS)

Malignant: liposarcomas: myxoid/round cell, pleomorphic, mixed, dedifferentiated

Fibroblastic/Myofibroblastic tumors

Benign: includes modular fasciitis, fibrous hamartoma of infancy, myofibroma/myofibromatosis, fibroma of tendon sheath, calcifying aponeurotic fibroma, and so forth

Intermediate (locally aggressive): superficial fibromatoses: palmar, plantar, Desmoid type fibromatosis, lipofibromatosis

Intermediate (rarely metastasizing): hemangiopericytoma/solitary fibrous tumor, inflammatory myofibroblastic tumor, infantile fibrosarcoma

Malignant: adult fibrosarcoma, myxofibrosarcoma, low-grade fibromyxoid sarcoma, sclerosing epithelioid fibrosarcoma.

"Fibrohistiocytic" tumors:

Benign: includes giant cell tumor of tendon sheath, diffuse giant cell tumor, benign fibrous histiocytoma

Intermediate (rarely metastasizing): plexiform fibrohistiocytic tumor

Malignant: malignant fibrous histiocytoma/undifferentiated pleomorphic sarcoma and its variants

Smooth muscle tumors:

Benign: deep leiomyoma, angioleiomyoma

Malignant: leiomyosarcoma, excluding skin

Skeletal muscle tumors:

Benign: includes rhabdomyoma, adult/fetal/genital

Malignant: rhabdomyosarcoma, embryonal/alveolar/pleomorphic

Vascular tumors:

Benign: includes hemangiomas, angiomatosis, lymphangiomas

Intermediate (locally aggressive): Kaposiform hemangioendothelioma

Intermediate (rarely metastasizing): Retiform hemangioendothelioma, composite hemangioendothelioma, Kaposi sarcoma

Malignant: epithelioid hemangioendothelioma, angiosarcoma

Pericytic (perivascular) tumors:

Glomus tumor and its variants, including malignant glomus tumor, myopericytoma

Chondro-osseous tumors:

Benign: soft tissue chondromas

Malignant: mesenchymal chondrosarcoma, extraskeletal osteosarcoma

Tumors of uncertain differentiation:

Benign: includes intramuscular myxoma, pleomorphic hyalanizing angiectatic tumor (PHAT)

Intermediate (rarely metastasizing): angiomatoid fibrous histiocytoma, ossifying fibromyxoid tumor, parachordoma

Malignant: synovial sarcoma, epithelioid sarcoma, alveolar soft parts sarcoma, clear cell sarcoma of soft tissue, extraskeletal myxoid chondrosarcoma, Primitive neuroectodermal tumor (PNET), extraskeletal Ewing sarcoma, neoplasms of perivascular cell differentiation (PEComa, clear cell melanocytic tumor)

IMAGING

A thorough clinical evaluation guides the best imaging strategy. The goals of imaging should be to potentially diagnose the lesion, evaluate the extent of the tumor, help determine the need and location of biopsy, and, in malignant tumors, help in the staging. Imaging can also guide preoperative planning, by illuminating proximity of neurovascular structures, underlying bone involvement, vascularity of the lesion, determining the plane of resection, and so forth. Imaging before biopsy is mandatory.

The evaluation of most soft tissue masses should include radiographs. Synovial sarcomas occasionally demonstrate amorphous calcification; the presence of phleboliths is diagnostic of a venous malformation. Pressure changes in the bone underlying a soft tissue mass implies slow growth and may give us a clue about the biology of the mass, whereas invasion of the underlying bone is strongly suggestive of an aggressive lesion. Bone involvement may also be seen in infants with infantile myofibromatosis and this finding on radiography can help narrow the differential.

Ultrasonography is frequently used in evaluation of superficial soft tissue masses in children. Although operator dependent, it has the advantage of not requiring sedation and is relatively quick. It is extremely useful in evaluation of vascular lesions, as it helps distinguish tumor versus malformation and the classification of malformations (high flow vs low flow). Ultrasonography is also useful in distinguishing cystic versus solid lesions and thus adds confidence to the clinical diagnosis of popliteal cysts. For me, it is the imaging modality of choice for superficial lesions. Ultrasound-guided biopsy of soft tissue lesions is an attractive alternative to computed tomography (CT)-guided biopsy, as it involves no radiation.

Magnetic resonance imaging (MRI) is the gold standard for evaluation of most soft tissue lesions. It has the advantage of not having any radiation, but younger children often need to be sedated for this procedure and the relative high cost is also a factor in considering its use. MRI is especially useful for evaluating deep (subfascial) soft tissue masses, which may be difficult to evaluate on clinical or ultrasonographic examination. Even though imaging appearance of most soft tissue tumors is relatively nonspecific, MRI may occasionally be diagnostic, for example, a lipoma has the same signal as subcutaneous fat on T1 and T2 pulse sequences and shows uniform suppression on fat-suppression sequences, as compared with a low-grade liposarcoma, which will demonstrate some high-signal areas on the fat-suppression sequences.

Soft tissue sarcomas grow in a centrifugal fashion, often "push" the surrounding tissues, and are usually well circumscribed. Infiltrative growth is often seen in fibromatosis (desmoid tumors), malignant peripheral nerve sheath tumors, epithelioid sarcomas, and granuloma annulare. The use of contrast helps delineate the degree of vascularity of a lesion and to differentiate cystic from solid areas. MR angiography is useful in evaluation of some vascular malformations and also to evaluate the vascularity of tumors in select situations.

MRI provides excellent detail of the soft tissue anatomy, location, proximity to vital structures, and is an excellent preoperative planning tool. MR-guided interventions (needle biopsies, injections, aspiration, drainage) are feasible and may become more common as technology improves.[4,5]

CT is rarely used for diagnostic purposes secondary to its high radiation doses. It is useful in patients with pacemakers and implants that are sensitive to magnetic force (such as the noninvasive expandable prostheses used in extremity limb salvage). The main role for CT is for guided biopsies of deep soft tissue masses.

Biopsy: Imaging by itself may be inadequate in establishing the diagnosis of soft tissue tumors. For more superficial lesions that are small (less than 3 cm), an excisional biopsy may be considered. For large or deep (subfascial) lesions a needle or incisional biopsy may be performed. Precision, especially for deep lesions, can be improved by using image guidance (US, CT, MRI). The use of immunohistochemistry has made it possible to more accurately diagnose as well as subclassify tumors. (**Table 1**) Principles of biopsy are outlined elsewhere.[6]

Some of the common soft tissue tumors seen in children are discussed in the following sections.

Vascular Lesions and Tumors

Vascular lesions are the most frequent soft tissue masses in children, especially in infants. The International Society for the Study of Vascular anomalies emphasizes the distinction between vascular malformations, which result from localized defects in development and grow commensurate with the child's growth, with vascular tumors (**Tables 1** and **2**).[7] Vascular tumors may be benign, such as hemangiomas (eg, infantile, epithelioid), or malignant, such as epithelioid hemangioendothelioma and angiosarcoma (very rare in children). Vascular

Table 1
Commonly used immunohistochemical markers and the tissues/tumors they are commonly associated with

Marker	Tumor Type
S-100	Neurogenic tumors, some fatty tumors, fairly nonspecific
Glut-1	Hemangiomas
Podoplanin 2	Lymphatic malformations, Kaposi sarcomas
CD 31, CD 34	Vascular lesions, CD 34 also in DFSP, spindle cell lipomas
Myogenin and MyoD1	Skeletal muscle, rhabdomyosarcomas
Smooth muscle actin	Leiomyosarcomas, myofibroblastic lesions
Caldesmon	Smooth muscles, GIST, glomus tumors
Beta catenin	Desmoid fibromatosis (nuclear staining)
Cytokeratin, epithelial membrane antigen	Carcinomas, synovial sarcomas, epithelioid sarcomas, myoepithelial tumors
TLE1 (transducin-like enhancer of split 1)	Synovial sarcomas

Abbreviations: DFSP, Dermatofibrosarcoma protruberans; GIST, Gastro-intestinal stromal tumor.

malformations may be simple (single type) or combined (eg, capillary–venous malformation) (**Fig. 1**).

The use of ultrasound, including Doppler for detecting flow, is critical in the evaluation of vascular lesions in children.[8] Infantile hemangiomas usually go through an initial proliferative phase followed by spontaneous involution (50% by age 5 years, 95% by adolescence). In the proliferative phase, they may compress vital structures, especially in the head and neck, and may need to be treated with propranolol, steroids, or surgery. Extremity involvement is seen in about a third of cases. Association with spinal and urogenital anomalies and so forth may be seen. The histologic hallmark of a hemangioma is proliferation of the endothelium; immunohistochemistry shows *GLUT-1* reactivity (**Fig. 2**). Kaposiform hemangioendothelioma is a rare, locally aggressive vascular

neoplasm, which is sometimes associated with consumptive coagulopathy (Kasabach-Merritt phenomenon), especially if larger than 8 cm.

There are significant differences in glomus tumors in children compared with those in adults. They are more frequently multifocal, infiltrative, and less frequently seen in subungual locations. The superficial soft tissues of the extremities are frequently involved and an autosomal dominant inheritance pattern may be seen (*glomulin* gene on 1p21-22), and some may be associated with neurofibromatosis type 1 (NF1). Treatment is local excision.

Epithelioid hemangioendothelioma is a low-grade malignant vascular tumor that is rarely seen in children. The soft tissues of the extremities (usually solitary) and the liver (often multiple) are the most frequent sites in children. These tumors

Table 2
Differences between hemangiomas and vascular malformations

Characteristic	Hemangioma	Vascular Malformation
Present at birth	Less than 50%	More than 90%
Growth pattern	Proliferation followed by involution	Growth commensurate with growth of the child, no involution
Clinical characteristics	Color changes, noncompressible	Color stable, compressible
Imaging	Well-defined mass, homogeneous, enhances with contrast	Poorly circumscribed, heterogeneous enhancement with contrast
Pathology	Proliferation of endothelial cells	No proliferation of endothelium
IHC (GLUT-1, WT-1)	Present	Absent

Abbreviations: IHC, immunohistochemistry; GLUT, Glucose transporter; WT, Wilm's tumor gene.

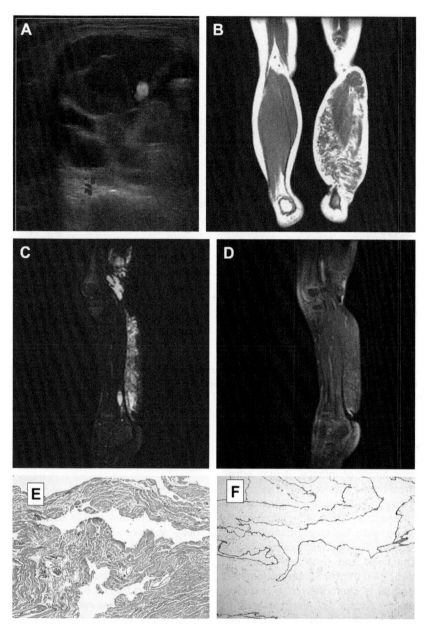

Fig. 1. Lymphatic malformation with macro and microcystic components. (*A*) US of the calf of a 2 year old boy demonstrates a multiloculated cystic lesion with no flow through it on color Doppler examination. (*B*) T2 weighted MR demonstrates an infiltrative soft tissue mass involving the muscle as well as the subcutaneous tissues. (*C*) STIR images demonstrate both a macrocystic component in the popliteal fossa and microcystic components in the leg. (*D*) Post contrast T1 fat saturated images do not demonstrate any significant contrast enhancement. (*E*) Photomicrograph (Hematoxylin & eosin stains, 10× magnification) demonstrates lack of endothelial proliferation which differentiates this lesion from a hamangioma. The lumina of the vessels lack red blood cells. (*F*) Immunohistochemical staining with D-2-40 shows immunoreactivity in the cells lining the walls of the cystic areas, indicating that this is a lymphatic malformation.

have the capacity to metastasize to multiple sites, including lung and bone, especially if larger than 3 cm. Treatment for solitary lesions is wide excision. The recurrence rate is approximately 10% to 15%, as is the mortality rate. Prolonged surveillance is recommended for late metastases.

Fibromatoses

These area a heterogeneous group of benign or intermediately aggressive, nonmetastasizing fibroblastic or myofibroblastic proliferations with variable clinical behavior.

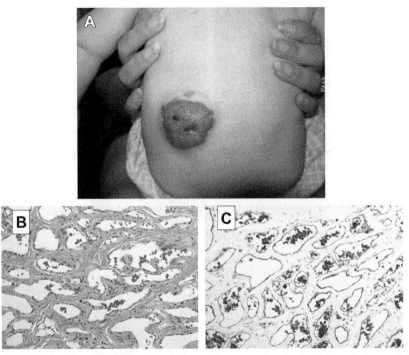

Fig. 2. (*A*) Clinical photograph of a child with a hemangioma over her back. The central area is beginning to ulcerate. (*B*) Photomicrograph (H&E) demonstrating the endothelial proliferation of the lining of the cavities. (*C*) Glut-1 (immunostain) highlights the endothelial cell proliferation.

Infantile myofibroma/myofibromatosis

Infantile myofibroma/myofibromatosis is the most common fibrous tumor of infancy. It may either be solitary (myofibroma, almost 80% of cases, may present later in childhood), multicentric, or generalized (present at birth, affecting viscera as well, poor prognosis). Solitary and multicentric lesions may involve skin, subcutaneous tissues, and bone. The head and neck are most frequently affected, then the trunk and extremities. The clinical course is characterized by spontaneous regression except in the generalized form, which is relentlessly progressive and frequently fatal. The symptoms depend on location, and large tumors may compress vital structures or restrict motion. Surgical treatment is indicated if they compress vital structures or restrict motion.[9]

Lipofibromatosis

Lipofibromatosis is an uncommon neoplasm, often seen in the distal extremities as a poorly circumscribed mass containing mature adipose tissue traversed by fascicles of fibroblasts and collagen with focal myxoid change (**Fig. 3**). It lacks the triphasic components of fibrous hamartoma of infancy, the neural elements of lipofibrous hamartoma, and the cartilage of a calcifying aponeurotic

fibroma. Recurrence/persistence of growth after resection is very common.

Desmoid fibromatosis

Desmoid fibromatosis is a fairly common benign tumor in children and is usually associated with deep aponeuroses. It may be sporadic or occur in association with familial adenomatous polyposis (*APC* gene mutation) or Gardner syndrome. The extremities and trunk are the most frequently affected and it can be solitary or multifocal. Clinically, these are slow-growing masses that can infiltrate into surrounding structures. These are often heterogeneous on MRI, with low-intensity areas on T1-weighted and T2-weighted sequences representing mature collagenous tissue (**Fig. 4**). Infiltrative growth, crossing fascial boundaries and lack of central necrosis, even in large lesions, helps differentiating desmoids from soft tissue sarcomas.[10] Histologically, these have variable cellularity, demonstrating uniform spindle cells arranged in fascicles or sheets and collagenous stroma. Immunoreactivity to vimentin and variable reactivity to smooth muscle actin is seen. Abnormal staining for beta-catenin (nuclear localization) and *CTNNB1* mutations in patients with desmoid tumors can help identify those at risk for familial adenomatous polyposis.

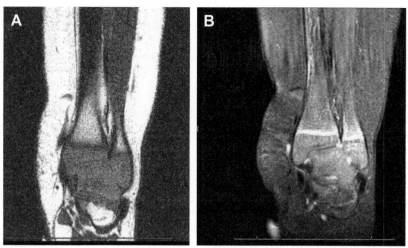

Fig. 3. (*A*) T1 weighted image of an infant with a poorly marginated soft tissue mass on the medial ankle. This shows predominantly high (fatty) signal. (*B*) STIR sequence demonstrates fat suppression for the most part within the lesion but does demonstrate higher signal areas (representing cellular and fibrous components).

Treatment traditionally has been resection with negative margins, when possible. Adjuvant radiation is used for inadequate margins. Aggressive surgery may be associated with functional deficits and, despite this, recurrence rates are high. Hence, observation for asymptomatic or slow-growing lesions and nonsurgical options are gaining popularity.[11] These include tamoxifen (estrogen receptor beta is expressed in 80% cases of desmoid fibromatosis) with sulindac, tyrosine kinase inhibitors, hydroxyurea, vinblastine, and methotrexate.

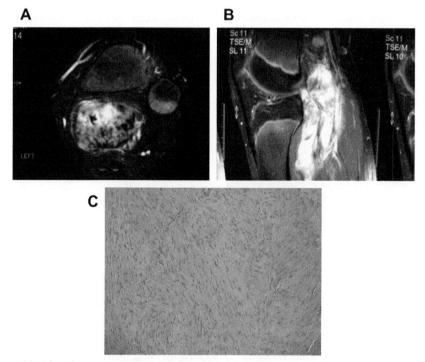

Fig. 4. 13 year-old girl with progressively enlarging relatively pain-free soft tissue mass in the calf. (*A, B*) Axial (5*A*) and sagittal cuts (5*B*) of the MRI demonstrate a heterogeneous soft tissue mass in the popliteal fossa as well as proximal calf. The higher signal areas represent more cellular areas within the tumor. (*C*) H&E photomicrograph demonstrates changes of fibromatosis with bland spindle cells, no mitotic figures. No atypia or pleomorphism noted.

Neurogenic Tumors

These include schwannomas, neurofibromas, and granular cell tumors.[12] Isolated neurogenic tumors are less common in children compared with adults. Schwannomas may be solitary or multiple, particularly in the setting of NF2. These are clinically characterized by a well-circumscribed, often painful mass with a positive percussion sign. MRI demonstrates a well-circumscribed, fusiform lesion that is isointense to hypointense on T1-weighted sequences and has variable hyperintensity on T2-weighted sequences. The periphery of the lesion usually shows a rind of hypointense signal on T2-weighted sequences due to the fibrous capsule. A *split fat sign* may be seen in intramuscular locations because of a small amount of surrounding fat. A *string sign* (entering and exiting nerve root), a *target sign* (low signal centrally and higher signal peripherally), and a *fascicular sign* (multiple ringlike structures within the lesion, possibly reflecting the fascicular bundles) may also be seen (**Fig. 5**).

Plexiform neurofibromas diffusely involve a long segment of nerve, often creating a "bag of worms" appearance as they extend along the branches of the nerve (**Fig. 6**). These are infiltrative lesions, poorly circumscribed, and extend into the surrounding soft tissues. These are often seen in the setting of NF1 and are difficult to differentiate from malignant peripheral nerve sheath tumors, which can arise within, especially in patients with NF1.

Histology in schwannomas demonstrates Antoni A (more cellular areas with spindled cells with elongated nuclei, nuclear palisading called Verocay bodies) and Antoni B (less cellular) areas. Schwannomas demonstrate diffuse S-100 immunoreactivity. Neurofibromas, on the other hand, are poorly encapsulated, do not show well-defined Antoni A and B areas, are more heterogeneous (fewer S-100 and calretinin-positive cells), and show intralesional nerve fibers.

Treatment is surgical excision of painful lesions, preserving as much of the parent nerve as possible. Schwannomas may be peeled away from the surrounding nerve fibers, but neurofibromas are much more intimately attached to the surrounding fibers.

Granular cell tumor

Granular cell tumor is an uncommon tumor of Schwann cell origin. In children, there is slightly increased incidence between 5 and 10 years of age, and female preponderance. It usually presents as a solitary, poorly circumscribed, and sometimes painful soft tissue mass often in the trunk or extremities, and is usually seen in the skin or subcutaneous tissues, but rarely in deeper tissues. The clinical behavior is quite variable.[13] Histologically, the tumors show large polygonal or spindled cells with abundant pale, granular cytoplasm arranged in sheets, nests, or cords with dense collagenous stroma (**Fig. 7**). Treatment is wide surgical excision.

Tenosynovial Giant Cell Tumors

Tenosynovial giant cell tumors (TGCTs) arise within joints, in tendon sheaths, or within periarticular soft tissues. They may present as a localized mass, giant cell tumor (GCT) of tendon sheath or nodular synovitis (within a joint), or may be more diffuse and infiltrative in nature (diffuse GCT, previously called pigmented villonodular synovitis). Diffuse TGCTs have been reported in association with NF1 and Noonan syndrome.

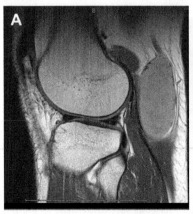
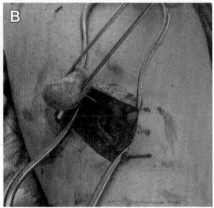

Fig. 5. Schwannoma. (*A*) Soft tissue mass in the popliteal fossa with an entering nerve root sign, suggestive of a peripheral nerve sheath tumor. (*B*) Intraoperative photograph after separating the lesion from the peroneal nerve.

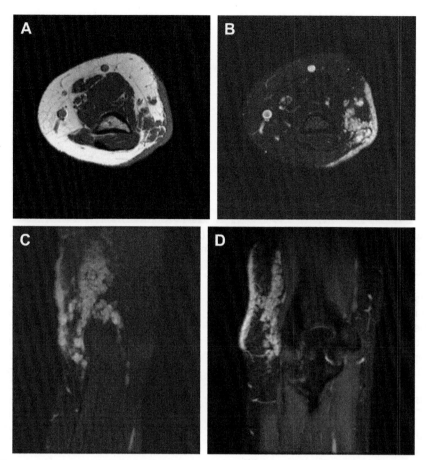

Fig. 6. Plexiform neurofibroma (*A*) T1 weighted sequence showing an infiltrative soft tissue mass on the medial aspect of the elbow. (*B*) STIR sequence demonstrates that the soft tissue mass infiltrates the soft tissue, subcutaneous fat as well as the skin. (*C*) Sagittal and (*D*) Coronal views on the MRI demonstrating the extent of the lesion.

TGCTs are fairly common and, in children, are most frequent in the second decade.[14] The most common type is a digital TGCT, seen as a firm, nontransilluminant, well-circumscribed nodule

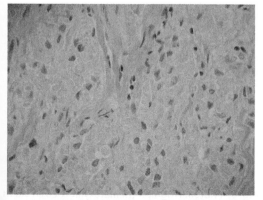

Fig. 7. Granular cell tumor. H&E photomicrograph (40×) demonstrates polygonal cells with finely granular pale eosinophilic cytoplasm.

within the soft tissues of the hands, feet, and wrist. This can also present in the periarticular soft tissue around larger joints, especially the knee. Joint involvement may be seen in the localized or diffuse versions. Diffuse TGCT (or pigmented villonodular synovitis) within joints can be a cause of pain, with recurrent synovitis and hemarthrosis eventually leading to cartilage damage and arthritis of the affected joint. Gradient echo sequences of MRIs are particularly useful in identifying the hemosiderin "blooming artifact" that is frequently seen in these tumors (**Fig. 8**).

Grossly villous or nodular hyperplasia of the synovium with or without pigmentation (brown from hemosedrin deposition) may be seen. Histology reveals lobules of polygonal mononuclear cells with multinucleated giant cells in a fibrous stroma. Chondroid metaplasia may be seen and may mimic synovial chondromatosis. Structural rearrangements of chr 1p21-p13 and translocations involving multiple partners have been reported.

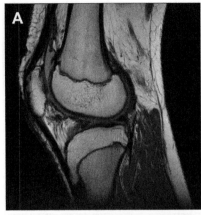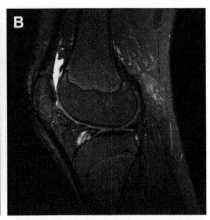

Fig. 8. Tenosynovial giant cell tumor (diffuse). Sagittal T1 (*A*) and T2 fat saturated (*B*) weighted MRI demonstrate fond like or villous structures projecting off the synovium. A moderate effusion is also noted in the knee.

The treatment is primarily surgical excision, with good results in localized TGCTs but high recurrence rates in diffuse TGCTs (up to 50%). Radiation has been used to minimize recurrences. Small molecule inhibition of the CSF1 tyrosine kinase receptor may be a potential therapeutic target in the future.

Lipomatous Tumors

Lipoma

Lipomas are relatively uncommon in children. Lipomatosis is a developmental abnormality in which mature adipocytes form an infiltrative or multifocal mass. Lipomas are well circumscribed and may be within the subcutaneous or deeper tissues. Intramuscular lipomas often splay muscle fibers and can reach large sizes. These often present as soft, often painless, nontransilluminant masses, and family history may be positive in about a third of cases. MRI is diagnostic. Variants of lipomas include angiolipoma (often painful, with capillary proliferation through it), fibrolipoma, hibernoma (tumor of brown fat, mostly seen around the shoulders), perineural lipoma (lipofibrous hamartoma, which often arises around the median nerve and is associated with macrodactyly), myolipoma, and chondroid lipoma. Treatment is marginal excision of symptomatic masses along with their pseudocapsule to minimize recurrences.

Lipoblastoma

Lipoblastoma is a benign tumor of embyronic white fat, mostly seen in infancy and early childhood and is capable of differentiation. Boys and the soft tissues of the trunk and extremities are more frequently affected. They can be either superficial and well circumscribed or deep and infiltrative. They may show rapid growth and can certainly be confused with liposarcomas on

clinical evaluation, imaging, and pathology. Histologically, lipoblastomas show lobules of mature and immature adipose tissue separated by fibrovascular septa (**Fig. 9**). The adipocytes show a spectrum of maturation, often with the more mature cells in the center of the nodule and the more immature myxoid cells at the periphery. Alteration/amplification of the *PLAG1* gene (chr 8q13) are seen in nearly 90% of lipoblastomas. Treatment is primarily complete, but conservative, surgical excision. Recurrences are frequent but may be successfully reexcised.[15]

ADVANCES
Imaging

Role of positron emission tomography
The role of positron emission tomography (PET) scans continues to evolve. The use of PET is standard for melanoma and lymphoma staging in adults, but its use is increasing in the pediatric

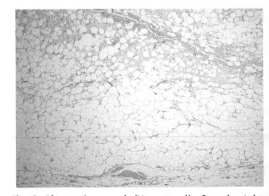

Fig. 9. Photomicrograph (Hematoxylin & eosin stains, 10× magnificaton) of a lipoblastoma showing a mix of mature fat cells, lipoblasts and myxoid tissue (basophilic).

population, especially in staging for rhabdomyosarcoma, assessment of response to chemotherapy,[16] and prediction of local control in rhabdomyosarcoma.[17] PET seems to be especially useful in detecting regional lymph node metastases and bone involvement, although it is inferior to standard CT for the detection of pulmonary metastases.[18] The use of PET-CT is therefore being recommended with increasing frequency. PET scans are also useful in the setting of neurofibromatosis to detect malignant change in plexiform neurofibromas (uptake more than that of the liver is often used as a diagnostic cutoff). They have high sensitivity but lower specificity in detection of MPNSTs (Malignant Peripheral Nerve Sheath Tumor) in the setting of plexiform neurofibromas.[19]

Role of whole-body MRI

Whole-body MRI for staging of malignant soft tissue tumors is becoming more common. Siegel and colleagues[20] reported the results of the American College of Radiology Imaging Network 6660 Trial. They found that there was improved accuracy in nonlymphomatous tumors and in the detection of skeletal metastases, but it was inferior to conventional imaging for detection of pulmonary metastases. It may also be used for screening in other disorders, such as infantile myofibromatosis.

Pathology

The increased use of immunohistochemistry, as well as flow cytometry and cytogenetic studies, has resulted in improved diagnosis and classification of tumors (**Table 1**). It has also helped us understand some of the pathways leading to tumorigenesis. This will likely only improve with increasing use of genomics and proteonomics. A better understanding of the pathways involved should then allow us to identify appropriate targets for therapy.

Treatment

Treatment of benign symptomatic lesions for the most part remains surgical. With malignant soft tissue tumors, adjuvant treatments, such as chemotherapy and radiation, are typically used. With improved understanding of pathways involved, there are now numerous Phase I and II trials using targeted therapies, but their efficacy remains limited for now.

ACKNOWLEDGMENTS

I would like to thank Katrina A. Conard, MD for providing some of the histologic images that are presented in this manuscript. I would also like to thank Kenneth Rogers, ATC, PhD for his help in preparing this manuscript.

REFERENCES

1. World Health Organization Classification of Tumors. Pathology and genetics of tumors of soft tissue and bone. Lyon (France): IARC Press; 2002.
2. Kransdorf MJ. Benign soft-tissue tumors in a large referral population: distribution of specific diagnoses by age, sex, and location. AJR Am J Roentgenol 1995;164(2):395–402.
3. Kransdorf MJ. Malignant soft-tissue tumors in a large referral population: distribution of diagnoses by age, sex, and location. AJR Am J Roentgenol 1995;164(1):129–34.
4. Carrino JA, Blanco R. Magnetic resonance–guided musculoskeletal interventional radiology. Semin Musculoskelet Radiol 2006;10(2):159–74.
5. Genant JW, Vandevenne JE, Bergman AG, et al. Interventional musculoskeletal procedures performed by using MR imaging guidance with a vertically open MR unit: assessment of techniques and applicability. Radiology 2002;223(1):127–36.
6. Thacker M. Musculoskeletal oncology. In: Fischgrund J, editor. Orthopaedic knowledge update. 9th edition. Rosemont (IL): American Academy of Orthopaedic Surgeons; 2008. p. 197–220.
7. Mulliken JB, Glowacki J. Hemangiomas and vascular malformations in infants and children: a classification based on endothelial characteristics. Plast Reconstr Surg 1982;69:412–22.
8. Restrepo R. Multimodality imaging of vascular anomalies. Pediatr Radiol 2013;43(Suppl 1):S141–54.
9. Levine E, Fréneaux P, Schleiermacher G, et al. Risk-adapted therapy for infantile myofibromatosis in children. Pediatr Blood Cancer 2012;59(1):115–20.
10. Lee JC, Thomas JM, Phillips S, et al. Aggressive fibromatosis: MRI features with pathologic correlation. Am J Roentgenol 2006;186:247–54.
11. Honeyman JN, Theilen TM, Knowles MA, et al. Desmoid fibromatosis in children and adolescents: a conservative approach to management. J Pediatr Surg 2013;48(1):62–6.
12. Murphey MD, Smith WS, Smith SE, et al. From the archives of the AFIP. Imaging of musculoskeletal neurogenic tumors: radiologic-pathologic correlation. Radiographics 1999;19(5):1253–80.
13. Thacker MM, Humble SD, Mounasamy V, et al. Case report. Granular cell tumors of extremities: comparison of benign and malignant variants. Clin Orthop Relat Res 2007;455:267–73.
14. Gholve PA, Hosalkar HS, Kreiger PA, et al. Giant cell tumor of tendon sheath: largest single series in children. J Pediatr Orthop 2007;27(1):67–74.

15. Coffin CM, Lowichik A, Putnam A. Lipoblastoma (LPB): a clinicopathologic and immunohistochemical analysis of 59 cases. Am J Surg Pathol 2009; 33(11):1705–12.

16. Eugene T, Corradini N, Carlier T, et al. (1)(8)F-FDG-PET/CT in initial staging and assessment of early response to chemotherapy of pediatric rhabdomyosarcomas. Nucl Med Commun 2012;33(10): 1089–95.

17. Dharmarajan KV, Wexler LH, Gavane S, et al. Positron emission tomography (PET) evaluation after initial chemotherapy and radiation therapy predicts local control in rhabdomyosarcoma. Int J Radiat Oncol Biol Phys 2012;84(4):996–1002.

18. Benz MR, Tchekmedyian N, Eilber FC, et al. Utilization of positron emission tomography in the management of patients with sarcoma. Curr Opin Oncol 2009;21(4):345–51.

19. Treglia G, Taralli S, Bertagna F, et al. Usefulness of whole-body fluorine-18-fluorodeoxyglucose positron emission tomography in patients with neurofibromatosis type 1: a systematic review. Radiol Res Pract 2012;2012:431029.

20. Siegel MJ, Acharyya S, Hoffer FA, et al. Whole-body MR imaging for staging of malignant tumors in pediatric patients: results of the American College of Radiology Imaging Network 6660 Trial. Radiology 2013;266(2):599–609.

Index

Note: Page numbers of article titles are in **boldface** type.

Orthop Clin N Am 44 (2013) 445–450
http://dx.doi.org/10.1016/S0030-5898(13)00070-9
0030-5898/13/$ – see front matter © 2013 Elsevier Inc. All rights reserved.

orthopedic.theclinics.com

Moving?

Make sure your subscription moves with you!

To notify us of your new address, find your **Clinics Account Number** (located on your mailing label above your name), and contact customer service at:

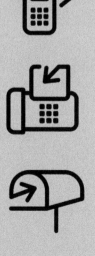

Email: journalscustomerservice-usa@elsevier.com

800-654-2452 (subscribers in the U.S. & Canada)
314-447-8871 (subscribers outside of the U.S. & Canada)

Fax number: 314-447-8029

**Elsevier Health Sciences Division
Subscription Customer Service
3251 Riverport Lane
Maryland Heights, MO 63043**

*To ensure uninterrupted delivery of your subscription, please notify us at least 4 weeks in advance of move.

Printed and bound by CPI Group (UK) Ltd, Croydon, CR0 4YY

03/10/2024

01040346-0004